Diagnostic Dermatopathology

A guide to ancillary tests beyond the H&E

Diagnostic Dermatopathology

A guide to ancillary tests beyond the H&E

Edited by

Gregory A. Hosler, MD, PhD

Dermatopathologist, Division of Dermatopathology and Molecular
Diagnostics, ProPath
Clinical Associate Professor of Dermatology and Pathology
The University of Texas Southwestern
Dallas, Texas
USA

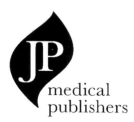

JP
medical
publishers

London • Panama City • New Delhi

© 2017 JP Medical Ltd.
Published by JP Medical Ltd,
83 Victoria Street, London, SW1H 0HW, UK
Tel: +44 (0)20 3170 8910   Fax: +44 (0)20 3008 6180
Email: info@jpmedpub.com Web: www.jpmedpub.com

ISBN: 978-1-909836-12-9

British Library Cataloguing in Publication Data
A catalogue record for this book is available from the British Library

Library of Congress Cataloging in Publication Data
A catalog record for this book is available from the Library of Congress

Publisher:	Richard Furn
Development Editor:	Gavin Smith
Editorial Assistant:	Katie Pattullo
Design:	Designers Collective Ltd

Foreword

Surgical pathology developed in departments of surgery primarily in Germany in the 19th century. Dermatopathology developed in dermatology departments, also in Germany, with Dr Paul Unna widely considered as the father of dermatopathology. However, many of the founding fathers of dermatopathology were cross trained in both dermatology and pathology. The first modern dedicated department of pathology was founded by Dr William Welch at the Johns Hopkins Hospital in 1884. Dermatopathology came into its own in the USA in 1962 with the founding of the American Society of Dermatopathology, the establishment of the certifying exam in 1973, and accreditation of fellowships by the ACGME in 1976.

For over a century, the hematoxylin and eosin (H&E) stained section has been the bedrock of diagnostic dermatopathology and it remains so today. Special stains were developed to aid in the detection of organisms, melanin and mucin, all important in dermatopathology. Electron microscopy and immunofluorescence became essential supplemental diagnostic techniques. In the late 1970s immunoperoxidase stains were first used in the diagnostic laboratory. The applications and the number of antibodies are now numerous. Molecular pathology techniques developed in research laboratories were well established in diagnostic laboratories by the 1980s.

I have been practicing dermatopathology for over 30 years. This period has seen rapid change and the development of tools which aid our ability to make more accurate and efficient diagnoses. While the H&E section remains center stage, these ancillary techniques have gained an increasingly important role. In this work, Dr Hosler has gathered authors who are expert in these subspecialty techniques. Each chapter goes in depth into a specific technique. For those interested in the history of our specialty, the introductory chapter is both enjoyable and enlightening. The rest of this work discusses the diagnostic methods which are increasingly important and go beyond the H&E.

Terry L. Barrett, MD
Clinical Professor of Pathology and Dermatology
University of Texas Southwestern Medical School
Dallas, USA

Preface

Dermatopathology has become an increasingly dynamic field. In my career I have seen dramatic shifts in how we diagnose dermatologic disease and how we teach dermatopathology; changes largely driven by technology.

The inspiration behind *Diagnostic Dermatopathology* came from observing dermatology and pathology residents and dermatopathology fellows. These trainees are bright and energetic people with a thirst to learn. The learning process has evolved over the generations, but whether methods have improved or declined in efficacy is debatable. Clearly there is more information and a need or desire to assimilate that information as quickly as possible. Rapid-fire unknowns and constant assessments have become an integral part of the learning process in dermatopathology for many trainees. In my opinion, however, assimilating quantity comes at the price of depth. 'What is the answer?' is the knee-jerk question at the expense of asking 'How?' or 'Why?'

The goal of this book is to round out the educational experience of the true dermatopathology disciple. I feel that those who truly wish to study the subject will be willing to dig deep. They will want to know where dermatopathology has been, where it is going, what tests are available and how to use them. The Introduction, Section 1, should satiate the first appetite by giving some background on the origins of our discipline, including a discussion on the person who in my opinion is the true founder of dermatopathology, Paul Unna, and the fascinating history behind our bread and butter assay, the H&E stain. Sections 2–6 explore dermatopathology in an unconventional manner, arranged not by diagnosis but by assay, providing the reader with insight on why these tests are performed and how to use and interpret them. I have decided to focus on techniques that have made a huge impact in diagnostic dermatopathology and, in most cases, are still used today. It should be recognized that many other technologies have come and since disappeared. The latter portion of the book (Sections 7 & 8) introduces the newest members to the dermatopathologists' test menu, the molecular assays, and outlines the direction in which dermatopathology is heading.

I want to thank JP Medical, my esteemed colleagues and authors, and my family for understanding this book's purpose and providing the necessary support.

Gregory A Hosler
October 2016

Contents

Contributors

Pamela M Aubert MD
Dermatopathologist
Department of Dermatology
Panorama City Medical Center
Panorama City, CA
USA

Ryan W Hick MD
Dermatopathologist
Division of Dermatopathology, ProPath
Clinical Assistant Professor of Dermatology
The University of Texas Southwestern
Dallas, TX
USA

Gregory A Hosler MD PhD
Dermatopathologist
Division of Dermatopathology and Molecular
Diagnostics, ProPath
Clinical Associate Professor of Dermatology and
Pathology
The University of Texas Southwestern
Dallas, TX
USA

Robert M Law MD
Dermatopathologist
Division of Dermatopathology, ProPath
Clinical Assistant Professor of Dermatology and
Pathology
The University of Texas Southwestern
Dallas, TX
USA

Marc R Lewin MD
Dermatopathologist
Division of Dermatopathology, ProPath
Clinical Assistant Professor of Dermatology
The University of Texas Southwestern
Dallas, TX
USA

Matthew Lewin MD
Surgical Pathologist
Division of Gastrointestinal and Renal Pathology,
ProPath
Dallas, TX
USA

Bahram Robert Oliai MD
Surgical Pathologist
Division of Immunohistochemistry, ProPath
Dallas, TX
USA

Travis Vandergriff MD
Dermatopathologist and Assistant Professor of
Dermatology
The University of Texas Southwestern
Dallas, TX
USA

Acknowledgements

I would like to thank the following for their contributions:

Authorship: I wish to thank my esteemed colleagues for donating their time and expertise in authoring sections of this book. In the order of their contributions: Terry Barrett, Ryan Hick, Marc Lewin, Bob Oliai, Travis Vandergriff, Rob Law, Matthew Lewin, Pamela Aubert

Graphics: I would like to thank Andrew Jenkins at ProPath for his dedication to this project.

Support: I wish to thank the Hosler family (Julie, Calvin, Quincy, Silas) for their sacrifices as I know that every minute I spent on this project was time away from them.

GAH

Dedication

This book is dedicated to all the disciples of dermatopathology. May we continue to perfect our craft and stay relevant as technology attempts to make us obsolete.

Section 1

Introduction

History of dermatopathology

Gregory A. Hosler

'And when we recognize what our teachers and leaders accomplished without present-day methods, we will do well to bow our heads deeply before them.'

Gierke, in *Färberei zu mikroscopischen Zwecken*
(Conn 1933; Gierke 1884)

Before venturing to discuss current dermatopathology and its associated technologies, it is important to understand where the field has been.

In many respects, modern dermatopathology was born in 1974, when the first trainees sat for an exam and became certified, providing the final stamp of approval and legitimizing dermatopathology as a subspecialty of medicine. If 1974 was its birth, dermatopathology incubated in the womb with a gestation period lasting for centuries, and, in some eyes, millennia. From its inception to the present, the study of cutaneous pathology has undergone a remarkable transformation, evolving from naked-eye examinations to the complete genetic analysis of patients and their afflicted skin.

Dermatopathology can be defined in different ways. Many consider dermatopathology synonymous with dermatohistopathology. This view may be too narrow. Dermatopathology, if defined as 'the study of cutaneous disease', existed prior to the microscope and will persist long after the microscope is finally laid to rest. As the scope of pathology broadened from autopsies to surgical pathology and laboratory and molecular medicine, so too will the scope of dermatopathology. Will we not still call ourselves dermatopathologists once we retire our microscopes? Using the broadest definition of dermatopathology makes pinpointing its origins challenging. Dermatohistopathology really took off in the 19th century, but individuals were investigating and diagnosing skin disease long before then.

As Pusey states in the introduction of his oft-cited *The History of Dermatology*,

'The beginnings of dermatology can hardly be less ancient [than the Cro-Magnon man, who trephined men's skulls 25,000 years ago], for skin diseases obtrude themselves upon the attention in a way that few others do, and none of man's medical efforts can have been much earlier than those to relieve his itching and to get rid of the sores and scabs and parasites that afflicted his skin.'

Pusey, in *The History of Dermatology*
(Pusey 1933)

Thus, the origins of dermatology, and, by extension, dermatopathology, arguably date back to the origins of medicine and, taken further, the origins of man.

The following history of dermatopathology (**Figure 1.1**) includes key names and discoveries to highlight how the field has been – and continues to be – shaped by the interwoven threads of dermatology and pathology.

Ancient medicine

The *Edwin Smith Papyrus* (17th century BC) and the *Ebers Papyrus* (16th century BC) are considered the earliest records of dermatologic disease and the oldest preserved medical literature. The *Ebers Papyrus* includes medical lore as old as 3000 BC, and a significant portion of this ancient document is devoted to the skin. Specifically, there are writings on cosmetics and the treatment of skin disease, citing the virtues of bandages, sunlight, and, of course, exotic animal parts. The Egyptians described many dermatologic conditions, including alopecia

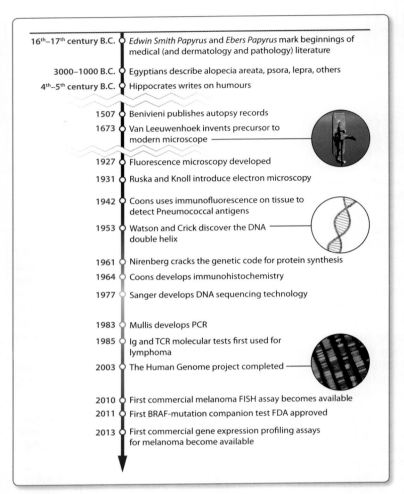

Figure 1.1 A timeline of significant events in the history of dermatopathology.

The timeline contents:

- **16th–17th century B.C.** Edwin Smith Papyrus and Ebers Papyrus mark beginnings of medical (and dermatology and pathology) literature
- **3000–1000 B.C.** Egyptians describe alopecia areata, psora, lepra, others
- **4th–5th century B.C.** Hippocrates writes on humours
- **1507** Benivieni publishes autopsy records
- **1673** Van Leeuwenhoek invents precursor to modern microscope
- **1927** Fluorescence microscopy developed
- **1931** Ruska and Knoll introduce electron microscopy
- **1942** Coons uses immunofluorescence on tissue to detect Pneumococcal antigens
- **1953** Watson and Crick discover the DNA double helix
- **1961** Nirenberg cracks the genetic code for protein synthesis
- **1964** Coons develops immunohistochemistry
- **1977** Sanger develops DNA sequencing technology
- **1983** Mullis develops PCR
- **1985** Ig and TCR molecular tests first used for lymphoma
- **2003** The Human Genome project completed
- **2010** First commercial melanoma FISH assay becomes available
- **2011** First BRAF-mutation companion test FDA approved
- **2013** First commercial gene expression profiling assays for melanoma become available

areata, psora, lepra, herpes zoster, scabies, impetigo, and others. While some of these conditions may not have been the same ones implied by current dermatologic vernacular, the contribution of the Egyptians in describing dermatologic disease is undeniable.

The ancient Greeks documented a similar breadth of dermatologic conditions as the Egyptians. The main advancement in this era was the shift in belief that these conditions were caused naturally and not the result of the wrath of the gods. Greek medicine cannot be discussed without mentioning Hippocrates (c.460–370 BC), who is considered the 'Father of Western Medicine', both for his more secular view on disease and for his teachings

on medical ethics. Hippocrates developed the view that the pathologic basis of disease is related to the imbalance in the patient's humours: black bile, yellow bile, phlegm, and blood. This author has his fair share of the third humour. The humoural theory was pervasive in medicine for the next 2000 years, until the mid-19th century. The Hippocratic Corpus (of which only part was written by Hippocrates) had a considerable component dedicated to dermatology. The understanding of the value of clinical inspection and observation can be traced back to Hippocrates. He understood that skin disease was often a manifestation of internal or systemic disease. He described the association between clubbed fingers and chronic pulmonary disease, and provided the first descriptions of many dermatologic diseases, including (arguably) melanoma (Rebecca et al. 2012).

During the height of Roman civilization, the 1st century AD is notable for *De Medicina (On Medicine)*, by Aulius Cornelius Celsus (c.25 BC–c.50 AD). He states, "For the signs of inflammation are four – redness (*rubor*) and swelling (*tumor*), with heat (*calor*) and pain (*dolor*)." This description, in largely its original form, is still included in *Robbins and Cotran Pathologic Basis of Disease* (Kumar et al. 2014), the bible of modern medical school pathology. Celsus is also credited with describing myrmecia and kerion, but overall, the Romans did not add much to the Egyptian and Greek dermatologic descriptions.

For the next 1500 years, there was little advancement of medicine. Leprosy outbreaks were described and became pandemic in medieval Europe, later subsiding by the latter half of the 15th century. Leprosy elevated the overall interest in dermatology among physicians during these centuries and dominated the dermatologic literature.

Renaissance dermatology and pathology

The Renaissance (15th–17th centuries) accelerated medical knowledge through scientific and evidence-based study. This was a time of inquisitiveness and some degree of intellectual freedom. Anatomic pathology began in Renaissance Italy, with physicians performing autopsies and reporting results to families (Rosai, 1997). Antonio Benivieni (1443–1502), a Florentine physician, is considered the 'Father of Pathologic Anatomy.' His autopsy records were published in 1507, titled *De Abolitis Normullis ac Mirandis Morborum et Sanation Causis (The Hidden Causes of Disease)*, and this work is considered the first anatomic pathology book with clinicopathologic correlation.

Jean Astruc (1684–1766) of France used the newly discovered microscope to study the skin, and described the features of epidermis, corium, mucous membranes, nerves, and adnexal units. Other notable cutaneous microanatomists of this time, many with recognizable names through their anatomic descriptions, include Gabriele Falloppio (1523–1562) and Marcello Malpighi (1628–1694) of Italy, Nicolas Steno (1638–1686) of Denmark, Abraham Vater (1684–1751) of Germany, and Frederik Ruysch (1638–1731) and Herman Boerhaave (1668–1738) of The Netherlands. The Renaissance was also a time of major advancements in the philosophy and practice of medicine, led by individuals such as the Swiss German physician and alchemist Paracelsus (1493–1541), the French physician and leader in physiology Jean Fernel (1497–1558), and the French barber surgeon and early forensic pathologist Ambroise Paré (1510–1590).

During this time, there were many monographs written on dermatologic disease. One of the first treatises on syphilis and venereal disease was written by no other than Jean Astruc. Dermatology shifted its focus from leprosy to syphilis, a new enigmatic disease possibly brought to Europe from the New World by Christopher Columbus (c.1450–1506). Syphilis dominated the dermatologic literature for centuries, as evident by the names of dermatologic organizations and journals (for example the American Board of Dermatology and Syphilology formed in 1932 and only changed its name to American Board of Dermatology in 1955).

Technological advancements

During this period, the microscope was invented, paving the way for modern dermatopathology and the histologic examination of skin disease. In 1590, Zacharias Janssen (c.1580–c.1632), a Dutch inventor, invented the compound microscope allowing for 9× magnification. This contraption consisted of several lenses placed inside a hollow tube. In 1609, The Italian Galileo Galilei (1564–1642) engineered the refracting telescope, which he modified in 1624 to a compound microscope for studying insects, among other subjects. Galileo referred to his invention as 'the little eye'. In 1625, the term 'microscope' was coined by Giovanni Faber (1574–1629) when describing his friend Galileo's invention. Antonie van Leeuwenhoek (1632–1723), another Dutch inventor, often credited with inventing the precursor to the modern microscope (**Figure 1.2**), experimented with grinding lenses and increased the total magnification to 300×, introducing a whole new world within a world.

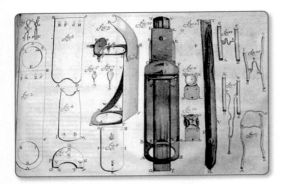

Figure 1.2 van Leeuwenhoek microscope (c.1673).

Also during this period, with the advent of the microscope, scientists begin experimenting with fixatives and stains in order to better view their subjects. The first stains were natural dyes derived from plant extracts, such as saffron (crocus), red cabbage, litmus, blueberry juice, alizarin/madder, purpurin, and indigo. In 1719, van Leeuwenhoek used saffron macerated in wine to study cow muscle. In 1770, Sir John Hill (1716–1775), an English botanist, used dyes (carmine) in the microscopic study of timber. Hill placed his stream-softened and macerated small branches into an alum solution, and then transferred them to spirits of wine. Hill is considered by most to be the first person to study the use of fixatives and dyes for the purposes of microscopic staining (Conn 1933).

Dermatology and pathology in the 1740s-1840s

Following the French Revolution (and changes in the political climate of France in its aftermath), the epicenter of dermatology moved to France. In the rest of continental Europe, Britain, and the United States, clinical specialization was not popular. The old L'Hôpital Saint-Louis became a dermatological hospital and home to the next generation of influential dermatologists. These included Jean-Louis-Marc Alibert (1768–1837), Laurent-Théodore Biett (1781–1840), Pierre François Olive Rayer (1793–1867), Alphée Cazenave (1795–1877), Camille-Melchior Gibert

(1797–1866), and Pierre-Antoine-Ernest Bazin (1807–1878). One of Alibert's most recognizable contributions was the Arbre des dermatoses (Tree of Dermatoses), which illustrated in cartoon form his view on the classification of skin disease: dividing them based on family, genus, and species (gradually smaller branches of the tree). Also in France during this period, in 1806, the French physician René Laennec, while a medical student, first reported on melanoma, which he termed 'melanose' (Rebecca et al. 2012). Other notable figures during this period include William Norris, the English physician who first published on the familial inheritance of melanoma, and Robert Willan (1757–1812), considered the founder of British dermatology and author of the 1808 treatise *On Cutaneous Disease*, a widely popular work due to its translation into many languages and its use of color plates. More landmark descriptions in cutaneous microanatomy were given by the Italian Filippo Pacini (1812–1883), the Czech Jan Purkinje (1787–1869), and the German Jakob Henle (1809–1885). While anatomy was increasingly studied during this period, pathology was not accepted as a part of medicine in all parts of the world. In fact, in the United States, the American physician and civic leader Benjamin Rush (1746–1813) once quipped 'simple anatomy is a mass of dead matter'.

Technological advancements

The technological advancements in this period, as they pertain to dermatopathology, were centered on the burgeoning field of microscopic anatomy. Microscopes continued to improve with the introduction of interchangeable objectives and improved focusing. In 1745, The Englishman John Cuff (1708–1772) created the 'Side-pillar' or 'double microscope', a popular and easy-to-use version with efficient focusing. Cuff's rival and competitor Benjamin Martin (1704–1782) reportedly opened his shop next door to Cuff's and drove him out of business. In 1780, Martin rolled out his finest work, a 2-foot-tall Grand Universal microscope, which featured focus adjustment knobs and an elaborate rack-and pinion gear mechanism for the mirrors and stage (**Figure 1.3**).

Primitive fixatives such as chromic acid were used but hampered by requiring up to six weeks to have their desired effect. By the mid-1800s,

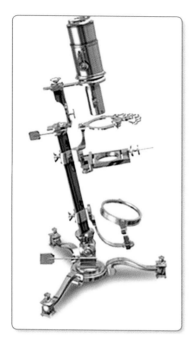

Figure 1.3
Benjamin Martin's Grand Universal microscope (c.1780). Courtesy of Molecular Expressions at Florida State University

'fed' indigo to his 'animalcules' (bacteria), and stained them with carmine, to study their digestive system. The end of this era marks the beginnings of histochemistry, led by the French chemist François-Vincent Raspail (1794–1878). Raspail's pioneering contributions between 1825 and 1834 have earned him the title 'Father of Histochemistry'.

The golden years of dermatohistopathology (1840s-1920s)

The people, their discoveries, and the technological improvements of this era shaped what we now consider modern dermatopathology, or dermatohistopathology. This era was host to the lives of legends, including the 'Father of Modern Dermatology', Ferdinand von Hebra, the 'Father of Modern Pathology', Rudolf Virchow, and the 'Father of Dermatopathology', Paul Unna. Cross-training was common, with clinicians studying microscopy (and vice versa), a philosophy of dermatopathology training maintained to the present. This era produced our first dermatopathology textbooks, written by, arguably, the first dermatopathologists, Gustav Simon and Paul Unna. The work of these individuals would not have been possible without the technological advancements and subsequent explosion in interest in microscopic anatomy. The advancements in the microscope and histology were so numerous and profound that these technologies deviate little from what we use today.

newer agents such as potassium dichromate, mercuric chloride, and alcohol were used to fix and harden tissue sufficiently to produce thin microscopic sections. In 1842, the German anatomist Benedikt Stilling (1810–1879) famously and accidentally left a tissue sample on his windowsill overnight, and discoved the utility of freezing samples. Most histologists were cutting tissue 'freehand' with a knife blade during this era. The English developed the first primitive cutting devices in the late 1700s, led by George Adams, Jr (1750–1795). In 1835, Andrew Prichard (1804–1882) developed a table-top model. As microscopy gained widespread use, various improvements were made with slides. The early English slides, made of ivory, were replaced with glass and became commercially available in the 1830s. In 1840, the Microscopical Society of London formally declared the standard slide as 3 × 1 inch, which remains the standard today. The use of coverslips began in 1843. Tissue was mounted using glycerin or clove oil, which were not ideal as they had a tendency to decolorize the tissue. The natural dyes were still the only available stains and only modest improvements were made in technique. For example, in 1838, Christian Gottfried Ehrenberg (1795–1876)

Microscopic anatomy was born in Germany and Austria in the mid-1800s, led by Rudolf Virchow (1821–1902) (see Box on next page) and Carl von Rokitansky (1804–1878). Both were anatomic pathologists, and most of their work was devoted to autopsy subjects. Virchow wrote on and popularized the cell theory 'omnis cellula e cellula (all cells rise from other cells)', challenging the then-current dogma. In 1858, he published one of his most influential writings titled *Die Cellularpathologie in ihrer Begründung auf physiologische und pathologische Gewebelehre (Cellular Pathology As Based Upon Physiological and Pathological*

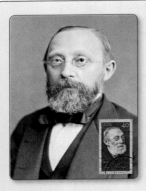

Rudolf Ludwig Karl Virchow (1821-1902). Courtesy of US National Library of Medicine.

Rudolf Ludwig Karl Virchow (1821-1902). Virchow was a German physician, pathologist, biologist, and anthropologist, among other things (Haas, 1989). He played a major role in the field of microscopic anatomy. He studied under Johannes Müller (1804-1858). Work by Müller, Theodor Schwann (1810-1882), Raspail and Virchow led to the cell theory 'omnis cellula e cellula (all cells rise from other cells), challenging other theories of life, including spontaneous generation. Virchow is often given the most credit for the development of this theory. In 1849, Virchow was named the first German Chair of Pathologic Anatomy at the University of Würzburg. This came at a time when pathology was not yet considered a separate, stand-alone specialty. In 1858, he published one of his most influential works, Die Cellularpathologie in ihrer Begründung auf physiologische und pathologische Gewebelehre (Cellular Pathology as Based upon Physiological and Pathological Histology). Virchow founded several journals, including one to (later) be named Virchows Archiv. He described numerous entities, including leukemia, ochronosis (and other pigments), myelin, and chordoma, to name a few, typically on autopsy material. He developed the first detailed autopsy protocol, which involved surgical dissection and histologic examination of all body parts. Interestingly, he had very little or no interest in surgical pathology. Reportedly, when serving under Kaiser Frederick III, he was asked to review the Kaiser's laryngeal biopsy, and misdiagnosed the laryngeal cancer as benign (later reports suggest this was a sampling error, not diagnostic error). The last autopsy Virchow performed was on the Kaiser himself. Due to all of Virchow's contributions to pathology, including his writings, his teachings, and innumerable influential students in pathology and clinical medicine, he is considered by many the 'Father of Modern Pathology'.

Histology) (Virchow, 1858). Both Virchow's and Rokitansky's teachings revolutionized thinking in Germany and Austria, and then the rest of the world. The list of Virchow's pupils is extensive, but two of the most well-known were Friedrich von Recklinghausen (1833–1910) and Paul Langerhans (1847–1888). Several prominent figures in dermatology, including Ferdinand von Hebra (1816–1880), Moriz Kaposi (1837–1902), and Heinrich Köbner (1838–1904), studied under Virchow and Rokitansky and translated their methods to the skin. Friedrich Sigmund Merkel (1845–1919) was another outstanding German anatomist and histologist. His father-in-law and mentor was Henle. At the University of Rostok, Merkel taught anatomy, histology, physics of the microscope, and histological techniques. He was a true disciple of pathology. In 1875, he published Das Mikroskop und seine Anwendung (The Microscope and its Applications) (Merkel, 1876). In the same year, Merkel published on the cutaneous touch-sensitive receptors, Tastzellen (Merkel cells). Another notable microanatomist of this era was the English comparative anatomist Thomas Huxley (1825–1895), who published on the Huxley layer of the hair root sheath in 1845.

In 1849, Virchow was named the first German chair of pathologic anatomy at the University of Würzburg at a time when pathology was not yet considered a separate, stand-alone specialty. In the mid-1800s, most of diagnostic pathology, if performed at all, was performed by surgeons and other clinicians. This practice continued until the mid-20th century. Examples include the English surgeon James Paget (1814–1899), who lectured on the importance of gross and microscopic examination and, in 1874, published on Paget disease, and another English surgeon, Jonathan Hutchinson (1828–1913), who described entities such as lentigo maligna (Hutchinson freckle), keratoacanthoma, Peutz-Jeghers syndrome, forms of melanonychia (Hutchinson sign), and the Hutchinson triad (peg teeth, keratitis, and deafness) of congenital syphilis. By the latter part

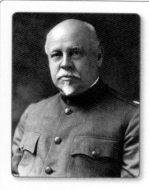

William Henry Welch (1850-1934). Courtesy of US National Library of Medicine.

William Henry Welch (1850-1934). Welch was an American pathologist (Carter, 1997). In 1877, after studying in Germany under Wilhelm von Waldeyer (1836-1921) and von Recklinghausen, among others, Welch returned to the United States and started a pathology laboratory at Bellevue Hospital in New York City, working under Francis Delafield. In 1884, he was recruited to Baltimore by Daniel Coit Gilman (1831-1908), becoming the first Professor of Pathology and first member of the faculty at The Johns Hopkins Hospital. Welch subsequently recruited the other three physicians immortalized in John Singer Sargent's (1856-1925) painting The Four Doctors. These included Physician in Chief William Osler (1849-1919), first Professor of Gynecology

Howard Kelly (1858-1943), and Professor of Surgery William Halstead (1852-1922). Together, these four doctors brought pathology to the forefront of medicine, emphasizing to their peers and pupils the importance of pathology in the care of patients. They were visionaries in the development of surgical pathology as a discipline, creating a dedicated laboratory of surgical pathology, using intraoperative frozen sections, creating tissue banks, and coining the term 'residents' for their boarding house staff. Welch embodied the 'triple threat' of academic medicine, stressing the importance of clinical service, teaching, and research. His main research interest was in bacteriology, which he learned under Robert Koch (1843-1910) while in Germany in 1884-1885. He established the first post-graduate training program for physicians in the United States, and trained such prominent figures as William Halstead, George Whipple (1878-1976), Simon Flexner (1863-1946), and Walter Reed (1851-1902). In 1893, Welch was named the first Dean of The Johns Hopkins School of Medicine. Welch also served in the United States Army Medical Corps in World War I, achieving the rank of Brigadier General, and received a Distinguished Service Medal. He died of prostate cancer at The Johns Hopkins Hospital in 1934.

of the 19th century, full-time pathologists were beginning to be hired in European and American academic institutions and, by the 1890s, surgical pathology became recognized as a stand-alone discipline (Rosai, 1997). In 1875, Francis Delafield (1841–1915), an American physician, was named Chair of Pathology and Practice of Medicine at the College of Physicians and Surgeons in New York. Delafield wrote several of the first American pathology textbooks, including, in 1885, *A Handbook of Pathological Anatomy and Histology* (Delafield & Prudden, 1885). He also developed a popular formula for hematoxylin staining. In 1877, William H. Welch (see Box above) started one of the first American pathology laboratories at Bellevue Hospital in New York City and, later, was a founding father (one of *The Four Doctors* – see Box above) of The Johns Hopkins Hospital. While at Johns Hopkins, Welch recruited other physicians, including William Osler (1849–1919), a Canadian physician who studied pathology

under Virchow and dermatology under Hebra. These new recruits shared Welch's vision of pathology playing a central role in the diagnosis of disease. Through Welch's development of the 'pathology culture' at The Johns Hopkins Hospital and his establishment of the first dedicated surgical pathology laboratory, he is considered by many to be the founder of modern surgical pathology.

Clinical dermatology did not begin in this era, as already discussed, but with new attention being made to microscopic anatomy, and new understanding of the pathologic basis for dermatologic disease, this era was the birth of modern dermatology. In Vienna, Ferdinand von Hebra (1816-1880) (see Box on next page) used the teachings of Virchow and Rokitansky to develop a new classification of skin diseases based on pathologic findings. In 1845, he published his *Versuch einer auf Pathologischer Anatomie Gegründeten Eintheilung der*

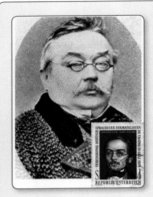

Ferdinand Ritter von Hebra (1816-1880). Hebra was an Austrian dermatologist (Holubar, 1981). Like Rokitansky, he came from The Allgemeines Krankenhaus, the general hospital in Vienna, considered one of the best centers of medical teaching. Hebra founded The School of

Ferdinand Ritter von Hebra (1816-1880). Courtesy of US National Library of Medicine.

Viennese Dermatology, arguably the most influential institution of dermatology in its era. In 1856, likely influenced by his studies with Virchow and Rokitansky, he wrote the widely circulated Atlas der Hautkrankeiten (Atlas of Skin Diseases) (von Hebra, 1856), which included a new classification of skin disease using a pathological basis. He had many contributions to dermatology, including discovering the cause of scabies, and original descriptions of erythema multiforme and lupus erythematosus. By some reports, Hebra had a unique lecturing style, peppered with sarcasm, which created a loyal following. Given his contributions to dermatology, punctuated by his creation of The School of Viennese Dermatology, Hebra is featured on a postage stamp and is considered by many the 'Father of Modern Dermatology'.

Hautkrankheiten (Classification of Skin Diseases Based upon Anatomical and Pathological Considerations). He followed this, in 1856, with his most influential piece titled *Atlas der Hautkrankheiten (Atlas of Skin Diseases)* (von Hebra 1856). Interestingly, Hebra abandoned histology later in his career. Hebra was an effective teacher, and perhaps his most important contribution was the founding of The School of Viennese Dermatology, which produced many subsequent leaders in the field, including Heinrich Auspitz (1835–1886), Isidor Neumann (1832–1906), Salomon Stricker (1834–1898) and Moriz Kaposi. Moriz (Kohn) Kaposi (1837–1902) was a Hungarian dermatologist and the son-in-law of Hebra. He succeeded Hebra in running The School of Viennese Dermatology (Holubar & Frankl 1981), and was also known as a tireless, excellent lecturer. In 1874, Kaposi co-wrote with Hebra *Lehrbuch der Hautkrankheiten (Textbook of Skin Diseases).* He complemented Hebra by adding detailed dermatohistopathology to Hebra's classic clinical descriptions. In 1880, he wrote *Pathologie und Therapie der Hautkrankheiten in Vorlesungen für praktische Ärzte und Studierende (Pathology and Therapy of the Skin Diseases in Lectures for Practical Physicians and Students),* which was widely circulated and firmly placed Kaposi among the dermatology greats. Kaposi created a

massive body of published work, writing on lupus erythematosus, syphilis, erythema multiforme, rhinoscleroma, cutaneous mycoses, and eczema, and is credited with first describing xeroderma pigmentosum, and, of course, idiopathic multiple pigmented sarcoma (Kaposi sarcoma).

The first two textbooks devoted to skin pathology appeared during the lives and teachings of Virchow and Hebra, both in 1848. Gustav Simon (1810-1857) published the comprehensive volume titled *Die Hautkrankheiten durch anatomische Untersuchungen erläutert (Skin Diseases Elucidated by Anatomic Investigation)* (**Figure 1.4**) (Simon 1848). By all accounts, including those by Unna (see below), Simon's was the first textbook devoted to histopathology of the skin. The American Journal of Dermatopathology paid homage to Simon in 1979–1980 with translations of excerpts from his book by S. Milton Rabson (King 1979). Included in Rabson's translations of Simon, '...I wanted to place in the student's hands a volume which would introduce him to the study of the skin diseases in a more simple fashion and one more appropriate to the present state of the science.' Simon was director of the Clinic for Cutaneous and Syphilitic Diseases at the Charité hospital in Berlin, and for many years, he devoted himself to the study of pathologic anatomy. He died of cerebral syphilis in 1857. Felix von

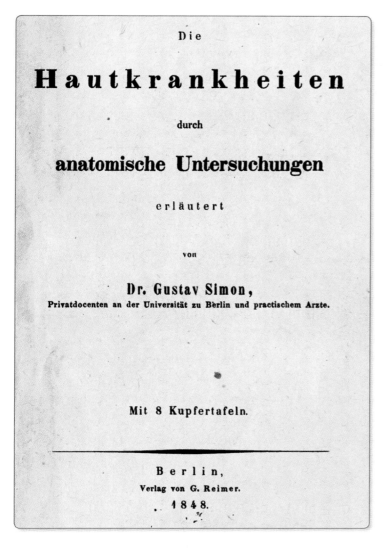

Die

Hautkrankheiten

durch

anatomische Untersuchungen

erläutert

von

Dr. Gustav Simon,
Privatdocenten an der Universität zu Berlin und practischem Arzte.

Mit 8 Kupfertafeln.

Berlin,
Verlag von G. Reimer.
1848.

Figure 1.4 Gustav Simon's title page for *Die Hautkrankheiten durch anatomische Untersuchungen erläutert (Skin Diseases Elucidated by Anatomic Investigation)*.

Bärensprung (1822–1864) published *Beiträge zur Anatomie und Pathologie der menschlichen Haut (Treatise on the Anatomy and Pathology of the Human Skin)*, the lesser known of the two texts, likely because it was not as comprehensive as Simon's (von Bärensprung 1848). Bärensprung is best known for his clinical and microscopic descriptions at autopsy suggesting herpes zoster originates in the spinal ganglia. Bärensprung jumped into the sea while suffering from neurosyphilis in 1864 (King 1982). How ironic is it that both of the original dermatopathology text authors would succumb to neurosyphilis?

Simon and Bärensprung set the stage for Paul Gerson Unna (1850–1929) (see Box on next page). Unna was a remarkable individual and, given his gifts and contributions in both clinical dermatology and microscopy, considered by many as the 'Father of Dermatopathology' (though some argue that this title should go to Simon). Unna was a German dermatologist who studied under Hebra, Kaposi, and Auspitz. Histology was not a mere hobby for Unna. He was a true microanatomist and histochemist, developing several widely-used stains in skin pathology, including orcein and the Pappenheim–

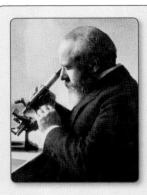

Paul Gerson Unna (1850-1929).

Paul Gerson Unna (1850-1929). Unna was a German dermatologist who studied under Hebra, Kaposi, and Auspitz (Hollander, 1980). He was also influenced by von Recklinghausen, Felix Hoppe-Seyler (1825-1895), Oswald Schmiedeberg (1838-1921), and Waldeyer. Unna served as a volunteer in the Franco-Prussian War and was severely wounded. In 1881, he opened a private clinic with Hans Hebra (son of Ferdinand) called 'Monatchefte fur praktische Dermatologie'. Unna was a so-called 'freelance' investigator, not an academician, funding his own work without the aid of grants or university support. In 1894, he wrote one of the seminal textbooks on dermatopathology, titled Die Histopathologie der Hautkrankheiten (The Histopathology of the Diseases of the Skin) (Unna, 1894). In this book, he acknowledges the work of Virchow and Hebra, but justifies writing a new textbook as Virchow did not devote enough to the skin and Hebra did not devote enough to histopathology. He writes, 'A summary of the literature soon made it evident to me that there was no real histopathology of the skin, that there was but little harmony between clinical and histological detail, and that to the clinician, microscopical observation had been more troublesome than useful.' As early as his M.D. thesis on Beiträge zur Histologie und Embryologie der menschlichen Oberhaut und ihrer Anhangsgebilde (Skin Development), Unna showed an aptitude and love for staining. He discovered plasma cells using polychrome methylene blue, decolorized with glycerine-ether, or with Pappenheim-Unna's methyl-green-pyronin and phenol. He characterized mast cells using polychrome methylene blue and developed the orcein method for elastic fiber detection. In 1921, he wrote Chromolyse, Sauerstofforte und Reduktionsorte (Chromolysis, Areas of Oxidation and Reduction) in the Manual of Practical Biology describing his theories on the constitution of various tissue structures based on how they stain and what solvents make them disappear. In 1928, he wrote Histochemie der Haut (Histochemistry of the Skin). Unna's excitement for histochemistry is palpable, 'With all these adjuvants [new staining methods], it is no longer remarkable that most skin diseases not only do not look alike, but even show such an abundance of histological peculiarities, that their explanation must be for the present postponed.' Unna's contributions to dermatology and dermatopathology include (but are not limited to) describing seborrheic eczema, a group of ulerythemas, senile purpura, ballooning degeneration (varicella infections), elacin, plasma cells, foam cells, mast cells as source of urticaria pigmentosa, the organism behind soft chancre (streptobacillus), impetigo, differences between acne and rosacea, Unna nevus, and palmoplantar keratoderma (Unna-Thost syndrome). He received numerous honors, including being elected to Chair of Dermatology at the University of Hamburg in 1919. Unna died of influenza in Hamburg in 1929. After Unna's death, Jean Darier stated in a memoir, 'When faced with histological problems of any description or – to give a concrete example – with puzzling tumor, e.g. a sarcoma, one would like to know of the correct working method of Unna's to be adopted for fixing, embedding, staining, and solution, the usual way of approaching the subject and the probable answer to the problem.' While some give the title to Gustav Simon, given Unna's early and massive contributions to dermatology, pathology, and histochemistry, many consider him the 'Father of Dermatopathology'.

Unna stain. In 1894, he wrote one of the earliest and most comprehensive dermatopathology textbooks, titled *Die Histopathologie der Hautkrankheiten (The Histopathology of the Diseases of the Skin)* (Unna 1894). While other textbooks preceded his, Unna incorporated gross and microscopic features, including information provided by histochemical stains, to describe and classify skin disease, providing a blueprint for dermatopathology text books for the next 100 years and more. In the preface to his text, the reader can feel his devotion for his craft.

'for...we have, in connection with the skin, two very great advantages. Firstly, we can always get fresh, living material for investigation; and secondly, we are able to observe the part, and to note its relation to the disease as a whole, before excision. ...For since it is possible to compare the clinical appearances with the histological details, it is our duty closely to analyse them, to investigate every apparent disharmony, and not to rest till we have brought the macro- and microscopical appearances into agreement one with the other.'

Paul Gerson Unna in *Die Histopathologie der Hautkrankheiten* (Unna 1894)

Unna also penned *Histochemistry of the Skin* in 1928. His ideas were so novel that they were slow to be accepted. Unna was a tireless investigator and writer. He funded his own research in his private clinic, without university support (not unlike many current dermatopathologists, including this author). Over his career, Unna had over 600 publications and innumerable other contributions to the field of dermatopathology.

Several of Unna's contemporaries shared his enthusiasm for dermatology and dermatopathology. Ferdinand-Jean Darier (1856–1938) was a French physician who often lectured on histology, once claiming 'biopsy is bound to expand and complete clinical examination.' Darier founded the Museum of Histology in L'Hôpital Saint-Louis. He provided descriptions for sarcoidosis, Paget disease, Bowen disease, eruptive hidradenomas, Darier sign (mastocytosis), and, of course, keratosis follicularis (Darier disease) (Civatte 1979). Interestingly, he incorrectly described the psorosperm (infectious parasite) as the cause of keratosis follicularis, and later retracted his inaccurate hypothesis. Darier was one of the 'big 5' at L'Hôpital Saint-Louis, along with Ernest Henri Besnier (1831-1909), Jean Alfred Fournier (1832–1915), Louis-Anne-Jean Brocq (1856–1928), and Raymond Sabouraud (1864–1938). Louis A. Duhring (1845–1913), an American dermatologist and student of Hebra, described dermatitis herpetiformis (Duhring disease), and in 1870, published on alopecia, marking the beginning of dermatopathology at the University of Pennsylvania. Other notable Americans of this period include James White (1833–1916), John Fordyce (1858–1925), and Samuel Becker (1894-1964). Albert Neisser (1855–1916) was a German

dermatologist and microbiologist. He discovered the organism later called Neisseria gonorrhoeae, among others. He is often named, with Unna, as a pre-eminent figure in the scientific advancement of histology and bacteriology. Josef Jadassohn (1863–1936) was another German dermatologist and assistant to Neisser. He introduced patch testing, understanding the immunologic contributions to disease, and described several entities, such as pachonychia congenita (Jadassohn–Lewandowsky syndrome) and Naegeli–Franceschetti–Jadassohn syndrome, which bear his name. Bruno Bloch (1878-1933) was a Swiss dermatologist, who worked under Jadassohn. In the 1920s in Basel, Bloch developed the Dopa reaction, an in situ enzymatic reaction, which stained cells that formed melanin (Sulzberger 1980). Interestingly, he lost the ability to repeat the stain when he moved to Zurich. After three years, he discovered that this was due to the differences in the Basel and Zurich tap water.

Technological advancements

The technological advances during this time period cannot be overstated. Improvements to the microscope and a massive body of work improving histologic stains set the stage for the marked contributions to dermatopathology discussed above.

In the late 1800s, the majority of microscopes were produced at the Zeiss Factory in Germany. The Optical Institute of Ernst Leitz (or Leitz, for short), was also a major player, also in Germany. The German physicist and entrepreneur Ernst Abbe (1840-1905) was the main intellectual force at Zeiss, developing new technologies, such as oil immersion lenses, apochromatic objectives, and substage condensers, all of which contributed to marked improvements in resolution (**Figure 1.5**). In 1920, The Japanese company Olympus manufactured their first microscope, named the Asahi. Merkel ponders the impact of the microscope in his textbook *Das Mikroskop und seine Anwendung (The Microscope and its Applications)* (Merkel 1876).

'...is it a *great* invention, comparable with the steam engine, the printing press, the powdergun, the compass—or is it only a invention of second degree, as for instance the pocket watch or the process of galvanization....?'

Friedrich Sigmund Merkel in *Das Mikroskop und seine* Anwendung (Merkel 1876)

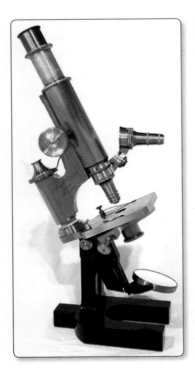

Figure 1.5
Early Zeiss microscope (c.1870).

developed a formula fixing carmine-glycerin prepared tissue with bichromate or picric acid, and then cutting after freezing. In 1869, the German-Swiss pathologist Edwin Klebs (1834–1913) discovered paraffin wax embedding, which was critical for cutting ribbons capable of tracing single cells, for example. Paraffin replaced celloidin. By 1881, histologists began infiltrating tissue with paraffin (processing), and then dissolving the paraffin on the slide with chloroform. Chloroform replaced turpentine at it caused less tissue damage. The most popular tissue mounting agents remained gum damar and Canada balsam. Regarding tissue cutting, the Swiss anatomist and embryologist Wilhelm His (1831–1904) improved upon Prichard's design and first used the term 'microtome' when he described his wooden contraption with a mounted blade in his 1870 work *Beschreibung eines Mikrotoms (Description of a Microtome)*. Cryostats were also available by the 1870s and the first frozen sections were performed adjacent to surgical suites in the 1890s, with mixed results. The modern microtome was available by 1900. This apparatus had mounted blades capable of generating ribbons that would fall over the blade under gravity. Automated stainers were available by the 1890s and automated processors by the 1900s. Paul Mayer (1848–1923), a German zoologist and botanist, was one of first to develop complete beginning-to-end (fixation-to-staining) procedures for preparation of tissue sections.

This time period was the era of histological stains. The enthusiasm during this period is captured by Otto Maschke (1824-1900), who writes.

'...staining solutions will, I am sure, become as indispensable in the future as iodine solutions and both will share the place of honor beside the microscope together with the dissecting knife'

Maschke in the journal *Botan Zeitg* (Conn 1933; Maschke 1859)

He goes on to conclude that it *is* great as 'the microscope opened a completely new, hitherto unknown world, and proved to be of invaluable use in almost every aspect of science and consequently to human life.'

Between 1875-1895, there were giant leaps in the understanding of the cell. These relied upon improvements in fixation, processing, embedding, cutting and mounting to generate ultra-thin, high-quality tissue sections, and better stains to visualize the tissue. The advances in staining were so vast that they will be considered separately (see below). By the 1870s, tissue was fixed using mixtures of chromic acid and osmium tetroxide. In 1893, the use of formaldehyde as a fixative was discovered by the German physician Ferdinand Blum (1865-1959), and Virchow began experimenting with various formaldehyde formulations. Freezing tissue was an alternative method. Nitrous oxide capsules were readily obtained from dentists, and, later, ether and ethyl chloride were used as freezing agents. Frozen tissue microtomes were developed in the 1870s. In 1877, Walther Flemming (1843–1905)

The development of these stains took a logical progression. Unna describes in his preface to *Die Histopathologie der Hautkrankheiten (The Histopathology of the Diseases of the Skin)* (Unna 1894),

'The oldest stains were nuclear, including mitosis detection, elucidating the reproduction of skin elements. Then came stains for intercellular substance, such as elastic tissue, then came stains for collagen, hyaline, mucinous, and fibrinoid substances.'

Unna in *Die Histopathologie der Hautkrankheiten* (Unna 1894)

This time period contributed many nuclear, intercellular substance, and bacterial stains.

Early pioneers in staining were mentioned previously in their appropriate time periods. During this period, a great leap was made in the field of histologic staining by Joseph von Gerlach (1820–1896), a German physician and professor of anatomy and physiology. He experimented for years with ammoniacal carmine. In a famous 'accidental experiment', he left cerebellum, fixed in potassium bichromate, in a dilute ammoniated carmine solution, eventually yielding excellent results, the nuclear staining allowing distinction between nerve cells and fibers. His techniques were published and subsequently followed and further refined. While amateur tissue-dyers preceded him (using carmine and other natural dyes), Gerlach's results were far superior and he is now considered the founder of staining techniques for human histology (von Gerlach 1858). Carmine was *the* dye of its time, used by most histologists, including Virchow. It is a cochineal dye derived from ground-up insects (*Coccus cacti*). In 1896, Mayer developed mucicarmine, which is one of the few carmine-based stains still used today (Titford 2009). The 'other' natural dye, hematoxylin, was the successor of carmine with an interesting history of its own (see Chapter 2). Like carmine, hematoxylin was used in various forms to stain tissue, but was ineffective until the discovery of mordanting in the textile industry. Mordanting combines the dye with a metal ion, markedly increasing its staining properties and longevity. In 1865, Franz Böhmer discovered alum as effective mordant, and this ultimately led to hematoxylin replacing carmine as the leading tissue stain by the early 1900s.

The late 19th century brought a wave of synthetic dyes, specifically the aniline (coal tar) dyes (Conn 1933). In 1854, the English chemist William Perkin (1838–1907), as a 15-year-old boy and amateur chemist, accidentally discovered aniline violet (or 'mauveine'), which became the first commercially prepared synthetic dye. Of course, numerous permutations, resulting in the entire spectrum of colors, soon followed, fueled by the textile industry. Histologists, mostly in Germany, quickly experimented with these 'new toys'. Some of the giants of the time included Dmitri Romanowsky (1861–1921), Paul Ehrlich (1854–1915), Carl Weigert (1845–1904), Waldeyer, Koch, Neisser, Merkel, and, of course, Unna. By 1880, there were numerous stains being used in histology, including methylene blue, crystal violet, orange G, acid fuschin, and eosin, to name just a few. Silver nitrate is not a dye, but its value in highlighting calcium, melanin, and microorganisms was recognized in this period. Oil red O (fat, 1926), orcein (elastic fibers, 1890), and Congo Red (amyloid, 1886) were also developed during this time. Many eponymic stains from this period are still used today: Perl's Prussian blue (iron, 1867), Gram (bacteria, 1884), Van Gieson (connective tissue, 1889), Ziehl–Neelson (acid fast, 1880s), Weigert (bacteria, 1887), Mallory (connective tissue, 1890s), Von Kossa (calcium, 1901), Verhoeff (elastic fibers, 1908), Masson–Fontana (melanin, 1914), and Warthin–Starry (syphilis, 1920) (Conn, 1933; Titford, 2009). Double-staining, such as hematoxylin and eosin, became routine by the end of the 19th century.

By 1900, skin biopsies were still rare and only carried out by surgeons with scalpels. Marion Sulzberger reminisces about a typical day in the laboratory of his mentor Bruno Bloch (Sulzberger, 1980) in the early 20th century.

'…Tissue from each inpatient or outpatient on whom a scalpel biopsy (never a punch biopsy) had been performed during the week had been cut and treated with a routine series of stains. These included hematoxylin-eosin, Van Gieson, elastic fiber stains, silver nitrate stain, and a Dopa preparation. …Quite often, Bloch… asked for additional sections and for special stains such as Ziehl–Neelsen or methylene blue and other stains for particular microorganisms or tissue elements (iron, glycogen, etc.). The new materials and findings were reviewed a week later.'

Sulzberger in *Three lessons learned in Bloch's clinic* (Sulzberger 1980)

Modern dermatopathology from 1920s to present day

While the previous era set the stage for modern dermatopathology, the field had some major paradigm shifts following 1930. Organized medicine played a major role in defining the specialty, establishing dedicated training programs, and providing a road map to certification. In many ways, certification legitimized the specialty and greatly increased its popularity among pathology and dermatology trainees. Recent technological advancements steered dermatopathology into new directions. The dermatopathology diagnostic arsenal extended beyond haematoxylin and eosin (H&E) and special stains to include electron microscopy, immunohistochemistry, immunofluorescence, and molecular assays. Moreover, the role of the dermatopathologist was elevated, providing not only diagnoses to clinicians but offering critical data on prognosis and therapeutic options for patients based on biopsy findings.

Organized medicine did not begin in this era, but organized dermatopathology did. The International Association of Medical Museums (IAMM) formed in 1906, with the help of Osler, and, in 1955, changed its name to the International Academy of Pathology (IAP). The United States and Canadian Academy of Pathology (USCAP) and similar societies in other countries were officially made divisions of the IAP in 1969. Other pathology societies that were formed in the United States include the American Society of Clinical Pathologists (ASCP, 1922), the College of American Pathologists (CAP, 1946), and the first and longest-standing state society, the Texas Society of Pathologists (TSP, 1921). The American Board of Pathology was established in 1936. The oldest dermatological society in the world is actually The New York Dermatological Society, founded in 1869. This was followed by dermatological societies in France (1884), Italy (1885) and Germany (1889). In 1932, The American Board of Dermatology and Syphilology was formed (now named the American Board of Dermatology). And 1938 marked the beginning of the American Academy of Dermatology (AAD), followed by the formation of the American Osteopathic College of Dermatology (AOCD) in 1957. Prior to the AAD, there were no national forums to discuss dermatopathology in the United States, only local meetings. The AAD not only offered a venue to learn dermatopathology, but introduced several critical programs: the Gross and Microscopic Dermatology Session, the Self-Assessment Course, the Clinicopathologic Conference, and the Dermatopathology Registry (at the Armed Forces Institute of Pathology, or AFIP). The AAD also supported the widely popular Osbourne Fellowship at the AFIP for training dermatopathologists. This training program was run by Elson Helwig (1907-1999) (**see Box on opposite page**), one of the greats of modern dermatopathology who in essence trained the next generation of dermatopathologists.

The American Society of Dermatopathology (ASDP) was founded in 1962 with its first meeting in 1963 (Freeman, 1984). The founding members were a 'Who's Who' of dermatopathology at the time, a mix of dermatologists and pathologists, and included the following: Herman Beerman (1901-1995), John R. Haserick (1915–2006), Elson B. Helwig (1907–1999), Arthur B. Hyman, Walter F. Lever (1909–1992), Herbert Z. Lund (1907–1996), Hamilton Montgomery (1898–1982), Walter Nickel (1907–1989), Hermann Pinkus (1905-1985), Frederick Szymanski (1915–2009), Louis H. Winer (1903–1990), and Richard K. Winkelmann (1924–2012). In 1973, the American Board of Pathology and the American Board of Dermatology formed the Joint Dermatopathology Committee, establishing a road to subspecialty certification. The first trainees sat for the first Dermatopathology Board Certification Exam in 1974, and most received certificates! A. Bernard Ackerman (1936–2008) (see Box on page 18) helped establish the International Society of Dermatopathology (ISDP) in 1979.

The dermatopathology lexicon is riddled with eponyms, many of which originated in the beginnings of the modern era. Examples include Breslow depth (Alexander Breslow, 1928–1980), Churg-Strauss disease (Jacob Churg, 1910–2005; Lotte Strauss, 1913–1985), poikiloderma of Civatte (Achille Civatte, 1877–1956), Clark level (Wallace Clark, 1924–1997), Erdheim-Chester disease (Jakob Erdheim, 1874–1937; William Chester, 1903–1974), Gottron papules (Heinrich Gottron, 1890–1974), Hailey–Hailey disease (Hugh Edward Hailey, 1909-1964; William Howard Hailey,

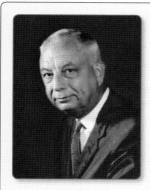

Elson Bowman Helwig (1907-1999). Helwig was an American pathologist, trained under Howard Karsner (1879-1970), Shields Warren (1898-1980), and Robert Moore (1901-1971), three giants of pathology (Lupton, 2002). In 1946, Helwig was appointed Chairman of the Department of Skin and Gastrointestinal Pathology at the Armed Forces Institute of Pathology (AFIP). He ran a very popular training program, training both pathologists and dermatologists (the latter as Earl D. Osborne Fellows, with support from the American Academy of Dermatology). Many current prominent figures in dermatopathology can be traced back to Helwig, both through the Osbourne Fellowship and though active duty pathology fellowships, defining Helwig as a true 'teacher of teachers.' In addition to his training program, Helwig was a giant in dermatopathology with numerous other contributions. He was registrar of the American Registry of Dermal Pathology (1947-1980). He was a leader of the panel that created the World Health Organization Histological Classification of Skin Tumors, published in 1974. He was a founding member of the American Society of Dermatopathology. President Lyndon B. Johnson awarded him the President's Award for Distinguished Federal Civilian Service in 1966. The list of published contributions to skin pathology is massive, mostly original extensive descriptions of tumors, including but not limited to atypical fibroxanthoma, eccrine spiradenoma, eccrine acrospiroma, chondroid syringoma, hidradenoma papilliferum, dermatofibrosarcoma protuberans, adenoid squamous cell carcinoma, and angiolymphoid hyperplasia with eosinophilia. By all accounts, Helwig was a grandfather figure and gentleman, widely loved and respected. One of his students, James Graham, writes, 'He loved the Lord, his family, country, the AFIP, dermatopathology, and Indiana basketball' (Lupton, 2002).

Elson Bowman Helwig (1907–1999). With permission from John Wiley and Sons.

1898–1967), the spongiform pustule of Kogoj (Franjo Kogoj, 1894–1983), Kyrle disease (Josef Kyrle, 1880–1926), Masson tumor (C.L. Pierre Masson, 1880–1959), Pautrier microabscesses (Lucien Pautrier, 1876-1959), Spitz nevus (Sophie Spitz, 1910–1956), and Wells disease (George Wells, 1914–1999). It is impossible, and somewhat uncomfortable, for this author to name all the contributors to modern dermatopathology, as many are still alive and many contributions are yet to be fully recognized. The contributions of women in dermatopathology must be noted, however, arguably led by the American pathologist Sophie Spitz and her 1948 original descriptions of 'juvenile melanoma', now known as the Spitz nevus. Currently, many women dermatopathologists occupy top leadership roles in academia, training programs, and professional societies, and their contributions are having a profound impact on the specialty.

Another group of individuals with great influence includes authors of textbooks widely used among trainees. Again, this is not a complete list. In the early part of the 20th century, Josef Kyrle (1880–1926), an Austrian dermatologist, wrote *Vorlesungen* über *Histo-Biologie der menschlichen Haut und ihrer Erkrankungen (Lectures about histo-biology of the human skin and its diseases)* (Volume I, in 1925), and Oscar Gans (1888–1983), a German dermatologist and student of Unna, wrote *Histologie der Hautkrankheiten. Die Gewebsveränderungen in der Kranken Haut Unter Berücksichtigung Ihrer Entstehung und Ihres Ablaufs (Histology of Skin Diseases. Tissue Changes in the Diseased Skin with Regard to Their Genesis and Their Course)* (Volume I, also in 1925). These were two of the main dermatopathology teaching tools of their day. Walter F. Lever (1909–1992), a German-born dermatologist, spent over 20 years in the pathology laboratories of the Massachusetts General Hospital and wrote the first edition of his textbook, *Histopathology of the Skin*, in 1947 (published in 1949). He specialized in bullous

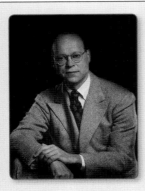

Albert Bernard Ackerman (1936-2008). 'Bernie' Ackerman was an American dermatologist and dermatopathologist, and graduate of Princeton University (Kerl & Burgdorf, 2009). He trained in dermatopathology at Massachusetts General Hospital. He was outspoken, gifted at language, and a controversial writer and speaker. He was prolific in publishing, with over 700 papers, contributions to over 60 books, and numerous editorials. He consistently challenged the current dogma and was often criticized for lack of supporting evidence for his claims. One of his most well-known controversial viewpoints was his belief that there was no clear link between ultraviolet light and melanoma. In 1978, he wrote Histologic Diagnosis of Inflammatory Skin Diseases: A Method by Pattern Analysis, in which he stresses pattern recognition 'by silhouette' and the value of scanning magnification. In 1979, he helped found the International Society of Dermatopathology (ISDP). He also founded two journals, including The American Journal of Dermatopathology and Dermatopathology: Practical and Conceptual. The American Academy of Dermatology honored Ackerman with the Master Dermatologist Award in 2004. He was involved in the training of thousands of residents and many dermatopathologists at his own Ackerman Academy of Dermatopathology, now owned by Quest Diagnostics, and has a very loyal following. Ackerman's reach spans the entire globe, through the ISDP and his many American and international students.

Albert Bernard Ackerman (1936–2008). With permission from Wolters Kluwer Health.

diseases and appendageal tumors. This book is now in its 11th edition. The American Arthur C. Allen was one of the first general pathologists to effectively tackle clinicopathologic correlation in dermatopathology with his *The Skin: a clinicopathologic treatise* in 1954. Pinkus wrote *A guide to dermatohistopathology* in 1969. The AFIP contributed several works, including a fascicle in 1962 entitled *Melanotic Tumors of the Skin* by Herbert Z. Lund and Jane M. Krause, and *Dermal pathology* by James Graham, Wayne Johnson, and Helwig in 1972. More recent comprehensive and influential dermatopathology textbooks include *Histologic Diagnosis of Inflammatory Skin Diseases: A Method by Pattern Analysis* by Ackerman, *Skin Pathology*, by the tireless Australian pathologist David Weedon (first in 1997, and now in its 4th edition), and *Pathology of the Skin with Clinical Correlation* by the Irish pathologist Phillip H. McKee (first in 1996, and now also in its 4th edition).

Technological advances

Technological advances to the microscope continued during this era. Olympus joined the German microscope makers as a global force, introducing versions with their own light source (ex. DF Biological, 1957), interchangeable modules for effective teaching (CH Series, 1976), and a new Y-shaped design (BX series, 1993). The latter series has a model this author uses today (**Figure 1.6**). Confocal microscopy was invented by the American scientist Marvin Minsky (1927–2016) in 1957. This technology allows for three-dimensional reconstruction imaging of its subjects at high resolution. It is extremely powerful but not widely used outside of the research setting due to cost. Slide scanning with virtual microscopy is also a new technology, rapidly increasing its practical applications and global reach.

In histology, new tissue stains continued to be developed (Titford 2009). In bacteriology, there were improvements made to the Gram stain (Brown & Brenn, 1931; Brown Hopps 1973), the acid fast stain (Fite 1947), syphilis stains (Steiner & Steiner 1944), and fungal stains (Grocott-Gomori 1955). Better tissue substance stains were also developed for the skin, including the Periodic Acid Schiff (PAS) stain for carbohydrates (McManus 1946), and Hales colloidal iron stain (1946) and Steedman's alcian blue stain (1950)

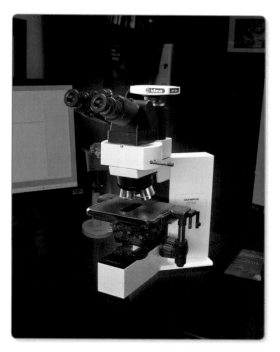

Figure 1.6 Modern Olympus microscope (BX series, 2016).

for mucin. The worlds of dermatology and cytopathology collided in this era with the work of Arnault Tzanck (1886-1954), a French physician and student of Darier who developed a modified Giemsa prep (Tzanck smear) to diagnose pemphigus, malignancies, and, of course, herpes infections. By the end of the 20th century, procedures which encompass the entire fixation → processing → embedding → cutting → staining process have been streamlined, optimized, and standardized. Automation is now routine. Today, a typical process for creating H&E stains includes the following:

- **Biopsy:** Specially designed blades and skin punch tools are routinely used. Clinicians from many specialties (surgeons, gynecologists, general practitioners), led by dermatologists, perform skin biopsies, including shaves, punches, and ellipses
- **Fixation:** 10% buffered formalin (40% formaldehyde) is the primary fixative
- **Processing:** The tissue is fixed, gradually dehydrated with alcohol, and cleared with xylene (which is miscible with both alcohol and paraffin). It is then infiltrated with paraffin
- **Embedding:** The processed tissue is embedded in paraffin wax molds to create paraffin blocks
- **Cutting:** Microtomes contain mounts, which are moved by a hand crank toward a stationary blade, creating paraffin ribbons (4–7 µM thick), which fall over the blade by gravity. Wrinkles are removed by floating the ribbons in a water bath. Select sections, to get adequate sampling from the block, are put on 3 × 1 inch positively charged slides
- **Staining:** Stainers are often automated. The tissue is dewaxed with xylene, hydrated with water, and stained with hematoxylin. The hematoxylin is pre-prepped with sodium iodate (an oxidizer or ripening agent) and aluminum potassium sulfate (mordant). Non-specific or over-staining is removed by differentiation with acid alcohol (in the commonly employed regressive method). Bluing of hematoxylin is achieved by using a weak base or alkaline tap water. The tissue is counterstained with eosin. The slides are then dehydrated and coverslipped using a mounting agent
- **Modern dermatopathology special stains:** A current, typical arsenal of special stains includes Periodic acid Schiff (PAS), mucin stains (alcian blue or colloidal iron), organism stains (Kinyoun's, Fite, PAS, GMS, Giemsa, Brown Hopps), Congo Red, Fontana-Masson, Perl's iron, Von Kossa, and Verhoeff Van Gieson

While histology of today maintained a striking resemblance to histology at the beginning of the 20th century, other emerging technologies allowed for great progress in research and diagnosis of dermatologic disease. Most of the technologies discussed in the following dedicated chapters were recent developments. The electron microscope was introduced in 1931 by Germans Ernst Ruska (1906-1988) and Max Knoll (1897-1969), providing new perspectives for the pathologic basis of disease. This tool was very popular in the mid-20th century, and while its use has faded, a few applications still remain. Fluorescence microscopy was developed around the same time (1927) and was necessary for current technologies such as immunofluorescence and fluorescence in situ hybridization (FISH). The fluorescence microscopy technology has improved (since the

1970s) with the use of ultraviolet mercury vapor bulbs for epiluminescence (or epifluorescence). Immunofluorescence was first used in 1942 by the American physician Albert Coons (1912–1978) in *Pneumococcus* research, with dermatopathology applications developing in the 1960s. Immunofluorescence remains the gold standard for diagnosis of immunobullous disease and has other applications including diagnosis of vasculitis and connective tissue disease. Immunohistochemistry is also accredited to Coons, who modified his immunofluorescence assay. Immunohistochemistry first appeared in the literature in the 1960s. This technique helped 'clean up' some nosologic nightmares in dermatology, such as nevocarcinoma and melanosarcoma, and is now a staple in the diagnostic workup of cutaneous tumors, among other applications.

Molecular diagnostics, including assays such as FISH, mutational analysis, and gene sequencing, is the fastest growing area of dermatopathology. These technologies became possible following decades of work by thousands of scientists, led by a few monumental events:

1. In 1953, James Watson (1928–), Francis Crick (1916–2004) and Maurice Wilkins (1916–2004) uncovered the structure of the DNA double-helix.
2. In 1961, Marshall Nirenberg (1927–2010) cracked the genetic code for protein synthesis.
3. In 1983, Kary Mullis (1944–) developed the polymerase chain reaction (PCR).
4. In 2003, the Human Genome Project was completed.

These building blocks provided the tools necessary to advance the understanding, classification, and diagnosis of disease. The first molecular assays in dermatopathology were developed in the 1970s and 1980s, including Ig/TCR gene-rearrangement molecular tests for lymphoma and mutational assays (by sequencing) for select genodermatoses. In the 1990s, more genetic mutations in dermatologic disease were uncovered leading to corresponding mutational assays, and FISH found some applications in soft-tissue dermatopathology. The 21st century brought more FISH applications, including aiding in the diagnosis of melanoma, and a whole new genre of tests – tumor somatic mutational assays (*BRAF*, for example), high throughput

sequencing, and gene expression profiling – to not only diagnose disease, but also aid prognosis and predict the responses to therapies, ultimately extending the role of the dermatopathologist. Molecular assays have introduced new challenges for the dermatopathologist, such as standardizing pre-analytic variables (such that fixation and processing do not impact molecular assay performance), determining appropriate use of tests (and communicating this with clinicians), controlling costs of healthcare, and getting appropriately reimbursed for performing these tests. Other technologies such as teledermatopathology and social media medicine have the potential for a massive impact on global medicine, and are already shaping the education and practice of the next generation of dermatopathologists.

Summary

The history of dermatopathology is riddled with giants of medicine, including physicians of national leaders (Virchow), the subjects of stamps (Hebra), innovators (Unna), and teachers of teachers (Helwig). The interlacing histories of dermatology and pathology are tightly woven, as attempts to separate them consistently break down. Today's tradition of cross-training pathologists in dermatology and dermatologists in pathology can be traced back to the likes of Virchow, Hebra, Welch and Osler.

Todays practice of dermatopathology has changed, led by technological advances. The litany of diseases described by dermatopathology's forefathers, without the aid of an Olympus microscope and modern stains, is staggering. However, ignoring the power of newer technologies that go beyond the H&E would be naïve and short sighted. Special stains, electron microscopy, immunohistochemistry, immunofluorescence, point of care testing, and molecular studies all have allowed dermatopathologists to refine their diagnostic abilities and elevate the care they provide to the dermatology patient. Newer molecular technologies are extending the dermatopathologist beyond dermatohistopathology, and will undoubtedly significantly shape future writings on the history of dermatopathology.

References

Carter D. Surgical Pathology at Johns Hopkins. In: J. Rosai, Ed. Guiding the Surgeon's Hand: The History of American Surgical Pathology. Washington, DC: The American Registry of Pathology, AFIP, 1997: pp. 23-40

Civatte J. Jean Darier: a memoir. Am J Dermatopathol 1979; 1:57-60.

Conn HJ, Ed. History of Staining, 1st ed. Geneva, NY: The W. F. Humphrey Press, 1933.

Delafield F, Prudden TM. A Handbook of Pathological Anatomy and Histology. New York: William Wood & Company, 1885.

Freeman RG. History of the American Society of Dermatopathology. Am J Dermatopathol 1984 6;1:25-33.

Gierke H. Färberei zu mikroscopischen Zwecken. Zits Wis Mikr, 1884;1:62-100.

Haas N. The man behind the eponym. Rudolf Virchow (1821-1902). A short overview of his work in dermatology. Am J Dermatopathol 1989 11;3:270-275.

Hollander A. Glimpses at the life and work of P. G. Unna. Am J Dermatopathol 1980; 2:137-142.

Holubar K. Ferdinand von Hebra 1816--1880: on the occasion of the centenary of his death. Int J Dermatol 1981; 20:291-295.

Holubar K, Frankl J. Moriz (Kohn) Kaposi. Am J Dermatopathol 1981; 3:349-354.

Kerl H, Burgdorf WA. Bernard Ackerman (1936-2008) the most important dermatopathologist of the 20th century, who transformed the world of dermatopathology. Am J Dermatopathol 2009; 31:734-739.

King DF. Gustav Simon. The father of dermatopathology. Am J Dermatopathol 1979; 1:225-228.

King DF. Felix von Bäerensprung (1822-1864): an early pioneer in dermatopathology. Am J Dermatopathol 1982; 4:39-40.

Kumar V, Abbas AK, Aster JC (Eds). Robbins and Cotran Pathologic Basis of Disease (9th ed.). Elsevier Ltd, 2014.

Lupton GP. Elson B. Helwig MD (1907-1999). J Cutan Pathol 2002; 29:129-134.

Maschke O. Pigmentlösung als Reagens bei mikroskopisch-physiologischen Untersuchungen. Botan Zeitg 1859;17: 21-27.

Merkel FS. Das Mikroskop und seine Anwendung. Oldenburg, Germany: Munchen, 1876.

Pusey WA. The History of Dermatology. Springfield, Il: Charles C. Thomas, 1933.

Rebecca VW, Sondak VK, Smalley KSM. A brief history of melanoma: from mummies to mutations. Melanoma Research 2012; 22:114-22.

Rosai J. Some Considerations on the Origin, Evolution, and Outlook of American Surgical Pathology. In: J. Rosai (Ed.), Guiding the Surgeon's Hand: The History of American Surgical Pathology (pp. 1-6). Washington, D.C.: The American Registry of Pathology (AFIP) 1997.

Simon G. Die Hautkrankheiten durch anatomische Untersuchungen erläutert. Berlin: Reimer, 1848.

Sulzberger MB. Three lessons learned in Bloch's clinic. Am J Dermatopathol 1980; 2: 321-325.

Titford M. Progress in the Development of Microscopical Techniques for Diagnostic Pathology. J Histotechnol 2009; 32:9-19.

Unna PG. Die Histopathologie der Hautkrankheiten. Berlin: A. Hirschwald, 1894.

Virchow R. Die Cellularpathologie in ihrer Begründung auf physiologische und pathologische Gewebelehre. Berlin: Verlag von August Hirschwald, 1858.

Von Bäerensprung F. Beiträge zur Anatomie und Pathologie der menschlichen Haut. Leipzig: Druck und Verlag von Breitkopf und Hartel, 1848.

Von Gerlach J. Mikroskopische Studien aus dem Gebiete der menschlichen Morphologie. Erlangen: Enke, 1858.

Von Hebra F (Ed). Atlas der Hautkrankheiten, Volumes 1-2. Erlangen: Aus der Kaiserlich-königlichen Hof- und Staatsdruckerei, 1856.

2 Hematoxylin and eosin

Gregory A. Hosler

Nothing in pathology has a better story than that of hematoxylin.Who or what else has had as rich a history, which is centuries old and includes the loss of many lives and the creation of nations? Who or what else has had as monumental an impact on the diagnosis of disease? While the diagnostic arsenal in dermatopathology, and indeed all fields of pathology, continues to increase, millions of hematoxylin and eosin (H&E) stains continue to be generated daily in laboratories throughout the world as first-line diagnostic tests. This chapter pays homage to what remains the true 'bread and butter' of pathology.

Hematoxylin is a natural dye. Natural dyes were the only dyes until the mid-to-late 19th century. Other natural dyes include other plant dyes (indigo, saffron, red cabbage, brazilein) and cochineal dyes (carmine, for example, derived from ground-up insects), but all natural dyes, with the exception of hematoxylin, largely have disappeared from histology. Hematoxylin is extracted from the heart wood of the logwood tree, *Haematoxylum campechianum*. Its name is derived from the Greek, meaning 'Campeche blood wood', referencing its origin in the Campeche region and the color of its wood upon oxidation. Logwood is native to the Campeche region of Mexico, on the Yucatan peninsula. It can now be found in its natural habitat, or by successful introduction, throughout Central America and the West Indies. Currently, the tree's primary use is in hedges and landscaping. The tree grows to approximately 40 feet with a crooked trunk and yellow flowers (Titford, 2005). Eosin is a synthetic agent. Its name is also derived from the Greek, meaning 'dawn' or 'morning red'.

History

The wood from *Haematoxylum campechianum* was recognized as a valuable resource by early inhabitants of the Campeche region (Allison, 1999; Smith, 2006; Titford, 2005). The Mayans and Aztecs used this wood and its coloring properties as a fabric dye, creating vibrant black, violet, and blue apparel. They also used it as a food additive and for medicinal purposes, specifically to treat dysentery. Unfortunately for the Europeans, the natives' dyeing methods were lost or destroyed, causing virtually a century-long delay in re-creating effective dyeing protocols.

In the 1500s, shortly after Spain discovered the New World, sailors used logwood as ballast. The name 'logwood' was given to this tree because the wood was shipped in 3-foot sections. The dyeing properties within the wood were quickly recognized, significantly increasing its value. Clashes developed between Spain and England, as Spain attempted to monopolize trade in the logwood-growing regions and England coveted the treasured cargo. Under Henry VIII (1491–1547) and later Elizabeth I (1533-1603), the English aggressively plundered the Spanish ships, leading to several wars.

Interestingly, the popularity of logwood/ hematoxylin in England quickly waned. This new dye initially competed with the indigo industry, but because the Europeans did not understand how to increase the lifespan of the dye (the dye was not 'colorfast'), the colors quickly faded. Queen Elizabeth I banned the 'deceitful dyeing wood' from England with the passage of an Act of Parliament in 1581. In 1620, the Dutch inventor Cornelis J. Drebbel (1572–1633) developed mordanting (while using cochineal dyes). This use of metal ions in combination with the dyes led to sustained coloration, or colorfastness, reinvigorating the appeal of logwood and the lifting of its ban in England in 1661.

In the aftermath of Drebbel's discovery, the renewed hunger for logwood led to more clashes between England and Spain, both on the seas and in New World settlements. During this time, around 1638, an English buccaneer named Captain Peter Wallace settled in the New World (British Honduras) to ambush Spanish ships for their logwood. He was called 'Ballis' (a local pronunciation of Wallace) by the Spanish-speaking inhabitants of the area, and his name subsequently evolved to 'Belize'. The Belize River and, later, the country were given his name. Today, Belize honors hematoxylin by featuring two logwood cutters on its flag (**Figure 2.1**) and some of its currency. In 1667, a treaty was signed among European powers to reduce piracy, but fighting continued regarding rights to settlements and the logwood trade. In the 18th century, both the Treaty of Paris marking the end of The Seven Years War in 1763, and The Treaty of Versailles officially marking the end of the War of American Independence in 1783, specifically addressed the rights to logwood. Hematoxylin has further ties to war as it was used in the uniforms of United States soldiers during The Civil War and both world wars.

This author was a little disappointed to learn that the wars over hematoxylin were fueled by the textile industry and not insatiable pathologists. Hematoxylin use in histology began during this era but really only flourished in the 19th century and beyond. There are mentions of the scientific use of hematoxylin by the English scientist and philosopher Robert Hooke (1635–1703) as early as the 1600s. Georg Christian Reichel (1721–1771), in 1758, and later John Thomas Quekett (1815-

1861), in 1848, described the use of hematoxylin to stain tissue (Quekett, 1848; Reichel, 1758). In 1863, Wilhelm von Waldeyer (1836-1921) used an aqueous extract of hematoxylin to study neural tissue (Waldeyer, 1863). Waldeyer is considered the first to actually study hematoxylin as a histologic stain, even though he later abandoned the technique. In1865, Franz Böhmer first used mordanting of hematoxylin (alum-hematoxylin), a technique taken from the textile industry, with great success (Böhmer, 1865). Once the value of mordanting was realized, many investigators – Paul Ehrlich (1854–1915), Francis Delafield (1841–1915), Paul Mayer (1848–1923), Carl Weigert (1845–1904), and H. F. Harris-refined the staining procedure (Titford, 2005). The Harris formula, developed in 1900, is still widely used today, with minor modifications (Harris, 1900). Later, other scientists recognized the value of hematoxylin as a nuclear stain and used it in their own specialized formulas. Examples include Verhoeff (1908, elastic fiber stain), van Gieson (1889, connective tissue), Weil (1928, myelin), Masson (1929, trichrome), and Papanicolau (1928, Pap smear) (Conn, 1933; Papanicolaou, 1941).

The history of eosin is not quite as exceptional as that of hematoxylin. Eosin is a synthetic dye and did not lead to any wars or naming of nations. In the mid-1800s, aniline (coal tar) dyes were discovered and quickly absorbed into the textile industry. Eosin is one of the many aniline dyes, first synthesized in 1871 by Adolf Baeyer

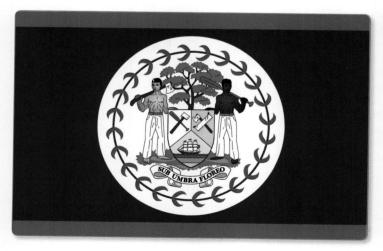

Figure 2.1 The Belize national flag featuring logwood cutters.

(1835–1917) (Baeyer, 1875). In 1876, Ernst Fischer (1854–1917) and Julius Dreschfeld (1845–1907) first described the use of eosin in staining tissue sections (Conn, 1933). Hematoxylin and eosin double staining was first reported by Wissozky (1876) (Wissozky, 1877). The rest, as they say, is history.

Histochemistry

Hematoxylin is a flavonoid, a phenolic compound related to flower pigments (**Figure 2.2**) (Horobin & Kiernan, 2002). It is extracted from the logwood by running hot water or steam over the heart wood chips, ultimately producing crystals or powder. This process is usually performed at the site of the logwood harvesting, which is now almost exclusively in Mexico. Hematoxylin is actually colorless, and must be oxidized to hematein, which is a red brown color. With further oxidation, hematein converts to oxyhematein, which is again colorless. Therefore, hematoxylin is not really a dye (hematein is), but by convention, hematoxylin is the preferred dye name within the industry. The pigment can be visualized in the heartwood from the cut surface of oxidized logwood (**Figure 2.3**). Oxidation can occur with atmospheric oxygen or by the use of a ripening agent (sodium iodate is the most common these days) or a mordant. Mordants are metal ions, and, depending on which one is used, can produce a different color. The most common mordants are alum (gray-violet) and ferric ion (gray-black). Other less-common ones are magnesium (yellow), copper (green), antimony (crimson), and gold (orange). In dermatopathology (and almost all H&E protocols), the alum mordant is used. Hemalum is the name of the alum-hematein complex. Mordants are required for colorfastness, or fade-resistance, of the stain. Hemalum stains nuclei red or dull-brown. Bluing of the hemalum is performed by exposing the stain to a slight alkaline solution, which may be alkaline distilled water, or most tap water. Blue is preferred over red since there are

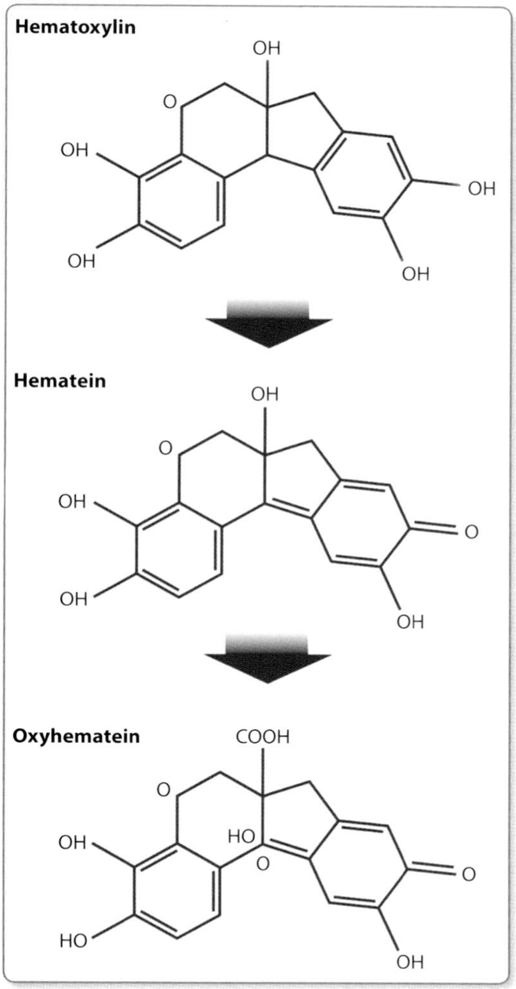

Hematoxylin

Hematein

Oxyhematein

Figure 2.2 The chemical structures of hematoxylin, hematein, and oxyhematein.

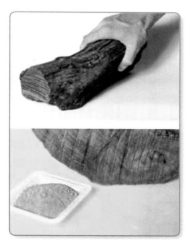

Figure 2.3 Pigment in the oxidized cut surface of the logwood heart wood. Logwood and powder from cut surface (With permission from Dr Gary Gill and Agilent Technologies Company).

readily available and effective red counterstains, such as eosin. The bluing procedure converts the red alum-hematein complex to blue polymers. On routine H&E tissue sections, the hemalum stains deep blue or black (or violet with an eosin counterstain). Interestingly, the mechanism of staining by hemalum is still unknown. It appears that hemalum is attracted to proteins in the nuclei, such as histones, and remains held there by van der Waals forces. It is not strictly an acid-base reaction, although it is convenient (for memorizing purposes) to recognize that hemalum will stain acids, such as DNA and RNA. In addition to nuclei, hemalum will also stain the cytoplasm of some cells with high levels of rRNA, such as plasma cells, and it will stain some mucins at a standard pH. Components that stain with hematoxylin (hemalum) are considered basophilic.

Eosin Y, or just 'eosin', is the potassium salt of tetrabromofluorescein (**Figure 2.4**). The 'Y' refers to a yellow tint (eosin B, for 'blue', also exists), and eosin Y is the most common form of eosin used in routine H&E stains. It is soluble in alcohol or water. It is an anionic, or acid, dye. Again, the mechanism of eosin staining is not fully understood, but it is thought that eosin is attracted to positively charged molecules by ionic forces, and held in place by van der Waals forces.

Many intracellular and extracellular proteins are positively charged, and, depending on their concentration, eosin will stain with a range of red, orange, and pink hues. For example, eosin stains nucleoli red, cytoplasm red or dark pink, and collagen pink (less protein and more water). It also makes hemalum appear more violet. Components that stain with eosin are considered eosinophilic.

The modern hematoxylin and eosin stain

Most modern H&E protocols use either a so-called 'progressive' or a 'regressive' staining method (progressive has slower uptake of dye, but doesn't require differentiation: see below). Differentiation refers to the de-staining of hematoxylin in the tissue, primarily leaving only nuclear staining. Clearing by xylene minimizes light diffraction, helping to optically improve the final product. The following steps are used in the more common regressive staining method:

- Water (hydrating)
- Hematoxylin (staining nuclei, mucins, etc.)
- Weak acid (0.5% HCl in 70% EtOH, differentiation, this step is skipped in the progressive method)
- Water (bluing and rinsing)
- Eosin (0.5% w/v, counterstaining)
- Water (rinsing)
- Ethanol (dehydrating)
- Xylene (clearing)

Because hematoxylin and eosin stain tissues through biochemical interactions, many pre-analytic and analytic variables can affect the final H&E product, both in terms of morphology and color. These variables include, but are not limited to, the condition of the tissue, tissue size, time delay prior to fixation, fixation, processing (dehydration, clearing), cutting (thickness), dewaxing, mounting, reagent list, quality of stains and solutions (purity, oxidation status, pH), temperature, and staining protocol. H&E is a morphologic stain and most pathologists have their own color preferences. Differences in H&E tinctorial qualities from different laboratories

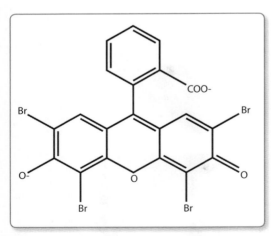

Figure 2.4 The chemical structure of eosin Y.

are quickly recognized when examining consult material. Every pathologist has their preferences, and as long as the product is considered 'useful for its intended purpose', it is considered satisfactory. But what is satisfactory for one pathologist may not be deemed so for another.

For dermatopathology specimens, this author prefers the following tinctorial qualities (**Figure 2.5**): the epidermis should be violet. The dermis should have orange-red collagen, with red pilar muscles and lighter pink neural bundles. The adnexal structures, including the follicles and secretory units (eccrine/apocrine glands) should have a slightly lighter shade of violet than the epidermis. The sebaceous units and subcutaneous fat should appear white. Basement membrane material should be red. Regarding cytological detail, the nuclear chromatin should be dark blue-black with a slight reddish hue for the nucleoli. Intracellular granules should vary from blue-black (keratohyaline/epidermal),

to dark violet (mast cells) and bright red (eosinophils).

The H&E stain is not infallible. Shortcomings not only include inconsistencies in coloration, but also poorly understood histochemical mechanisms, lack of discernment for cytoplasmic structures, variable quality of reagents (purity variation, quality not regulated), and a limited supply (Mexico has a virtual monopoly on logwood extract and a recent shortage occurred when the main supplier decided to swap logwood extract manufacture for the production of more lucrative skin care products). For these reasons, there have been previous attempts to replace the H&E stain with alternatives. Alternatives do exist, some of which have excellent results, but most pathologists are unwilling to relinquish the familiar H&E stain. Most of the diagnostic shortcomings of the H&E stain can be addressed using the methods described in the following chapters.

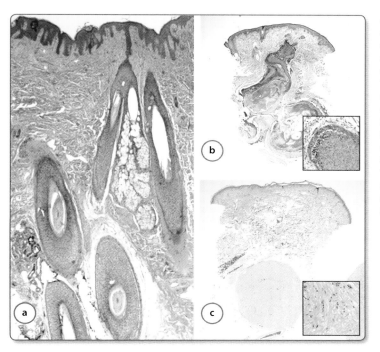

Figure 2.5 The hematoxylin and eosin (H&E) stain. (a) An example of a routine H&E stain of skin reveals different shades of pink, red, purple, and blue (40×). (b, c) Tumors have varying degrees of red and blue hues at low power (20×). (b, inset) Tumors with higher degrees of cellularity and high nuclear:cytoplasmic ratios appear more basophilic, or blue (pilomatricoma 400×). (c, inset) Tumors with lower cellularity or low nuclear:cytoplasmic ratios appear more eosinophilic, or red (angioleiomyoma 400×).

References

Alliso RT. Haematoxylin – from the wood. J Clin Pathol 1999; 52:527–528.

Baeyer A. Zur geschichte des Eosins. Berichte Der Deutschen Chemischen Gesellschaft 1875;8:146–148.

Böhmer F. Zur pathologischen Anatomie der Meningitis cerebromedullaris epidemica. Aerztl Intelligenzh Munchen 1865;12:539–550.

Conn H J, ed. History of Staining Geneva, NY: The W. F. Humphrey Press, 1933.

Gill GW. Gill hematoxylins: first person account. Biotech Histochem 2010;85:7–18.

Harris H. On the rapid conversion of haematoxylin into haematein in staining reactions. J App Micr 1900;3:770–780.

Horobin R, Kiernan J, Eds. Conn's biological stains: a handbook of dyes, stains, and fluorochromes for use in biology and medicine, 10th ed. Oxford: BIOS Scientific Publishers, 2002.

Papanicolaou G. Some improved methods for staining vaginal smears. J Lab Clin Med 1941; 26: 1200–1205.

Quekett J. A Practical Treatise on the Use of the Microscope, Including the Different Methods of Preparing and Examining Animal, Vegetable and Mineral Structures. London: Bailliere, 1848.

Reichel C. Das vasis plantarum spiralibus. Lipsine: Breitkopf, 1758.

Smith C. Our debt to the logwood tree: the history of hematoxylin. MLO: Medical Laboratory Observer 2006;38: 20–22.

Titford M. The long history of hematoxylin. Biotechnic & Histochemistry. 2005; 80:73–78.

Waldeyer W. Untersuchungen uber den Ursprung und den Verlauf des Axencylinders bei Wirbellosen und Wirbelthieren sowie uber dessen Endverhalten in der quergestreiften Muskelfaser. Henle U Pfeufer Z Ration Med 1863; 20:193–256.

Wissozky N. Ueber das Eosin als Reagens auf Hämoglobin und die Bildung von Blutgefässen und Blutkörperchen bei Säugethier- und Hühnerembryonen. Archiv Für Mikroskopische Anatomie 1877; 13:479–496.

Section 2

Special stains

3 Special stains: background

Ryan W. Hick

For over a century, pathologists have relied on routine hematoxylin and eosin (H&E) staining in the primary interpretation of tissue specimens. For just as long a variety of alternative staining methods, also known as 'special stains' in the jargon of histotechnologists and pathologists, have been used to demonstrate cell structure, foreign organisms, and other tissue structures. In many instances, these special stains depend upon affinities of dyes to particular macromolecules within tissue sections. Other special stains rely on chemical reactions to produce a visible color change against a background stain. With the advent of relatively newer immunohistochemical techniques with high specificity and sensitivity, some of these special stains have fallen by the wayside (i.e. consider the detection of *Treponema pallidum* by immunohistochemistry versus the Warthin–Starry silver stain). However, many of these older special stains remain comparatively inexpensive, sensitive and specific methods to assist the process of making a diagnosis. This is especially true in cases of infectious diseases and deposition disorders.

An understanding of the basic biochemical underpinnings of these special stain techniques will assist the aspiring or already experienced dermatopathologist in deciding which stains to use, in knowing the optimal circumstances for their use, and in recognizing the shortcomings of some stains or the possible sources of error in interpretation. This chapter places the development of special stains in a historical context relative to the development of other stains and ancillary tissue techniques.

Carbohydrates

Periodic acid–Schiff

The first histologic application of the periodic acid–Schiff (PAS) technique was published in 1946 by McManus (McManus, 1946; Titford, 2009). This method for detecting various carbohydrates and glycoproteins in histologic sections has become one of the most commonly used complements to routine H&E staining in the anatomic pathology setting. It is most routinely used by dermatopathologists as an adjunct to H&E for the detection of fungal organisms; however, it has other important, albeit less frequently utilized, applications.

The PAS technique relies upon a two-step process that allows for detection of carbohydrates composed of monosaccharides with 1,2-glycol bonds. In the first step, periodic acid (metaperiodic acid [HIO_4] or orthoperiodic acid [H_4IO_5]) cleaves the carbon bond between 1,2-glycols in an oxidation reaction that results in the formation of two aldehyde moieties (**Figure 3.1**). While other oxidants may be used, they may result in further oxidation of aldehydes to carboxylic acids, limiting the effectiveness of the second step in the reaction (Suvarna, 2013).

The second step relies upon a technique developed in the late 19th century by German-Italian chemist Hugo Schiff for the detection of aldehydes. This step involves the preparation of Schiff reagent from the magenta-hued basic fuchsine dye (a triarylmethane dye also referred to as pararosanaline) and aqueous sulfurous acid. The conjugation of a sulfonic acid group with the central carbon atom of the basic fuchsine results in loss of the dye's color in solution. However, when Schiff reagent is applied to tissue sections that have been treated with periodic acid, the highly concentrated aldehyde groups of structures rich in carbohydrates and proteoglycans remove the sulfonate group from basic fuchsine and restore the quinoid structure of the dye as well as its rich magenta color within those target tissue structures (**Figure 3.2**). Periodic acid oxidizes other alcohol groups including the terminal

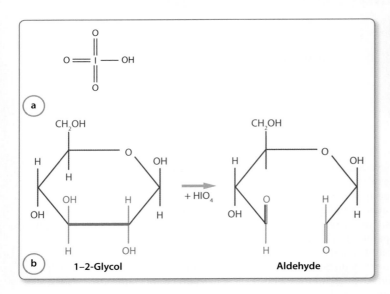

Figure 3.1 Periodic acid conversion of 1,2-glycol bonds in polysaccharide monomers to aldehyde moieites. (a) Periodic acid. (b) Periodic acid converts the 1,2-glycol bond within the monosaccharide to two aldehyde moieties.

amino alcohols of serine and threonine. Given the relatively low concentrations of these groups in tissue, the reactions are mostly insignificant (Suvarna, 2013).

The PAS stain is most frequently used by dermatopathologists to exclude the presence of fungal organisms. The stain targets the polysaccharide mannan in the cell wall of yeast, dermatophytes, and other fungi. The PAS stain also highlights the polysaccharide molecule glycogen, which often appears in mucosal epithelium, inflamed reactive epidermis, clear cell acanthoma, eccrine glands, and normal outer root sheath or tumors with outer root sheath differentiation (**Table 3.1**). Pretreatment with the enzyme diastase removes glycogen but the use of diastase may be more useful in cases where PAS is employed to detect neutral mucins in simple epithelia, and differentiation from glycogen is required. This application is not routine in the interpretation of skin specimens. Sulfated mucins and acid mucins, such as hyaluronic acid, are PAS-negative. The PAS stain is sometimes used to evaluate thickening of the basement membrane zone in cases of presumed connective tissue disease, such as discoid lupus erythematosus, as well as in conditions that cause thickening of the vascular basement membrane, such as

porphyria cutanea tarda, lipoid proteinosis and erythropoietic protoporphyria. The thickened basement membrane zone is associated with increased numbers of glycoproteins, which can be detected with the PAS technique.

Hematoxylin and Fast Green FCF are counterstains most frequently used in conjunction with the PAS technique to provide a contrasting background. The former is useful for highlighting nuclear features of the surrounding tissue, whereas the latter may provide better contrast with some targets of the reaction, such as fungal organisms (**Figure 3.3**).

Alcian blue

Alcian blue was used as a textile dye well before its application as a histologic stain. The name 'alcian' likely represents a corruption of the chemical name phthalocyanine (who wants to be adding extra 'phth' at the beginning of words anyway?). The dye is a large molecule composed of a phthalocyanine ring with four linked isothiouronium groups. There is a central copper ion that imbues the blue color observed on microscopy (**Figure 3.4**). The isothiouronium groups are cationic bases that can bond with polyanionic groups of sulfated and non-sulfated mucins (Suvarna, 2013). For most skin applications, skin specimens are treated with alcian blue at pH 2.5 because the usual target substance is hyaluronic acid. Alcian blue fails to stain hyaluronic acid when used at pH 1.0.

The combination alcian blue-PAS (AB-PAS) stain is used most commonly in gastrointestinal pathology to differentially stain acid and neutral mucins, with alcian blue staining the former

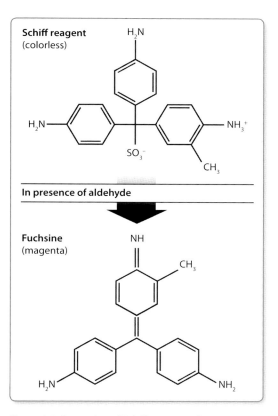

Schiff reagent (colorless)

In presence of aldehyde

Fuchsine (magenta)

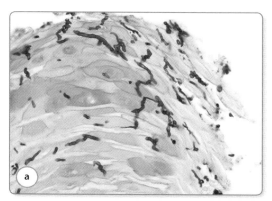

a

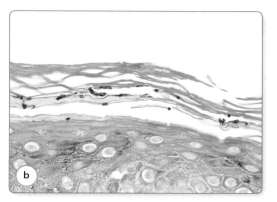

b

Figure 3.2 Conversion of Schiff reagent to basic fuchsine. Upon exposure to the aldehyde moieties of polysaccharides previously treated with periodic acid, Schiff reagent is converted back to magenta-hued basic fuchsine.

Figure 3.3 PAS stain for fungal organisms. (a) PAS stain of onychomycosis with hematoxylin counterstain (PAS 400×). (b) PAS stain of dermatophytosis with Green FCF counterstain (PAS-G, 400×). Melanin is often accentuated on PAS stain with either countertstain.

	PAS	PAS-D	Alcian blue 2.5	Mucicarmine	Colloidal iron
Table 3.1 Special stains for carbohydrates and mucopolysaccharides					
Glycogen	+	-	-	-	-
Hyaluronic acid	-	-	+	-	+
Neutral mucin	+	+	-	-	-
Sialomucin	+/-	+/-	+	+	+
Sulfomucin	-	-	+	+	+
PAS, Periodic acid–Schiff; PAS-D, Periodic acid–Schiff following diastase					

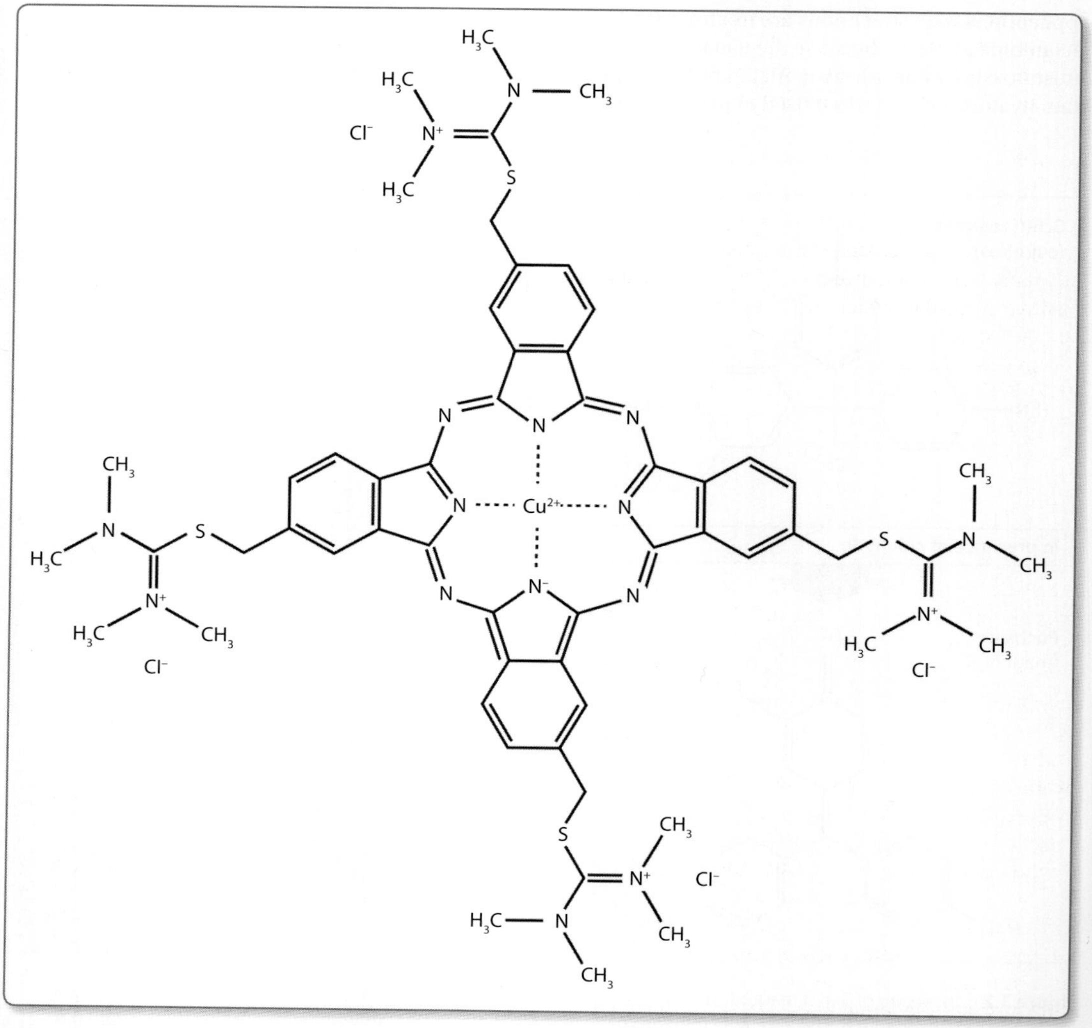

Figure 3.4 Alcian blue dye. The copper molecule at the center of the phthalocyanine ring imbues a blue color to the dye, which deposits in areas rich in sulfated, and acid mucopolysaccharides.

and PAS staining the latter. This combination may also be useful in cutaneous specimens. In cases of suspected connective tissue disease, AB-PAS may demonstrate increased dermal hyaluronic acid deposition and basement membrane zone thickening. The stain can also differentially highlight the mucinous capsule of *Cryptococcus neoformans* (blue) and the yeast form (magenta).

Colloidal iron

Hale published the initial application of a colloidal iron method for the detection of acid mucopolysaccharides in 1946 (Hale, 1946). The technique involves a two-step process. Firstly, a colloidal suspension of ferric oxide is applied to tissue sections allowing ferric ions (Fe^{3+}) to conjugate with carboxyl and sulfate anionic groups on acid mucopolysaccharides and proteoglycans. Secondly, the Perls reaction of potassium ferrocyanide with the tissue now infused with an excess of ferric ions is carried out, forming ferric ferrocyanide, a bright blue stain known as Prussian blue (**Figure 3.5**).

In the skin, this reaction primarily highlights hyaluronic acid, comprising the ground substance of the dermis. The papillary dermis, normally rich in acid mucins, serves as an internal positive control to which the amount of staining between collagenic bundles in the dermis or within the follicular epithelium can be compared. Perifollicular and perivascular zones, similar to the papillary dermis, are rich in hyaluronic acid and should not be confused for 'positive' staining. The presence of excess interstitial hyaluronic acid deposits between collagenic fibers in the dermis is considered abnormal and indicative of a pathologic process. Increased mucin deposition is also abnormal with the epidermis and adnexal epithelium (**Figure 3.6**). The staining pattern must be considered in the context of the tissue reaction pattern. In the setting of an interface dermatitis, increased interstitial dermal mucin supports a differential diagnosis that includes a connective tissue disease process. Increased interstitial hyaluronic acid deposition must be distinguished from solar elastosis in anatomic sites chronically exposed to ultraviolet radiation. Hyaluronic acid, due to dehydration during tissue processing, has a wispy appearance with beads along thin fibrils of material on both H&E and colloidal iron staining. On the contrary, solar elastosis appears merely as pale blue fibers of roughly the same caliber and thickness as adjacent collagen of the superficial reticular dermis.

Mucicarmine

The mucicarmine method was first published by Mayer in 1896 and later modified by Southgate in

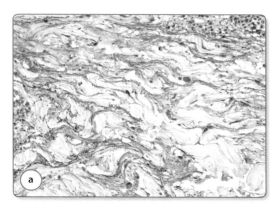

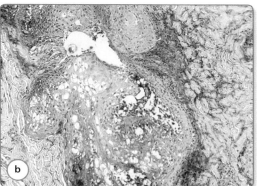

Figure 3.6 Colloidal iron stain. (a) In tumid lupus erythematosus there is an abundance of interstitial hyaluronic acid deposited between collagen bundles (colloidal iron, 200×). (b) In follicular mucinosis hyaluronic acid is deposited within follicular epithelium (200×).

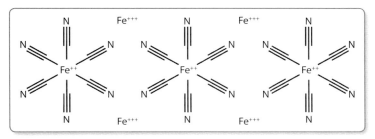

Figure 3.5 Ferric ferrocyanide. In the colloidal iron method, ferric ferrocyanide (Prussian blue) is produced by reaction of potassium ferrocyanide solution with ferric ions taken up by mucopolysaccharides from a colloidal iron solution.

1927. Carmine is a naturally derived pigment that comes from crushed, desiccated female cochineal scale insects (*Dactylopius coccus*) (**Figure 3.7**). The mucicarmine stain remains, along with hematoxylin, one of the few naturally derived dyes still used in modern dermatopathology. The pigment is formed from an aluminum salt of carminic acid, a red glucosidal hydroxyanthrapurin (**Figure 3.8**). Indigenous people of Central America used carmine to dye textiles prior to European colonization but its use increased substantially following colonization. In addition to applications in medical diagnostics and biologic research, the pigment is used on a large scale in the cosmetics and food industries. As an example, the author recently noted carmine listed as an ingredient in his strawberry yogurt. Cochineal and carmine made news headlines when a prominent purveyor of coffee beverages announced it would no longer be using the insect-derived dye in its products because its consumption is prohibited by a number of vegetarian and religious groups. The use of carmine to stain animal tissue dates to the mid-19th century. Later modifications resulted in an application that is useful today as a stain to highlight epithelial mucins.

In tissue reactions the aluminum-carmine complex bonds with negatively charged acid mucins including epithelial mucins (i.e. sialomucins found in tumors such as Paget disease and low grade mucoepidermoid carcinoma, among others) and the mucinous capsule of *Cryptococcus neoformans*. The primary component of the capsule is the complex polysaccharide glucuronoxylomannan (Zaragoza 2009). Neutral mucins and sulfated mucins either stain poorly or do not stain at all. A blue counterstain, such as alum hematoxylin, is typically used in order to differentiate nuclei.

Gomori/Grocott methenamine silver

Gyorgy Gomori first published a methenamine silver technique for detection of fungal organisms in 1946, followed by Grocott's modification in 1955 (Titford 2009; Suvarna 2013). The cell wall of fungi is primarily composed of the polysaccharide mannan. The mannose monosaccharides

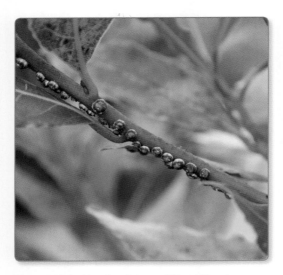

Figure 3.7　Cochineal scale insect. The cochineal scale insect is the source of carminic acid used in the mucicarmine stain.

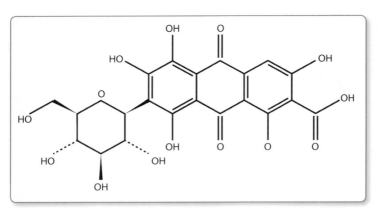

Figure 3.8　Carminic acid. This naturally produced red dye is useful in detecting epithelial mucins, as well as the mucinous capsule of *Cryptococcus neoformans*.

comprising these long carbohydrate chains include a 1,2-glycol bond that can be oxidized into two aldehyde moieties.

In contrast to the periodic acid–Schiff method, the GMS technique utilizes chromic acid to carry out the oxidation of the 1,2-glycol bond to two aldehydes moieties. A silver solution composed of silver nitrate, borax, and methenamine is applied at high temperature to the tissue. Under these conditions, the aldehyde component reduces silver nitrate to metallic silver, which deposits in the tissue and appears black on microscopy (Suvarna, 2013). The tissue is typically counterstained light green (**Figure 3.9**). Since it is a natural reducing agent that is not readily soluble and complexes with constitutive proteins of basal keratinocytes and melanocytes, melanin pigment also appears black with this technique. Neutrophils and neutrophil debris, which frequently also stain black, may be misinterpreted as organisms by less-experienced dermatopathologists.

Melanin

Fontana–Masson

When present in sufficient quantities, melanin is readily identified in histologic sections of skin by its color (brown) and its typical distribution (overlying the nuclei of basal keratinocytes). It is important to identify abnormal distribution of melanin pigment. The Fontana–Masson technique remains useful as a fairly precise method of highlighting the distribution of melanin pigment and its relative quantity. The most common dermatoses for which this stain finds important application today include vitiligo, drug pigmentation, pigmentation of the nail unit (i.e. melanonychia), and post-inflammatory pigment alteration.

The Fontana–Masson staining method relies on the argentaffin reaction. (*Argentum* is Latin for silver, so argentaffin literally means 'affinity for silver'). In this reaction, a silver salt solution is converted to elemental silver. The Fontana–Masson technique involves application of ammoniacal silver solution (Fontana's silver solution) to tissue sections followed by counterstaining with nuclear fast red. Melanin is a strong reducing agent that converts the ammoniacal silver to metallic silver. Impregnated in the tissue, elemental silver turns the already brown melanin pigment black (**Figure 3.10**) (Suvarna, 2013). The Fontana–Masson method is a very promiscuous stain that reacts with other tissue elements, including argentaffin, chromaffin, lipofuscin and fungi (**Table 3.2**).

Schmorl

As a strong reducing agent, melanin can reduce ferric ions (Fe^{3+}) to ferrous ions (Fe^{2+}). A subsequent reaction with potassium ferricyanide results in the production of ferrous ferricyanide (Turnbull blue or Prussian blue) similar to the colloidal iron and Perls staining methods discussed elsewhere in this chapter. This technique is used less commonly than the Fontana–Masson method for the detection of melanin.

Metal ions

Perls Prussian blue

Distinguishing among various pigments in histologic sections of skin is not always a simple task. The practiced eye can often discern subtle differences between endogenous and exogenous pigments, but in many instances it can be difficult to definitively differentiate melanin pigment from iron pigment. Hemosiderin is the hemoglobin-derived, iron-containing pigment most frequently encountered in skin biopsies. It generally appears

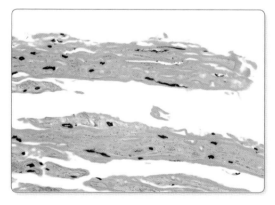

Figure 3.9 Grocott methenamine silver stain for fungal organisms. Silver nitrate is reduced to elemental silver in the presence of borax and methenamine after oxidation by chromic acid of 1,2-glycol moieties in the cell wall of fungal hyphae in onychomycosis (GMS, 400×).

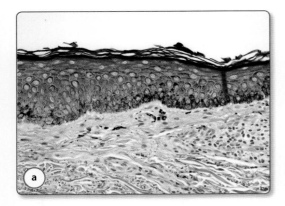

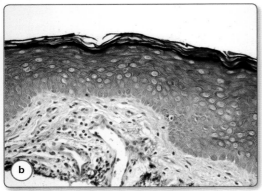

Figure 3.10 Fontana–Masson stain. (a) Fontana–Masson stain of normal uninvolved skin of a patient with vitiligo (FM, 200×). (b) Fontana–Masson stain of lesional skin of a patient with vitiligo (FM, 200×).

Table 3.2 Silver stains
Dieterle
Fontana–Masson
Gomori/Grocott methenamine silver
Steiner stain
von Kossa
Warthin-Starry

as slightly coarse, variably sized, refractile, golden-brown granules on H&E staining. Hemosiderin is present as ferric hydroxide $(Fe(OH)_3)$. It forms complexes with proteins typically in an intracellular location (i.e. within macrophages). Formalin-based tissue fixation renders hemosiderin somewhat soluble in weak acid solutions, whereas ferric and ferrous forms

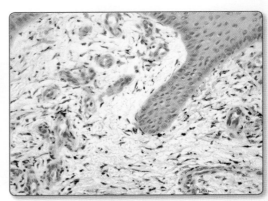

Figure 3.11 Perls Prussian blue iron stain in stasis dermatitis. In stasis dermatitis there is deposition of hemosiderin pigment within the dermis, predominantly in a perivascular distribution (Perls, 200×). Iron in hemosiderin reacts with the Prussian blue iron stain, whereas iron in hemoglobin is insufficiently soluble to react.

of iron in hemoglobin complexes are insoluble and will not react with staining solutions for iron pigment (Suvarna, 2013).

The Perls Prussian blue reaction allows demonstration of ferric iron ions (Fe^{3+}) in tissue sections. Treatment of tissue sections with a combination of dilute hydrochloric acid and potassium ferrocyanide allows the release of ferric hydroxide $(Fe(OH)_3)$ from hemosiderin-protein complexes and subsequent conversion to ferric ferrocyanide $(Fe_4[Fe(CN)_6]_3 \cdot \times H_2O)$ (i.e. Prussian blue). Ferric ferrocyanide is an insoluble blue pigment that is detected on light microscopy. The root word cyan (i.e. cyanide) is derived from the Greek *kyanos* meaning dark blue. Counterstaining for the Perls Prussian blue method is typically performed with nuclear fast red (**Figure 3.11**). Of note, the Prussian blue pigment has been used as a pigment in art since at least the early 18th century in Europe and perhaps in the well-known Japanese painting *The Great Wave Off Kanagawa* by Hokusai (c. 1830).

Von Kossa

Inorganic calcium salts in sections of skin are typically deposited as calcium phosphate or calcium carbonate salts. While free ionic calcium (Ca^{2+}) is to all intents and purposes not detectable using histochemical techniques, inorganic salts of calcium in tissue sections (i.e. calcium phosphate) can be demonstrated directly or indirectly. The dermatopathologist may find this stain most useful in identifying or confirming the presence of subtle calcification, as in calciphylaxis or pseudoxanthoma elasticum, as opposed to more grossly evident cases of calcinosis cutis.

The von Kossa method employs a silver staining technique, in which silver nitrate is applied to tissue sections. Silver cations (Ag^{1+}) precipitate with the phosphate and/or carbonate anions of the calcium salts (Suvarna, 2013). The stain is considered more sensitive but less specific than the alizarin red S method. For example, silver nitrate will stain melanin in treated sections in addition to the calcium salts. Given that melanin and calcium deposits are not frequently collocated, this does not typically cause significant errors of interpretation. Skin sections are typically counterstained with nuclear fast red (**Figure 3.12**).

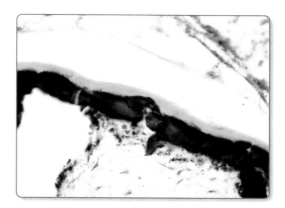

Figure 3.12 Von Kossa silver stain of calcinosis cutis. Calcium deposits in calcinosis cutis are demonstrated by precipitation of silver nitrate with phosphate and carbonate from calcium salts and subsequent reduction to elemental silver.

Alizarin red S

In contrast to the von Kossa method for the detection of inorganic calcium salts, alizarin red S represents a dye that directly stains calcium within tissue sections (**Figure 3.13**). Alizarin red S forms a chelate complex with calcium that appears red and is often paired with fast green FCF as a counterstain. A pH of 4.2 may improve the stain's ability to detect smaller particulate deposits of calcium.

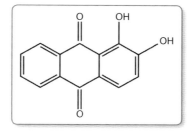

Figure 3.13 Alizarin red dye. This dye demonstrates calcium salt deposition directly through a chelation process.

Connective tissue

Verhoeff

The Verhoeff technique is a widely accepted method for detecting elastic fibers in formalin-fixed paraffin-embedded tissue sections. First published in 1908 by Frederick H. Verhoeff, this method permits the visualization of fine oxytalan fibers of the papillary dermis and elaunin fibers of the deeper reticular dermis (Titford, 2009).

The Verhoeff staining method takes advantage of the disulfide crosslinking between elastic fibers. These disulfide bonds are oxidized in the presence of iodine to anionic sulfonic acid. The iodine is applied in solution with alcohol hematoxylin and ferric chloride. The anionic sulfonic acid moieties have a higher affinity to iron and hematoxylin in the solution than the surrounding tissue during the subsequent decolorization step. So, as the dye is removed more readily from adjacent collagen and cellular elements, the result is deep blue or black staining of elastic fibers (Suvarna, 2013).

The van Gieson technique is commonly used as a counterstain with the Verhoeff method. This step employs picric acid with acid fuchsine resulting in black staining of nuclei and red staining of collagen (**Figure 3.14**) (Suvarna, 2013). Because of the frequent use of the van Gieson counter stain, this two-step process is typically known as the Verhoeff–van Gieson (VVG) or elastin–van Gieson (EVG) stain.

Masson trichrome

On routine H&E staining, the connective tissue comprising the dermis, including collagen,

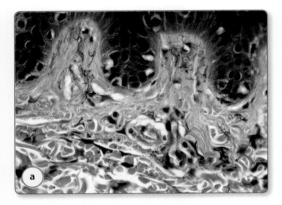

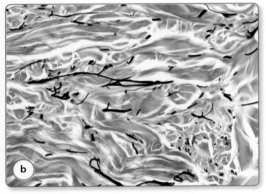

Figure 3.14 (a) Verhoeff-van Gieson stain. Verhoeff-van Gieson stain of normal papillary dermal elastin fibers (VVG, 400×). (b) Verhoeff-van Gieson stain of thicker elastin fibers in the reticular dermis (VVG, 200×).

smooth muscle, and nerve fibers, all appears in various shades of pink. Trichrome stains allow for differential staining of connective tissue structures. The Masson trichrome technique produces a very distinctive contrast between muscle (red) and collagen (blue/green). Historically, this stain was very useful for determining the lineage of soft tissue tumors, but that role has since been ceded to immunohistochemistry. In the skin, this is specifically useful for differentiating smooth muscle from collagen or for detecting collagen fibers entering the epidermis. The role of this technique is now somewhat limited to the confirmation of collagen fibers penetrating the epidermis in reactive perforating collagenosis. Some may still find it useful in the diagnosis of smooth muscle neoplasms and hamartomas as well. The stepwise application of various solutions

is required to allow for differential staining of the tissue sections.

The Masson trichrome method begins with hematoxylin staining of nuclei, which will be resistant to subsequent applications of acidic solutions in preparation for other dyes to adhere to other tissue structures. Next, an acid fuchsine solution stains the tissue red. Phosphomolybdic acid or phosphotungstic acid are used to decolorize collagen fibers, but muscle tissue, fibrin, cytoplasm, and erythrocytes retain the red acid fuchsine stain. Finally, aniline blue (a mixture of methyl blue and water blue dyes) is applied, staining collagen fibers blue (Suvarna, 2013). Because of retention of the red acid fuchsine stain, the other structures are unaffected by the blue dye (**Figure 3.15**).

Several other histochemical techniques allow differential staining of additional connective tissue structures, including the van Gieson stain, phosphotungstic acid-hematoxylin (PTAH), Gomori trichrome, and Russel–Movat pentachrome. Other than the van Gieson stain, these additional methods are employed to detect finer details in nerve and muscle tissue. They are less frequently utilized in the realm of dermatopathology.

Amyloid
Congo red

Congo red is a long, symmetrical, sulfonated azo dye that was first used as a textile dye (**Figure 3.16**). The name of the dye was chosen not because of some exotic source in central sub-Saharan Africa, but rather because it served as a catchy name that might attract the interest of textile manufactures in the nineteenth century (Steensma, 2001). The molecular structure of Congo red permits situation of the dye between the anti-parallel strands of β-pleated sheets comprising amyloid fibrils. The linear arrangement of the dye confers the property of dichroism upon polarization microscopy. In other words, light with different polarization is differentially absorbed by the Congo red dye (Suvarna, 2013). Typically, Congo red-stained amyloid tissue appears brick red on routine light microscopy but can appear yellow-green (or 'apple green') with polarized light. Hematoxylin is used as a counterstain so that nuclei appear blue (**Figure 3.17**).

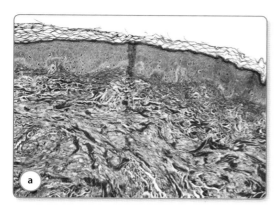
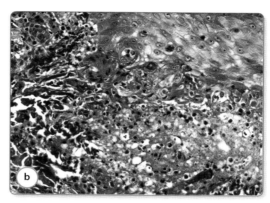

Figure 3.15 Masson trichrome stain. (a) Masson trichrome stain highlighting pink smooth muscle and adjacent blue collagen bundles in leiomyoma (Masson trichrome, 100×). (b) Masson trichrome stain demonstrating blue collagen fibers extending into pink epidermis (Masson trichrome, 200×).

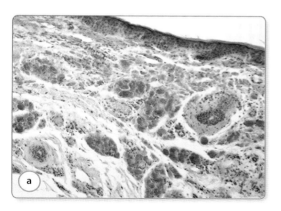

Figure 3.16 Congo red dye. The molecular structure of the Congo red dye allows for situation between the anti-parallel strands of β-pleated sheets of which amyloid deposits are composed.

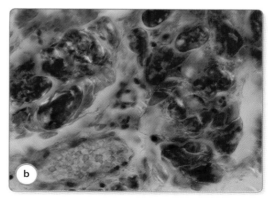

Figure 3.17 Congo red stain of amyloidosis. (a) Congo red staining of amyloid appears brick red with non-polarized light (Congo red, 100×). (b) However, with polarized light in the appropriate orientation amyloid deposits appear yellow-green (400×).

It is important to recognize that in some cases collagen fibers or other structures may also pick up the Congo red dye. Because of false positive and false negative results, interpretation should be performed with adequate positive tissue controls and in conjunction with routine tissue staining with hematoxylin and eosin.

Lipids

The routine processing of skin biopsies received in neutral buffered formalin limits demonstration of lipids on paraffin embedded tissue. Processing through steps of dehydration with alcohols, acetones and xylene allows the diffusion of endogenous lipids from adipocytes, as well as interstitial injected lipids and lipid-like materials, out of the tissue. On routine H&E staining, the clear spaces observed within subcutaneous adipose tissue, matures sebocytes, and xanthomatized histiocytes result from this loss of lipids. Therefore, optimal demonstration of lipids in tissue sections demands the use of unfixed frozen tissue that has not been dehydrated with alcohols, xylene or paraffin. Some application of formalin-containing solution is sometimes required to allow fixation of the protein comprising the surrounding tissue. Lipids are not fixed in neutral buffered formalin. Aqueous mounting medium, and not xylene, should be used for coverslipping.

Oil Red O and Sudan Black B are both fat-soluble diazo dyes (**Figure 3.18**). Their use involves application of the dye dissolved in a hydrophobic solvent. When the dye solution is applied to the tissue, the dye migrates to lipid-rich areas in the tissue. This is followed by application of a hematoxylin counterstain. Oil red O application results in bright red fat; Sudan black B application results in blue-black triglyceride staining and gray staining of phospholipids (Suvarna, 2013). Practical applications of these lipid stains in routine dermatopathology are limited.

Infectious disease

Gram stain for bacteria

The Danish bacteriologist Hans Christian Gram published a technique for the visualization of bacteria under microscopy in 1884 (Titford, 2009). Because of differences in the composition of bacterial cell walls and membranes there is differential staining in different types of bacteria. Bacterial species are broadly divided into Gram-positive and Gram-negative categories based on their differential staining using this method. Techniques adapting the Gram stain for use on formalin-fixed paraffin-embedded tissue were published in the 1960s and 1970s and have subsequently been modified. Two of the more

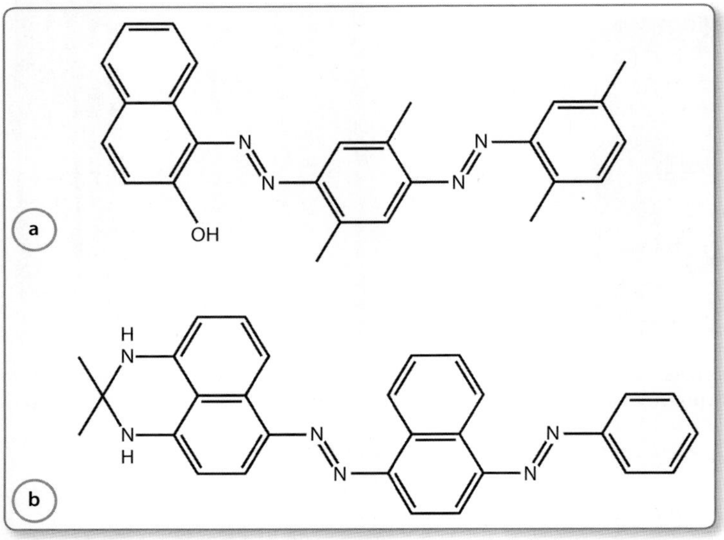

Figure 3.18 Oil red O and Sudan black dye. (a) Oil red O and (b) Sudan black are dyes that are used to highlight lipids in unprocessed tissue.

commonly used of these tissue-based techniques include the Brown and Brenn method and the Brown-Hopps method (the Brown is a different individual in each and, conventionally, the latter is hyphenated and the former is joined by a conjunction).

The Gram stain and subsequent modifications rely on similar principles. A crystal violet solution is applied to the tissue staining the thick outer peptidoglycan layer of Gram-positive bacteria and the lipopolysaccharide layer of Gram-negative bacteria (**Figure 3.19**). Next, an iodine solution causes fixation of crystal violet to the peptidoglycan layer of Gram-positive bacteria. Decolorizing with alcohol-acetone solution follows, removing crystal violet from the lipopolysaccharide layer of Gram-negative bacteria. The tissue is then counterstained with magenta-hued basic fuchsine, which highlights the peptidoglycan layer of Gram-negative bacteria. Due to prior fixation of crystal violet with iodine, Gram-positive bacteria do not take up the basic fuchsine counterstain (Suvarna, 2013). Additional steps allow for staining of the background tissue with picric acid, which results in a yellow color (**Figure 3.20**).

Ziehl–Neelsen and Kinyoun for acid-fast bacilli

The German bacteriologists Franz Ziehl and Friedrich Neelsen introduced the use of carbol fuchsine dye for detecting acid-fast bacilli in 1882. The stain's use allowed detection of the tuberculosis bacillus. In 1915 Joseph Kinyoun (K) published a modification of the Ziehl–Neelsen (ZN) method that allowed staining without the application of heat (Titford, 2009).

Carbol fuchsine is composed of a mixture of basic fuchsine and phenol. This red dye has a high affinity for hydrophobic mycolic acid in the fatty capsule surrounding the cell membranes of mycobacteria species and is not easily removed by application of acid alcohol (thus 'acid-fast') (Suvarna, 2013). A counterstain of methylene blue is typically employed, allowing the detection of red bacilli on a blue background (**Figure 3.21**). In addition to mycobacteria, the stain can detect some fungal organisms and filamentous bacteria (i.e. *Nocardia* and *Actinomyces* species) and often reacts with keratin in hair shafts and in the stratum

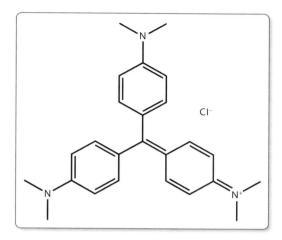

Figure 3.19 Crystal violet dye is used in bacterial Gram stain. Crystal violet binds to the peptidoglycan layer surrounding Gram-positive bacteria and the lipopolysaccharide layer of Gram-negative bacteria. The crystal violet dye is retained by Gram-positive organisms following iodine fixation, but is removed from Gram-negative bacteria during a decolorization step.

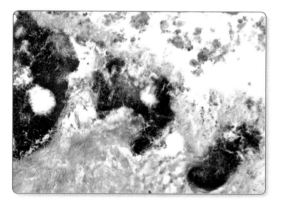

Figure 3.20 Brown-Hopps tissue Gram stain with Gram-positive and Gram-negative organisms. The Brown-Hopps tissue Gram stain allows the dermatopathologist to distinguish Gram-positive (purple) and Gram-negative (red) bacteria (B-H, 400×).

corneum. In skin specimens, this latter finding can be used as an internal positive control.

Fite for acid-fast bacilli

Sometimes called the Fite–Faraco or Wade–Fite method depending on the procedure followed,

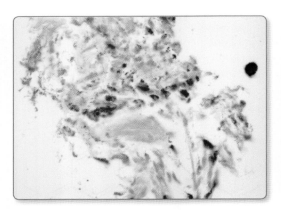

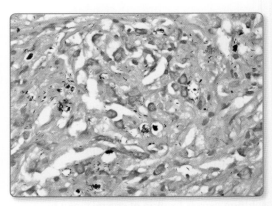

Figure 3.21 Kinyoun stain for acid-fast bacilli in an atypical mycobacterial infection. Most acid-fast bacilli and other bacteria (i.e. *Nocardia* spp.) are demonstrated by Kinyoun and Ziehl-Neelsen stains for atypical mycobacteria (Kinyoun, 400×).

Figure 3.22 Fite stain for acid-fast bacilli in leprosy. The acid-fast bacilli *Mycobacterium leprae* is demonstrated in this biopsy from a leprosy skin lesion (Fite, 400×).

but often shortened colloquially to Fite, this method is exceptionally useful in detecting *Mycobacterium leprae* and other atypical mycobacteria in paraffin-embedded tissue sections.

This method differs from the other methods for staining acid-fast bacilli (Ziehl–Neelsen and Kinyoun) in two important regards. Firstly, deparaffinization is performed using xylene and peanut oil. The peanut oil allows better preservation of the far more fragile fatty acid layer surrounding the organisms, as *M. leprae* is much less acid-fast than other mycobacterial organisms. Secondly, rather than an acid alcohol solution, sulphuric acid is employed as a decolorizer. Methylene blue is also used as a counterstain with this method (**Figure 3.22**) (Suvarna, 2013). In the author's experience, the Fite method is more commonly used alone or in combination with the Ziehl-Neelsen or Kinyoun methods, as the former will detect both *M. leprae* and other mycobacterial organisms in cutaneous specimens.

Warthin–Starry, Dieterle, Steiner and Steiner

A method for detecting spirochetes, such as *Treponema pallidum* and *Bartonella henselae*, was first published in 1920 by Aldred S. Warthin and Allen C. Starry (Titford, 2009). A solution of silver nitrate is applied and taken up by

spirochetes or other reactive bacteria. A reducing reaction, commonly using hydroquinone, allows conversion of the silver ions to elemental silver. In the Dieterle (1927) and Steiner (1944) methods, the specimen is pretreated with uranyl nitrate prior to application of a silver nitrate solution and gum mastic (Titford, 2009; Suvarna, 2013). The sections are then developed in a reducing solution with hydroquinone. On microscopy, the target organisms are stained black on a golden-yellow background (**Figure 3.23**). Because of a similar affinity for silver ions, melanin granules that have also reduced silver nitrate to elemental silver may obscure spirochete staining at the dermal-epidermal junction in secondary syphilis. The development of immunohistochemical stains for spirochetes such as *T. pallidum* has largely supplanted the use of these stains for cutaneous applications, although other applications for detection of *Legionella pneumophila*, *Bartonella henselae*, and *Borrelia burgdorferi*, remain.

Metachromatic stains

Metachromatic dyes, such as toluidine blue and methylene blue, are defined by their ability to change color in the presence of certain tissue components. The color change is most characteristically induced by closely grouped polyanionic moieties on carbohydrates, such as

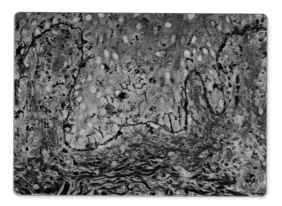

Figure 3.23 Warthin-Starry silver stain. Treponemal spirochetes in syphilis take up silver nitrate, which is reduced to elemental silver in a reaction with hydroquinone (W-S, 400×).

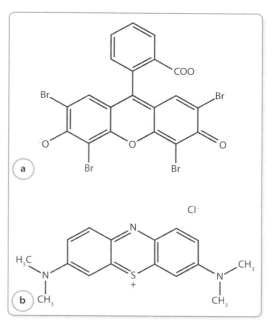

Figure 3.24 Giemsa stain. Giemsa solution is a mixture of (a) Eosin Y and (b) metachromatic methylene blue dyes.

long-chain proteoglycans. When the sulfate and carboxylate polyanionic moieties of proteoglycans have a charge and repeat at regular intervals, the positively charged metachromatic dyes aggregate. The positioning of the dye molecules allows polymeric binding between them, altering the absorption and emission spectra from the background dye monomers in the remainder of the tissue.

Giemsa

In 1904, the German bacteriologist Gustav Giemsa published a modification of Dmitri Romanowsky's previously published method for differentially staining cells in tissue sections (Titford, 2009). The Giemsa technique and subsequent modifications involve staining by a stock solution composed of a mix of eosin Y (an acid dye) and methylene blue (a basic dye) (**Figure 3.24**) (Barcia, 2007). This method is useful in detecting mast cells through metachromatic staining of mast cell granules rich in the glycosaminoglycan heparin (**Figure 3.25**). The Giemsa stain has also been used for detecting parasitic organisms such as *Leishmania*, *Entamoeba* and *Toxoplasma* species. Tzank is a modified Giemsa, often used in dermatology. Other modifications of the original Romanowsky method, including the Wright, Leishman and Jenner methods, are more commonly used for blood smears because of the nuclear detail provided and their ability to detect hematogenous parasites.

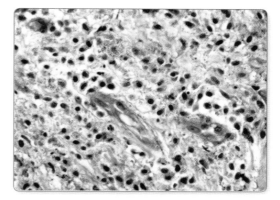

Figure 3.25 Giemsa stain of mastocytosis. Heparin within mast cell granules stain metachromatically in this example of cutaneous mastocytosis.

Toluidine blue

The metachromatic dye toluidine blue, also known as tolonium chloride, is a basic thiazine dye with limited application in routine dermatopathology (**Figure 3.26**). Like the

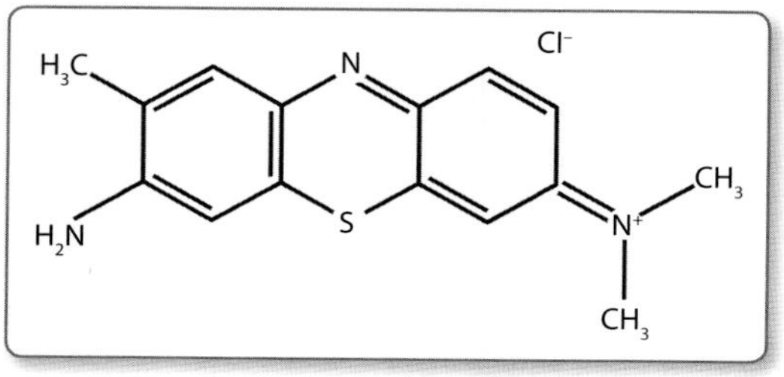

Figure 3.26 Toluidine blue dye. Toluidine blue stains mucopolysaccharides metchromatically and may have utility in Mohs surgery for basal cell carcinoma.

methylene blue used in the Giemsa method, toluidine blue appears red-purple in mast cell granules due to metachromatic properties (Sridharan, 2012). The proteoglycan hyaluronic acid is weakly metachromatic with toluidine blue staining and may be accentuated in the fibromyxoid stroma surrounding basal cell carcinoma. Toluidine blue also has a high affinity for nucleic acids, without metachromasia. These properties together may explain why some groups have found that toluidine blue may be useful as a stain in Mohs micrographic surgery for removal of basal cell carcinoma (Humpherys, 1996).

Miscellaneous

Leder

The Leder method relies on the retention of enzymatic activity of chloroacetate esterase in granulocyte and mast cell granules in formalin-fixed, paraffin-embedded tissue. The tissue is incubated in a solution containing naphthol AS-D chloroacetate and basic fuchsine. Chloroacetate esterase reacts with naphthol AS-D chloroacetate releasing naphthol, which subsequently acts on basic fuchsine to produce a bright magenta color (Patterson, 2016). The technique is both time- and resource-intensive. This method has been largely replaced by other special stains, like Giemsa and toluidine blue, or the immunohistochemical stain for mast cell tryptase. The method finds greater application today in hematopathology, but may be useful on occasion for the evaluation of leukemia cutis along with immunohistochemical stains for myeloperoxidase and lysozyme.

References

Barcia JJ. The Giemsa Stain: its history and applications. Int J Surg Pathol 2007;15:292–6.

Hale CW. Histochemical demonstration of acid polysaccharides in animal tissues. Nature 1946; 157:802.

Humpherys TR, Nemeth A, McCrevey S, Baer SC, Goldberg LH. A pilot study comparing toluidine blue and hematoxylin and eosin staining of basal cell and squamous cell carcinoma during Mohs surgery. Dermatol Surg 1996; 22:693–7.

McManus JFA. Histological demonstration of mucin after periodic acid. Nature 1946;158:202.

Patterson JW. Weedon's Skin Pathology, 4th ed. London: Elsevier, 2016.

Sridharan G, Shankar AA. Toluidine blue: A review of its chemistry and clinical utility. J Oral Maxillofac Pathol. 2012;16:251–5.

Steensma DP. 'Congo' red: out of Africa? Arch Pathol Lab Med 2001;125:250–2.

Suvarna SK, Layton C, Bancroft JD. Bancroft's Theory and Practice of Histological Techniques, 7th Ed. London: Churchill Livingstone, 2013.

Titford M. Progress in the development of microscopical techniques of diagnostic pathology. J Histotechnol 2009;32:9–19.

Zaragoza O, et al. The capsule of the fungal pathogen *Cryptococcus neoformans*. Adv Appl Microbiol 2009; 68:133.

4 Applications in dermatopathology

Ryan W. Hick

Special stains permit investigation of tissue structure beyond the findings of routine hematoxylin and eosin (H&E) staining. H&E allows visualization of protein and nucleic acid components of tissue sections. In most instances, this is sufficient to make a diagnosis. However, the addition of special stains allows detection of typically invisible or barely visible tissue elements on H&E (**Table 4.1**).

Table 4.1 Expected stain results			
Stain	**Target structures**	**Target color**	**Counterstain (background color)**
Alcian blue	Sulfated and acid mucopolysaccharides	Blue	Nuclear fast red
Alizarin red S	Calcium	Red	Green FCF
Brown-Hopps Brown and Brenn tissue Gram stain	Bacteria	Gram-positive: purple Gram-negative: red	Picric acid (yellow)
Chloroacetate esterase	Mast cells, neutrophils	Magenta	Hematoxylin (blue)
Colloidal iron	Sulfated and acid mucopolysaccharides	Blue	Nuclear fast red
Congo red	Amyloid	Brick red (non-polarized) Yellow-green (polarized)	Hematoxylin (blue)
Dieterle	Spirochetes	Black	(Yellow)
Fite	*Mycobacterium leprae* and other mycobacteria	Red	Methylene blue
Fontana-Masson	Melanin	Black	Nuclear fast red
Giemsa	Mast cells	Mast cell granules: purple Nuclei: blue	Eosin Y (red)
Grocott /Gomori methenamine silver	Fungi	Black	Light green
Kinyoun/Ziel-Neelsen	Mycobacteria, other acid-fast bacteria	Red	Methylene blue
Masson trichrome	Connective tissue	Muscle, cytoplasm: red Collagen: blue	N/A
Mucicarmine	Epithelial mucin: *Cryptococcus neoformans* capsule	Red	Hematoxylin (blue)
Periodic acid-Schiff	Carbohydrates: glycogen, fungal cell wall, proteoglycans	Magenta	Hematoxylin (blue)
Perls Prussian blue	Iron	Blue	Nuclear fast red
Steiner	Spirochetes, other bacteria	Black	(Yellow)
Toluidine blue	Mucin		N/A
Verhoeff-van Gieson	Elastin fibers	Dark blue	Van Gieson (red)
von Kossa	Calcium	Black	Nuclear fast red
Warthin-Starry	*Treponema pallidum*, other spirochetes, bacteria	Black	(Yellow)

The previous chapter outlined the mechanisms by which the stains work. This chapter will present, mostly in tabular form, various applications of the more common special stains used in dermatopathology.

Carbohydrates (Table 4.2)

The periodic acid–Schiff (PAS) method for detecting carbohydrates is one of the most, if not *the* most, commonly ordered special stain in dermatopathology. The stain is routinely ordered to rule out dermatophyte infection in the setting of spongiotic, pityriasiform, psoriasiform and superficial perivascular inflammatory reaction patterns. It is probably more cost effective than using the Grocott methenamine silver (GMS) stain. The sandwich sign (parakeratosis between layers of orthokeratosis) and 'neuts in the horn' are clues that may indicate a higher probability that the stain will find dermatophyte hyphae. Caution is warranted as serum in the stratum corneum can simulate hyphae. Dead dermatophyte hyphae may be impossible to identify in nail plate on PAS stained sections and GMS staining may be of value in cases with a high index of suspicion. Deep fungal infections require caution when evaluating with PAS or GMS as neutrophil granules are strongly positive. In tinea versicolor (or severe dermatophyte or candidiasis) PAS or GMS staining may not be necessary: *Malassezia* appears pale blue in the stratum corneum. Other infections, especially superficial bacterial infections caused by corynebacteria, are readily identified with a PAS stain.

Colloidal iron and alcian blue (pH 2.5) (mucin stains) are frequently used by dermatopathologists in the evaluation of interface dermatitis and superficial/deep perivascular lymphocytic dermatitis (without eosinophils). The presence of increased staining for hyaluronic acid between collagen fibers of the reticular dermis (interstitial mucin) may favor a diagnosis of cutaneous lupus erythematosus, dermatomyositis, or other connective tissue diseases. Increased hyaluronic acid is often well visualized on routine H&E. However, this is not a specific finding and can be found in other inflammatory dermatoses. Basement membrane thickening with PAS stain is helpful when present, but this finding is often restricted to advanced cases of discoid lupus erythematosus where other prominent histologic features on routine H&E mitigate its importance. The papillary dermis serves as a helpful internal control. Perifollicular, perivascular and perieccrine hyaluronic acid is also present constitutively and should not be misinterpreted as positive staining. Prominent intrafollicular hyaluronic acid is almost always pathologic and points to a diagnosis of follicular mucinosis or folliculotropic mycosis fungoides. A positive mucin stain is often helpful in the setting of a granulomatous dermatitis sampled by the shave biopsy technique because the characteristic palisade of histiocytes around areas of necrobiotic collagen in such specimens is difficult to discern or absent. Given the abundance of hyaluronic acid in primary mucinoses, mucin stains do not add very much in reaching a diagnosis.

Table 4.2 Stains for carbohydrates	
Stain	**Application**
Periodic acid-Schiff	Normal skin: • Glycogen in superficial keratinocytes of skin and mucosa • Basement membrane zone • Perifollicular, perieccrine, perivascular basement membrane • Eccrine glands • Neutrophil granules Organisms: • Bacteria • Fungi • Protozoa • Algae Basement membrane: • Discoid lupus erythematosus (thickened) • Epidermolysis bullosa simplex (base of blister) • Dystrophic epidermolysis bullosa (roof of blister) • Epidermolysis bullosa acquisita (mostly roof) • Diabetic dermopathy (capillary BM thickened) Deposition and metabolic disorders: • Erythropoietic protoporphyria • Lipoid proteinosis • Porphyria cutanea tarda • Pseudoporphyria (usually less than porphyria cutanea tarda) • Waldenstrom macroglobulinemia • Juvenile colloid milium • Infantile systemic hyalinosis • Juvenile hyaline fibromatosis • Fabry disease • Mucolipidosis II (foamy dermal spindle cells) • Neuronal ceroid lipofuscinosis (eccrine deposits) • Lafora disease (eccrine & apocrine deposits) • Alpha-mannosidosis (gingival histiocytes) Neoplasms: • Clear cell acanthoma (glycogen) • Clear cell papulosis (diastase resistant) • Eccrine poroma (glycogen) • Dermal duct tumor (glycogen) • Hidradenoma (glycogen) • Porocarcinoma (glycogen) • Spiradenoma (hyaline material) • Cylindroma (hyaline droplets & bands around islands; lost in malignant cylindroma) • Apocrine adenocarcinoma (diastase resistant) • Mucinous carcinoma • Acrosyringeal nevus (acrosyringeal keratinocytes); eccrine syringofibroadenoma negative • Hidradenoma papilliferum (apical) • (Extramammary) Paget disease (intra-epithelial mucin) • Adenosquamous carcinoma (sialidase labile) • Syringoid eccrine carcinoma (luminal material diastase resistant) Pigment: • Melanin • Amiodarone (lipofucsin granules in histiocytes) Miscellaneous: • Membranous lipodystrophy

Table 4.2 (*continued*)

Stain	Application
Alcian blue, pH 2.5 Colloidal iron	Normal skin: • Papillary dermis • Perifollicular fibrous sheath • Perivascular stroma
	Deposition: • Lipoid proteinosis • Erythropoietic protoporphyria • Polyvinylpyrrolidone storage disease (histiocytes)
	Neoplasms: • Clear cell papulosis • Hidradenoma papilliferum (spaces) • Mucinous carcinoma • Extramammary Paget disease • Ossifying fibromyxoid tumor (stroma)
	Primary mucinoses: • Pretibial myxedema • Scleredema • Severe generalized myxedema • Papular mucinosis • Acral persistent papular mucinosis • Cutaneous mucinosis of infancy • Nephrogenic systemic fibrosis • Reticular erythematous mucinosis • Focal dermal mucinosis • Digital mucous cyst • Mucocele • Nevus mucinosis • Follicular mucinosis • Mucopolysaccharidoses
	Secondary mucinoses: • Lupus erythematosus • Dermatomyositis • Degos disease (malignant atrophic papulosis) • Jessner lymphocytic infiltrate • Granuloma annulare
Mucicarmine	Organisms: • Cryptococcosis
	Neoplasms: • Clear cell papulosis • Mucinous carcinoma (sialidase labile) • Extramammary Paget disease • Adenosquamous carcinoma
	Deposition: • Polyvinylpyrrolidone disease (histiocytes)
Grocott methenamine silver	Normal skin: • Neutrophil granules
	Organisms: • Bacteria • Fungi • Protozoa
	Pigment: • Melanin

Table 4.3 Stains for melanin	
Stain	**Application**
Fontana-Masson	Normal skin: • Melanin pigment overlying basal keratinocyte nuclei • Hair shaft • Hair matrix cells
	Pigmentary disorders: • Vitiligo (absent staining in lesional skin) • Hypomelanosis of Ito (decreased staining in lesional skin) • Melasma • Post-inflammatory pigment alteration • Idiopathic guttate hypomelanosis • Dowling-Degos disease (pigment localized to rete ridges, decreased between) • Pigmented pretibial patches (diabetic dermopathy)
	Pigmentation secondary to medication: • Amiodarone • Methacycline • Minocycline • Omeprazole
	Melanocytic neoplasms: • Primarily historical use • Desmoplastic Spitz nevus (differentiates from dermatofibroma) • Hypomelanotic blue nevus
GMS and other silver stains	Not primarily for melanin but often may be useful because of argentaffin reaction
PAS	Not primarily for melanin but often accentuated

Table 4.4 Stains for metal ions	
Stain	**Application**
Perls Prussian blue	• Pigmented pretibial patches (diabetic dermopathy) • Pigmented purpuric dermatosis • Iron-containing foreign body • Minocycline pigmentation
Von Kossa Alizarin red S	• Calcinosis cutis • Calciphylaxis • Pseudoxanthoma elasticum • Malakoplakia (Michaelis–Gutman bodies)

Melanin (Table 4.3)

The Fontana–Masson silver stain is a very sensitive stain for melanin. It is not a very specific stain. A biopsy from the edge of a hypopigmented or depigmented skin macule may allow visualization of partial or complete loss of melanin pigment within the epidermis. It is sometimes useful to complement this stain with a MART-1 immunohistochemical stain to evaluate whether melanocytes are completely lost along the dermal–epidermal junction.

Metal ions (Table 4.4)

The Perls Prussian blue iron stain detects ferric and ferrous ions in the heme breakdown product hemosiderin. Typical uses in the skin include differentiation of hemosiderin from dermal melanin pigment in venous stasis dermatitis and pigmented purpuric dermatoses (capillaritis). Iron and melanin stains may both be positive in cases of dermal pigmentation due to medication deposition such as minocycline. Other iron deposits, including shrapnel and material from BBs, will also stain with this method. Von Kossa and alizarin red S stains are infrequently used because calcium in the skin is rarely difficult to identify. The stains may be useful if only trace deposits of calcium are present, as in some cases of calciphylaxis or pseudoxanthoma elasticum.

Connective tissue (Table 4.5)

Another infrequently ordered, but occasionally very helpful stain, is the Verhoeff–van Gieson (VVG) stain. The author finds this stain most useful in situations where it fails to find its target, similar to the Fontana-Masson stain for melanin. Reduced staining with thickened collagen fibers arranged in somewhat circumscribed bundles may be seen in connective tissue nevus (collagenoma). Reduced staining may be found in anetoderma. Absent, highly fragmented, and/or attenuated fibers are reported in mid-dermal elastolysis and Perifollicular elastolysis. So-called bramble bush elastic fibers that also stain for calcium are present in pseudoxanthoma elasticum. Comparison with a biopsy from normal, uninvolved skin is ideal when available.

Table 4.5 Connective tissue stains	
Stain	**Application**
Verhoeff–van Gieson	Normal skin: • Fine, thin elastin fibers in papillary dermis • Thick elastin fibers in reticular dermis • Connective tissue nevus • Mid-dermal elastolysis • Perifollicular elastolysis • Anetoderma • Elastofibroma • Pseudoxanthoma elasticum • Elastosis perforans serpiginosa
Masson trichrome	• Reactive perforating collagenosis • Leiomyoma • Smooth muscle hamartoma • Becker nevus • Supernumerary nipple

Table 4.7 Stains for lipids	
Stain	**Application**
Sudan Black or Oil red O (Fresh frozen sections or formalin-fixed unprocessed)	• Fabry disease • Lipoid proteinosis • Erythropoietic protoporphyria • Membranous lipodystrophy • Necrobiosis lipoidica • Granuloma annulare • Amiodarone pigmentation (lipofucsin granules in histiocytes) • Sebaceous neoplasms • Xanthogranuloma • Reticulohistiocytoma • Other xanthomas & lipidized histiocytoses • Lipidized (xanthomatized) dermatofibroma

The Masson trichrome stain is used very infrequently in modern dermatopathology. The author finds it very satisfying, however, to see blue, vertically-oriented collagen fibers pushing through epidermis in reactive perforating collagenosis.

Amyloid (Table 4.6)

Congo red dye stains keratin- and light chain-derived forms of amyloid in the skin. In most instances of macular and lichen amyloidosis, special stains are not necessary to arrive at the correct diagnosis. False negative results may occur in macular amyloidosis. Deposition of amyloid around vessels in the deeper dermis in systemic amyloidosis or nodular amyloidosis may be more difficult to distinguish from collagen. False positive results may occur in a background of solar elastosis.

Table 4.6 Stains for amyloid	
Stain	**Application**
Congo red	Amyloidosis (may have false negative result in macular amyloidosis) (may have false positive in background of solar elastosis) Polyvinylpyrrolidone storage disease (histiocytes)

Lipids (Table 4.7)

Oil red O and Sudan black stains are rarely performed for routine dermatopathology specimens. Without significant preoperative suspicion of a condition for which the stains might be helpful, routine skin specimens submitted in formalin are processed through steps in which lipids are removed from tissue sections. The most commons dermatoses in which lipids might be found can be diagnosed through other means without lipid stains.

Metachromatic (Table 4.8)

The Giemsa method is uncommonly used for routine dermatopathology given the availability of sensitive and specific immunohistochemical stains for mast cells (i.e. mast cell tryptase).

Table 4.8 Metachromatic stains	
Stain	**Application**
Giemsa	Organisms: Fungi Protozoa Algae Mast cells (metachromatic): Urticaria Mastocytosis
Toluidine blue	Mast cells (metachromatic) Hyaluronic acid (weakly metachromatic) Basal cell carcinoma

Though reportedly useful for detecting amastigotes in leishmaniasis, this author has not found Giemsa staining to be superior to routine H&E. Toluidine blue may have a place in Mohs micrographic surgery for basal cell carcinoma.

Table 4.9 Stains for detecting micro-organisms

Stain	Category	Diseases
Periodic acid–Schiff (PAS)	Fungi	Dermatophytosis Onychomycosis Tinea versicolor Pityrosporum folliculitis Chromomycosis Phaeohyphomycosis Blastomycosis Histoplasmosis Lobomycosis Sporotrichosis Candidiasis Coccidioidomycosis (stronger in sporangiospores than spherule) Paracoccidioidomycosis Cryptococcosis Trichosporonosis Eumycetoma Mucormycosis
	Bacteria	Erythrasma Pitted keratolysis Staphylococcal, streptococcal impetigo Nail unit pseudomonal infection Rhinoscleroma (Russell bodies) Malakoplakia (histiocytes inclusions)
	Protozoa/Algae	Bradyzoites of toxoplasmosis Amebiasis (viable forms) Protothecosis
Gomori/Grocott methenamine silver	Fungi	See PAS May be better for dead dermatophyte
	Bacteria	*Actinomyces* infection *Mycobacteria* infection Erythrasma Pitted keratolysis
	Protozoa	Cyst wall of Balamuthia
Kinyoun or Ziehl-Neelsen AFB	Mycobacteria	Tuberculosis Atypical mycobacterial infection
	Bacteria	Nocardia weakly acid fast
Fite AFB	Mycobacteria	Mycobacteria leprae Other mycobacterial infections
Warthin-Starry Dieterle Steiner	Bacteria	Syphilis Borreliosis Cat-scratch disease
Giemsa	Fungi	Histoplasmosis
	Bacteria	Granuloma inguinale (Donovan bodies)
	Protozoa	Leishmaniasis Toxoplasmosis Acanthamoebiasis Balamuthia Toxoplasmosis
	Algae	Protothecosis
Brown and Brenn Brown-Hopps	Bacteria	Gram-positive: purple Gram-negative: red
Mucicarmine	Fungi	Cryptococcosis capsule

Additional micro-organism stains (Table 4.9)

The Brown-Hopps or Brown and Brenn methods of tissue Gram stain may be useful for some bacterial infections such as impetigo, folliculitis, and mycetoma. Organisms remain difficult to detect despite the use of this technique. Tissue cultures in suspected cases of bacterial infection provide more meaningful results relatively rapidly.

Nothing brings a smile to the dermatopathologists face like a positive stain for acid-fast bacilli by whatever method (Kinyoun, Ziehl–Neelsen, or Fite). While frequently futile, hunting for acid-fast organisms is an important exercise in mixed suppurative and granulomatous dermal infiltrates. While tissue culture provides information regarding speciation, the AFB stain may allow earlier empiric therapy given the length of time required for culture results. Keratin and hair shafts may serve as a positive internal control. Given the possibility of contamination from water bath during slide preparation, comparison with areas of the slide away from tissue sections is important. If acid-fast bacilli are present away from tissue or out of the tissue plane, repeating the stain should be considered.

Silver stains (Warthin–Starry, Dieterle, Steiner) for spirochetes, especially *Treponema pallidum*, are relatively insensitive and non-specific in comparison with the newer immunohistochemical techniques of detection. Their use in skin specimens is probably unnecessary in most cases.

Conclusion

Special stains have played an important role in dermatopathology since their first development along the side of routine H&E staining in the late nineteenth century. Despite the development of new immunohistochemical and molecular methods for evaluating cutaneous disorders, special stains will continue to play an important part in making diagnoses in dermatopathology. Mastering their appropriate use and interpretation requires experience, practice and patience.

Further reading

Bolognia JL, Jorizzo JL, Schaffer JV. Dermatology, 3rd edn. Philadelphia: Elsevier/Saunders, 2012.

Patterson JW. Weedon's Skin Pathology, 4th edn. Philadelphia: Elsevier, 2015.

Suvarna SK, Layton C, Bancroft JD. Bancroft's Theory and Practice of Histological Techniques. 7th Ed. London: Elsevier/Churchill Livingstone, 2013.

Section 3

Immunohistochemistry

5 Immunohistochemistry: background

Marc R. Lewin, Robert Oliai

History

Immunohistochemistry (IHC) is an invaluable tool used by the practicing dermatopathologist on a daily basis. Pathologists routinely utilize IHC to classify tumors with ambiguous ontogeny and poorly differentiated malignant tumors, to identify the site of origin of metastatic tumors, to classify hematopoietic neoplasms (especially in cases in which material has not been submitted for flow cytometric analysis), to assess prognostic factors which may guide therapy, and finally to identify infectious agents in tissue sections. The great benefit of IHC is that it allows real-time, direct visualization of the cells bearing (or lacking) the marker, or antigen, of interest, permitting direct correlation with the histopathologic features of the diagnostic material. In this sense, it often has an edge over even exquisitely sensitive molecular and flow cytometric techniques.

Most consider the father of IHC to be Albert H. Coons, a former professor at Harvard Medical School. While on holiday in Berlin in 1939 he had a self-proclaimed scientific epiphany (**Figure 5.1**). While contemplating the Aschoff nodule, Dr Coons formulated the idea of labeling antibody molecules with a visible label to detect antigen tissues. He went on to publish a paper in 1941 demonstrating this ability to locate antigens in tissue by labeling fluorescein antibodies against *Streptococcus pneumoniae* and visualizing the reaction by fluorescein microscopy (Coons et al, 1941). This led to the development of diagnostic immunofluorescence microscopy (*see* Chapter 9). The next large leap in the science of IHC occurred in the 1960s when P. K. Nakane

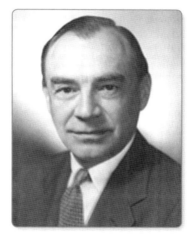

Figure 5.1
Albert H. Coons, MD. Coons is considered the father of immunohisto-chemistry (Photo by Bachrach).

introduced the use of enzymes as marked antibodies. This advent meant that specialized fluorescence microscopes were no longer needed, and the use of IHC could now be employed by the pathologist using routine light microscopy (Matos et al, 2010). The application of IHC continued to expand as methods such as antigen retrieval and secondary antibody detection systems allowed IHC to be applied not only to fresh frozen tissue, but also to formalin-fixed paraffin sections. This last step led to IHC becoming widely used in routine anatomic pathology practice in the 1980s. IHC remains one of the most invaluable and commonplace tools at the disposal of the practicing dermatopathologist, as it greatly enhances the practitioner's specific diagnostic ability. As the next chapter demonstrates, from infection to neoplasia, IHC plays a critical role in the evaluation of skin biopsies.

Principles

While a number of different methods may be used, the best of these at the present time is the polymer-based detection method. After placing the tissue section on an adhesive glass slide, the tissue is prepared using a variety of techniques known as 'antigen retrieval', which improve the ability to detect antigens of interest. Such methods may involve treatment of the slide with enzymes or a variety of solutions and heating in a vegetable steamer or pressure cooker. At this point, the primary antibody (which is selected to specifically bind to the antigen of interest) is placed on the slide. After rinsing the unbound primary antibody off the slides, the detection complex is then added. This detection complex consists of a polymer backbone that has another antibody (referred to as the 'secondary' or 'link' antibody) bound to the polymer backbone, along with an enzyme (most commonly peroxidase) that serves as the 'marker' enzyme (**Figure 5.2**). The secondary or link antibody bound to the polymer is selected for its ability to bind the primary antibody. For example, if the primary antibody is made in mouse (i.e. mouse anti-S100), the secondary antibody may be made in rabbits and raised against mouse immunoglobulin, i.e. a rabbit anti-mouse immunoglobulin antibody. At this point, we have the polymer backbone specifically bound to the antigen of interest, with multiple peroxidase ('marker') enzyme molecules present on this polymer. After rinsing the unbound secondary, the final step in the procedure involves placing the slides in a solution of diaminobenzidine (called the chromogen) which turns brown in the presence of peroxidase enzyme. As such, the presence (or absence) of the antigen in the tissue can be established by the presence (or absence) of the colored (brown)

reaction product observed when viewing the completed stain under a light microscope.

In many laboratories, the above steps have now been automated. Although automated immunostainers have improved the quality of immunostains in many laboratories, the machines used are not flawless, and it is naive to assume that obtaining an automated instrument will guarantee quality and reproducibility. An unfortunate by-product of automation is the ease with which pathologists can view the IHC laboratory as a 'black box', leading to insufficient understanding of the technical aspects involved to consistently avoid pitfalls and misinterpretation.

Finally, since key diagnostic decisions are often based on the results of IHC stains, it is very important to be absolutely certain that every antibody utilized has been appropriately optimized with respect to dilution (i.e. titer) and antigen retrieval method, to ensure the highest sensitivity and specificity. The appropriate use of control tissues is an integral step in ensuring that all of these techniques lead to consistently reliable and reproducible tissue stains. Control tissues with a known staining pattern to the antibody of interest are used for this purpose. While control tissues may be placed on separate slides from the patient's tissue, it is optimal to have the control tissues on the same slide as the patient's tissue to further ensure that all the tissues have been exposed to an identical staining environment. At ProPath, for example, this is accomplished through the use of multi-tissue 'sandwich' blocks, a technique developed by Rodney Miller, in which samples from multiple (up to 80) different tissues (both normal and neoplastic) are arranged in a grid-like fashion into a single paraffin block, with strips of amnion and chorion separating rows of different tumors. For most antibodies, these blocks

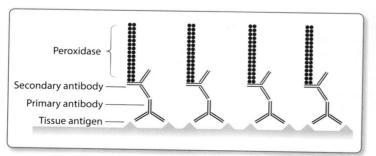

Figure 5.2 Schematic of primary and secondary antibodies with polymer backbone binding to tissue antigen.

Peroxidase

Secondary antibody
Primary antibody
Tissue antigen

will contain expected negative and expected positive tissues of varying antigen density, and their use allows efficient selection of the optimal antigen retrieval method and best primary antibody dilution (i.e. titer). Parenthetically, it is worth mentioning that relying solely on so-called 'pre-dilute, ready-to-use' antibodies is strongly discouraged, since this is a very common reason for suboptimal stains. Sections from these multi-tissue blocks are routinely placed on the same slide as the patient material, where they effectively serve as multiple external-tissue positive and negative control samples, enabling rapid and thorough assessment of the behavior of every stain performed. As such, they serve as a continuous monitor of quality, where sensitivity and specificity can be readily assessed on any stain that is performed by simply viewing the stained multi-tissue block on the same slide as the patient tissue. In assessing IHC staining, it is also very useful to use internal controls within the patient tissue itself. For example, when ordering a Mart-1 stain on a tumor, one can use the presence of normal junctional melanocytes as an internal positive control.

Interpretation

Accurate interpretation of IHC is essential, and the assessment of an IHC stain is not as simple as seeing brown or red staining on a slide and equating it to a positive result. Just like any other laboratory test, one must be aware that false positive staining may occur, and this is where the dermatopathologist's skill and knowledge enter into the equation. False positive staining may be easy to identify when the entire tissue sections (both tumor and background non-neoplastic structures) are covered by a 'muddy' haze. However, problems may arise when false positive staining is limited only to the tumor cells of interest, as this may lead to interpretation errors if the pathologist is not aware of the appropriate staining patterns. In these instances of false positive staining, the tumor cells often stain with a uniform 'blush' cytoplasmic stain that lacks cell-to-cell heterogeneity. This cell-to-cell heterogeneous staining is thus an important aspect to look for, as it is an indicator of true positive staining. Knowledge of the appropriate staining pattern for a particular IHC antibody is also crucial to avoid diagnostic pitfalls.

Different IHC markers display varying staining patterns, as they can be cytoplasmic, membranous, nuclear and cytoplasmic, granular, or even present in a peri-nuclear dot-like pattern (**Figure 5.3**). For example, Beta-catenin, a marker useful in the setting of desmoid fibromatoses, will have strong cytoplasmic staining in a variety of lesions, but it is only considered to be positive if nuclear staining is observed. Another example of a false positive result has been reported with CD20, a marker with membranous and cytoplasmic staining, which may sometime erroneously stain non-B cells in a nuclear pattern. Thus, a dermatopathologist must be aware of the expected staining pattern in order to avoid diagnostic errors.

In summary, IHC has established itself over the years as a great diagnostic aid to the practicing pathologist and remains one of the pathologist's greatest ancillary tools in the establishment of correct and specific diagnoses.

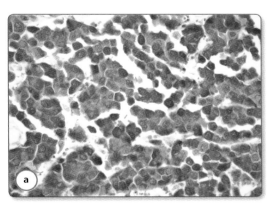

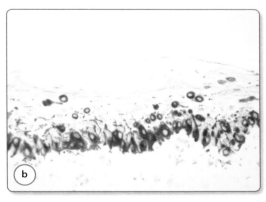

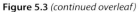

Figure 5.3 (continued overleaf)

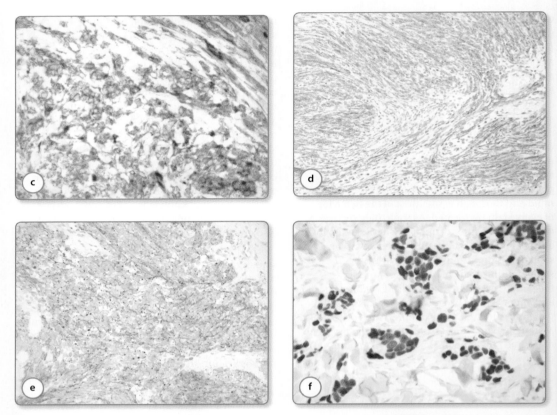

Figure 5.3 *continued*. Staining patterns in IHC. (a) Nuclear and cytoplasmic (S-100, melanoma, 200× original magnification). (b) Cytoplasmic (MART-1 stain, 200×). (c) Granular cytoplasmic (NKI-C3, cellular neurothekeoma, 200×). (d) Membranous (EMA, perineurioma, 100×). (e) Peri-nuclear dot like (CK20, Merkel cell, 200×). (f) Nuclear (GATA-3, breast carcinoma, 200×).

References

Coons AH, Creech HJ, Jones NR. Immunological properties of an antibody containing a fluorescent group. Exp Biol Med 1941; 47:200–202.

Matos LL de, Trufelli DC, de Matos MGL, da Silva Pinhal MA. Immunohistochemistry as an important tool in biomarkers detection and clinical practice. Biomark Insights 2010; 5:9–20.

Immunohistochemical markers

Marc R. Lewin

This chapter will discuss the specifics of the more commonly used immunohistochemical (IHC) markers at the disposal of the practicing dermatopathologist. As new markers and new applications of current markers are continually being developed and employed, this chapter is not intended to be a complete list of all available IHC markers, but a summary of the most commonly used markers and their primary associated applications in the field of dermatopathology. These markers will be divided into five sections:

1. Epithelial/neuroendocrine
2. Hematolymphoid
3. Melanocytic
4. Soft tissue
5. Infectious immunohistochemistry

Of note, some IHC antibodies may have a variety of uses and fall into one or more of these categories. In these instances, some of these markers will be included in more than one section, and in other cases, the marker will be discussed under its most commonly used application.

Epithelial/neuroendocrine tumor markers

Cytokeratins

Background: Cytokeratins (CKs) are intermediate filament proteins which make up the cytoskeletal structure of all epithelial cells. Epithelial cells contain from 2 to 10 different types of CKs. The CK family is a highly complex multigene family with molecular weights ranging from 40 to 68 kDa. The main CKs are expressed in pairs and numbered 1-20 based on their molecular weights and isoelectric points. There are different CK classification schemes, with the most famous being the Moll classification. In this scheme, the main CKs are generally classified into two groups: Class I/acidic type A group comprised by CK9-CK20, CKs which generally have a low molecular weight (LMWCK); Class II/basic type B group comprised by CK1-CK8, which have a higher molecular weight (HMWCK) (Franke et al. 1981). Within cells, each Class I/Type A CK forms a complex with a specific Class II/Type B CK.

Another way to classify CKs is to separate them into CK of simple epithelia (CK7, CK8, CK18, and CK20) and CK of stratified epithelia (CK1, CK5, CK10 and CK14). A somewhat confusing point is that pathologists tend to refer to cytokeratins as low or high molecular weight cytokeratins (LMWCK;HMWCK). However, as opposed to referring to the Moll Class I (LMWCK) or Class II (HMWCK) when giving this designation, pathologists generally refer to the simple epithelia CKs as the LMWCKs and the stratified/complex keratins as the HMWCKs. For example, while CK7 and CK8 are technically HMWCKs according to the Moll classification, they are simple epithelia keratins, and thus designated as LMWCKs in pathology. For the purpose of this chapter we will use this latter convention in designating cytokeratins, i.e. LMWCK=simple epithelia keratins and HMWCK=stratified/complex keratins. In general terms, HMWCKs are commonly expressed in skin epithelia (epidermis and adnexae) and their respective tumors. LMWCKs are commonly expressed in visceral epithelia and tumors which metastasize to skin. Of course, there is marked overlap.

Uses: Cytokeratins are used as markers for epithelial differentiation. However, it is important to realize that several non-epithelial tumors can stain with cytokeratins, and that CK expression is not pathognomonic for an epithelial origin of a tumor (**Table 6.1**). In addition, different CK profiles are variably expressed by different epithelial tumors, allowing pathologists to discern the origin of different tumors by their varying CK profiles.

Staining pattern: Cytoplasmic.

Specific cytokeratins useful in dermatopathology

High molecular weight cytokeratins (HMWCK)

CK5 or CK5/6
- In normal skin stains basal cells of squamous and glandular epithelium and myoepithelial cells
- Stains squamous cell carcinoma (SCC), Bowen's disease, basal cell carcinoma (BCC) and sebaceous carcinoma
- Also may be positive in epithelioid sarcoma and epithelioid angiosarcoma
- May be used to stain papillary dermal amyloid deposits in macular or lichen amyloid
- A potential pitfall to note is CK5 may sometimes stain colloid bodies or show 'bleeding artifact' and stains superficial elastin tissues. This should not be interpreted as invasive SCC (**Figure 6.1**)

Table 6.1 Non-epithelial tumors which may express cytokeratins on IHC

Epithelioid angiosarcoma
Anaplastic large cell lymphoma (ALCL)
Epithelioid sarcoma
Leiomyosarcoma
Melanoma
Synovial sarcoma

- Negative in mammary and extramammary Paget's disease (EMPD)
- Clones: 34BEH12; CK 05; RCK103; XM26

Low molecular weight cytokeratins (LMWCK)

CK7
- In normal skin, CK7 will stain eccrine and other ductal epithelial cells, but not stratified squamous epithelium. Also normally found in transitional epithelium of urinary tract as well as both lung and breast epithelial cells
- Stains adnexal tumors; Paget's disease, EMPD
- Useful in differentiating cutaneous Merkel cell carcinoma (CK7 -) from metastatic small cell lung carcinoma (CK7+)
- Generally negative in SCC, but small percentage of SCC in situ (SCCIS) will be +. This may lead to diagnostic confusion between EMPD and SCCIS. In this instance, SCCIS will always be CK5/6 +, while EMPD will be negative
- Used in combination with CK20 to evaluate the site of origin for metastatic adenocarcinomas (**Table 6.2**)
- Clones: KS7.18; LDS-68; CK 07; K72.7; BC1; EPR1619Y; LP5K; RN7; OVTL 12/30

CK20
- CK 20 is less acidic than other type 1 cytokeratins and is unique in its restricted range of expression, and in normal tissues it is expressed only in gastrointestinal epithelium, urothelium and Merkel cells
- Stains Merkel cell carcinoma in a perinuclear dot like pattern (**Figure 6.2**)
- Useful in the differential diagnosis (ddx) of desmoplastic trichoepithelioma (DTE) vs BCC, as CK20 + merkel cells are present in DTE and not BCC

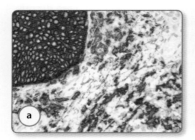
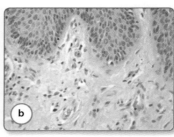

Figure 6.1 (a) Cytokeratin 5 IHC with marked 'bleeding artifact' in the dermis (CD5, 100×). (b) H&E demonstrates no atypical dermal cells (H&E, 100×).

Table 6.2 CK7/CK20 expression in evaluation of metastatic adenocarcinomas of unknown primary			
CK7+/CK20- tumors	**CK7-/CK20+ tumors**	**CK7+/CK20+ tumors**	**CK7-/CK20- tumors**
Breast	Colorectal	Gastric	Hepatocellular
Endometrial		Ovarian, mucinous	Prostate
Gallbladder		Pancreatic	Renal cell
Lung		Urothelial (transitional cell)	
Mesothelial			
Non-mucinous ovarian			
Pancreaticobiliary tract			
Small bowel			
Thyroid			

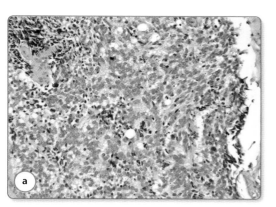 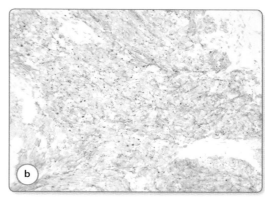

Figure 6.2 Cytokeratin 20. (a) Merkel cell carcinoma (MCC) (H&E, 100×). (b) CK 20 perinuclear dot-like pattern in MCC (CK20, 100×).

- Used in combination with CK7 to determine origin of metastatic adenocarcinomas (**Table 6.2**)
- Clones: KS7.18; LDS-68; CK 07; K72.7; BC1; EPR1619Y; LP5K; RN7; OVTL 12/30

CK15

- CK15 is present in follicular stem cells
- Along with p63 and D2-40, CK15 may be used to differentiate between primary cutaneous adnexal tumors and metastatic lesions (**Table 6.3**)
- Clones: CK15; LHK15

Cytokeratin cocktails

34betaE12/CK903

- HMWCK cocktail which detects CKs 1,5,10 and 14
- Stains squamous, ductal, and complex epithelia in normal skin

Table 6.3 Metastatic adenocarcinoma vs primary cutaneous adnexal carcinoma		
Stain	**Metastasis**	**Primary adnexal**
D2-40	-	+
P63	-	+
CK15	-	+

- Similar role and staining patterns as CK5/6.
- Clones: 34BE12; MA-903

CAM 5.2

- LMWCK cocktail
- Originally was thought to recognize CK8 and CK18, but is now known to recognize CK8 and CK7, and not CK18
- In normal skin, labels eccrine and apocrine secretory units and non cornifying stratified squamous epithelium

- Stains most adenocarcinomas and SCC
- Negative in SCC from cervix, vagina and esophagus
- Clones: Zym5.2; CAM 5.2; 5D3; KER 10.11

AE1/AE3

- So called 'pan-cytokeratin cocktail'
- Very broad reactivity and stains all types of epithelia
- AE1 directed to acidic types CK9, 10, 13, 14, 15, 16 and 19
- AE3 directed to neutral-basic types CK1-8
- In our experience, AE1/AE3 is not the best immunostain for SCC. Therefore, it may not be as useful as a screening immunostain to evaluate for epithelial derivation, and we prefer to use CK903 and a LMWCK cocktail for screening purposes (**Figure 6.3**)

Other epithelial markers

Adipophilin

Background: Adipophilin, also known as perilipin 2 (PLIN2) or adipose differentiation-related protein, is a 48.1 kDa protein found on the surface of intracellular lipid globules. It is normally found in a variety of tissues including cells of the adrenal gland, testis, ovary, muscle, lactating mammary glands, as well as in cells of the gastrointestinal tract and skin. It has a globular to membranous staining pattern.

Uses: Adipophilin is most commonly used to differentiate between sebaceous tumors, such as poorly differentiated sebaceous carcinomas, from other basaloid neoplasms. Sebaceous neoplasms have a characteristic membranous staining for adipophilin (Ostler et al. 2010). Other tumors generally in the differential diagnosis, including basal cell carcinomas, are negative for adipophilin. Adipophilin will stain xanthomas/xanthelasma and metastatic renal cell carcinomas in a globular pattern.

Staining pattern: Membranous.

Clones: AP125

Androgen receptor (AR)

Background: AR is a 90 kDa nuclear receptor involved in the binding of androgenetic hormones such as testosterone. In normal skin, AR is localized to both the basaloid and mature sebocytes of sebaceous lobules.

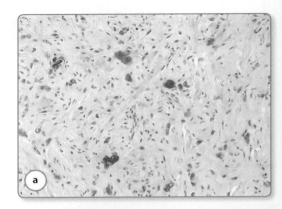

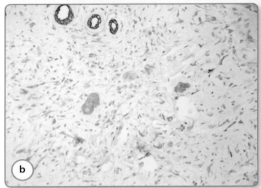

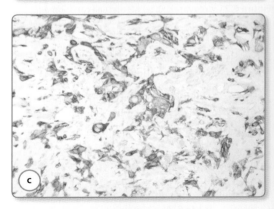

Figure 6.3 AE1/3 vs. cytokeratin 5. (a) Poorly differentiated SCC (H&E, 200×). (b) Negative AE1/A3 in large atypical cells (AE1/3, 200×). (c) Strong CK5 in atypical cells (CK5, 200×).

Uses: AR is strongly and diffusely positive in most sebaceous adenomas and carcinomas. It is very helpful in differentiating sebaceous neoplasms

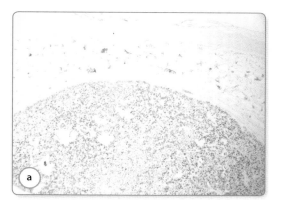

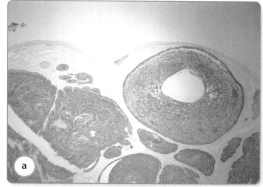

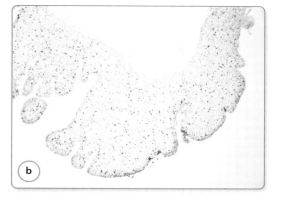

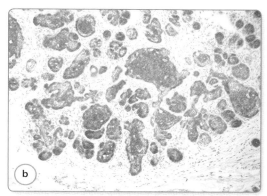

Figure 6.4 (a) Androgen receptor (AR) with diffuse nuclear positivity in sebaceous carcinoma (AR, 100×). (b) AR with focal nuclear staining (approx. 5%) in BCC (AR, 100×).

Figure 6.5 (a) BER-Ep4 in BCC (BER-Ep4, 100×). (b) BER-Ep4 in trichoepithelioma (BER-Ep4, 200×).

from BCCs (**Figure 6.4**). While, 60% of BCC may show some AR reactivity, this positivity is usually focal and faint (<5% of cells staining), in comparison to the diffuse, strong AR expression seen in sebaceous lesions (Bayer-Garner et al. 1999). In some studies, the focal AR positivity of BCCs may be helpful to differentiate them from DTE, which are completely AR-negative (Izikson et al. 2005). AR is positive in apocrine neoplasms, including mucinous carcinomas of the eyelid, and thus AR positivity on the eyelid is not synonymous with sebaceous differentiation.

Staining pattern: Nuclear.

Clones: AR27; AR441; AR-N20; F39.4.1

BER-Ep4

Background: Ber-EP4 is a monoclonal antibody against 34 kDa and 39 kDa cell surface glycoproteins, which are broadly distributed in epithelial cells (Ansai et al. 2012).

Uses: In the skin, Ber-EP4 is localized in basaloid epithelial cells, and as such, is found in BCC as well as follicular neoplasms, such as trichoblastomas and trichoepitheliomas (Ozawa et al. 2004) (**Figure 6.5**). In contrast, Ber-Ep4 is predominantly negative in squamous cell carcinomas, sebaceous carcinomas, and microcystic adnexal carcinomas; therefore, it is useful in differentiating basal cell carcinomas from these entities. Of note, peri-anal basal cell carcinomas are negative for Ber-EP4 (Alvarez-Cañas et al. 1996). Ber-Ep4 is positive in EMPD, but is negative in SCC with pagetoid spread, and as a subset of SCCs may stain positively with CK 7, Ber-Ep4 may be a useful adjunct to the workup of neoplasms with pagetoid spread

(Sellheyer & Krahl 2008). In this setting, it is important to note that Ber-EP4 may also stain cutaneous neuroendocrine carcinomas (Merkel cell carcinomas) with pagetoid spread (Smith et al. 1993).

Staining pattern: Membranous.

Clones: HEA125; EPCAM; BER-EP4; C10; AUA1; VU-1D9; MOC-31

Carcinoembryonic antigen (CEA)

Background: CEA consists of a 180 – 200 kDa heterogeneous family of related oncofetal glycoproteins which are part of the immunoglobin superfamily. This family of glycoproteins includes CEA-180, biliary glycoprotein (BGP), and non-specific cross reacting antigens (NCA). In normal tissues, CEA is the columnar cells of colon, small intestine, stomach, pancreatic ducts, secretory epithelia of sweat glands, squamous epithelial cells of the tongue, esophagus, uterine cervix, and urothelium.

Uses: In the skin, CEA has a relatively limited role, but can be used to highlight ductal differentiation in eccrine/apocrine adnexal tumors. In the setting of metastatic adenocarcinomas, CEA is relatively non-specific and is positive in a variety of lesions including carcinomas of the colorectum, salivary gland, esophagus, stomach, biliary tract, pancreas, small intestine, lung, uterine cervix, medullary thyroid and ovary (mucinous type). CEA is usually negative in breast carcinoma as well as mammary Paget's disease. It is generally positive in EMPD.

Clones: CEA-P; 11-7; 12.140.10; A115; A5B7; AF4; CEA-M; CEJ065; CEM010; COL-1; D14; IL-7; M773; PARLAM 1; T84.66; TF3H8-1; ZC23; 0062; alpha-7; CEA 41; CEA-GOLD 4; CEA-GOLD 1; T84.6; CEA 11;CEA-GOLD 2; CEA-B18; T84.1; CEA-GOLD 5; CEA-M431_31; CEA-D14; CEA 27; CEA-GOLD 3; CEA88

DNA mismatch repair proteins

Background: Mismatch repair (MMR) genes perform critical functions by repairing DNA mismatches that may occur during cell replication. The gene products of normal mismatch repair genes can be detected in the nuclei of normal cells by IHC, using antibodies directed against the normal gene products. Mutations in these genes often lead to an inability to detect the normal gene product in the nuclei of cells by IHC. As such, the absence of nuclear staining with the antibodies to the gene products has been found to correlate well with the presence of mutations in the corresponding mismatch repair gene (Orta et al. 2009).

Uses: In the skin, IHC for the MMR proteins MLH-1, MSH-2, MSH-6, and PMS-2 is used in the setting of sebaceous neoplasms in order to evaluate for the possibility of underlying gene defects associated with Muir-Torre syndrome. Muir-Torre syndrome is a genetic disorder thought to be a subtype of hereditary non polyposis colorectal cancer (HNPCC)/ Lynch syndrome. It is characterized by the presence of multiple cutaneous sebaceous neoplasms in association with underlying visceral malignancies, especially colorectal and genitourinary carcinomas. It is the result of mutations in various DNA mismatch repair (MMR) genes including *MLH1*, *MSH2*, *MSH6*, and *PMS2*. As stated above, normal tissues will have preserved staining of these MMR IHC markers, while mutations in these genes will lead to a loss in immunohistochemical expression of the corresponding markers (**Figure 6.6**).

Staining pattern: Nuclear (nuclear expression loss correlates with underlying mutation).

Clones: MSH-2: HMSH2; FE11; G219-1129; Ab-2; 25D12; MSH-6: GRBP.P1; HMSH6; MSH6; PU29; clone 44; BC/44 MLH-1: G168-15; HMLH1; G168-728; ES05; M1; PMS-2: PMS2; A16-4-PMS2; MRQ-28; EPR3947

Epithelial membrane antigen (EMA)

Background: EMA, also known as MUC-1, is one of the several transmembrane glycoproteins which were originally isolated from human milk fat globule proteins (HMFGP) membranes. It is found on most epithelial surfaces and is a useful marker in establishing the epithelial nature of neoplastic cells (Pinkus & Kurtin 1985). EMA is also found on non-epithelial cells including perineural cells as well as plasma cells. The most commonly used monoclonal antibody used for EMA detection is E29, a 450 kDa glycoprotein.

Uses: In the setting of epithelial cutaneous neoplasms, EMA is strongly positive in squamous cell carcinomas as well as sebaceous carcinomas. In sebaceous carcinomas, EMA staining of the sebocytes often displays a

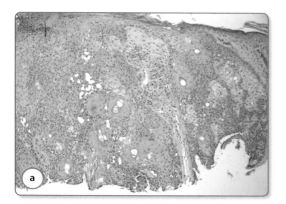

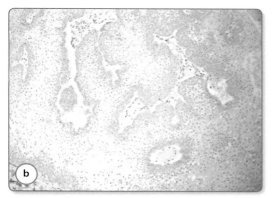

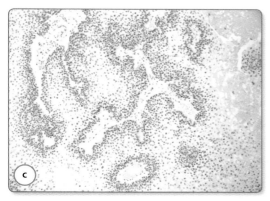

Figure 6.6 MSI staining in a sebaceous carcinoma associated with Muir Torre syndrome. (a) Sebaceous adenoma (H&E, 100×). (b) Loss of nuclear expression of MSH2 (abnormal) (MSH2, 100×). (c) Preserved MLH1 nuclear expression (normal) (MLH1, 100×).

foamy or bubbly type pattern (**Figure 6.7**). EMA is also expressed in high percentages of malignant eccrine carcinomas, but is often

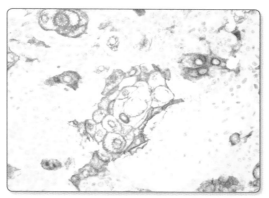

Figure 6.7 EMA with foamy membranous staining in a sebaceous adenoma (EMA, 200×).

negative in benign eccrine neoplasms such as eccrine spiradenomas (Swanson et al. 1987). EMA is generally negative in basal cell carcinomas, and thus, along with Ber-Ep4, may be useful in differentiating between squamous cell carcinomas, basal cell carcinomas and basosquamous carcinomas (Beer et al. 2000). Within the differential diagnosis of pagetoid spread, in addition to squamous carcinoma and sebaceous carcinoma, EMA is also expressed within EMPD. EMA is positive in perineuriomas.

Other: EMA may be expressed in wide variety of lesions which may present in the skin, including lymphomas, synovial sarcomas, myoepithelial neoplasms, plasmacytomas, ectopic meningioma, and epithelioid and angiomatoid fibrous histiocytomas. EMA has also been reported in low grade fibromyxoid sarcomas, a lesion which may mimic perineurioma histologically.

Staining pattern: Cytoplasmic staining is often present but is nonspecific, and for true EMA positivity, membranous staining must be present.

Clones: EMA, VU3D1; BC3; DF3; LICR-LON-M8; MA552; MUSEII; RD-1; MA695; 214D4; MC5; E29; GP1.4; ZCE113; MUC1

p63 (and p40)
Background: p63 is a member of the p53 gene family, which is involved in cell cycle arrest and apoptosis in response to DNA damage. p63 is a nuclear stain; thus, blush cytoplasmic staining should be interpreted as negative staining. In normal tissues, expression is restricted to

epithelial cells of stratified epithelia, such as skin, esophagus, exocervix, tonsil, and bladder, myoepithelial cells, and to certain subpopulations of basal cells in glandular structures of prostate and breast, as well as in bronchi.

Uses: In the skin, p63 is helpful in the differential diagnosis of poorly differentiated spindle cell neoplasms, as p63 positivity is an indication of squamous cell differentiation. In particular, p63 positivity argues against the diagnosis of atypical fibroxanthoma (AFX), and is supportive of a diagnosis of poorly differentiated squamous or spindle cell carcinoma (Gleason et al. 2009). P40, a p63 isoform, has recently been reported to have the same sensitivity but greater specificity than p63 for distinguishing between spindle cell squamous carcinomas and AFX (Henderson et al. 2014).

P63 is also a marker of myoepithelial cells, and as well as staining myoepithelial neoplasms such as myoepitheliomas and myoepithelial carcinomas, it may be used to highlight a myoepithelial layer in various adnexal neoplasms (such as apocrine hidrocystomas). As mentioned, along with markers such as D2-40 and cytokeratin 15, p63 may have some use in distinguishing primary adnexal carcinomas from metastatic visceral malignancies to the skin as primary adnexal carcinomas are generally p63 positive while the majority of metastatic lesions are p63 negative (Ivan et al. 2007)(Mahalingam et al. 2010). P63 may also be used in differentiating pagetoid squamous cell carcinoma in situ (positive) versus EMPD (negative). P63 stains a subset of Merkel cell carcinomas, and p63 expression within these lesions may indicate a more aggressive clinical behavior (Asioli et al. 2007). P63 will also stain basal cell carcinomas as well as follicular and sebaceous neoplasms. Of note, p63 may also stain striations in skeletal muscle cells.

Staining pattern: Nuclear.

Clones: 63PO2; 7JUL; H-137; P63; 4A4; BC4A4

Neuroendocrine markers

CD56 and CD57

Background: CD56 (neural cell adhesion molecule/N-CAM) and CD57 (HNK1;Leu-7) are natural killer associated antigens with molecular weights of 140 kDa and 95 kDa respectively. CD56 is normally expressed on natural killer cells, as well as neural and neuroendocrine tissues, and can be found normally in peripheral nerves, cerebral cortex synapses, follicular thyroid epithelium, renal tubules, parietal cells and pancreatic islet cells. In normal skin, CD56 expression can be seen in basal epidermal cells, sweat glands, and the outer root sheath of follicles. CD57 is found on a subset of peripheral lymphoyctes as well as myelin and schwann cells. It is also expressed in prostate epithelium, pancreatic islets, and gastric chief cells.

Uses: In addition to being markers for natural killer cells, CD56 and 57 can be used as neuroendocrine markers and as such will be positive in neuroendocrine neoplasms, such as Merkel cell carcinomas. However, given the lack of specificity, these markers are generally not used in isolation for neuroendocrine differentiation. CD56 is useful in the differential diagnosis of small round blue cell tumors as CD56 is positive in: neuroblastoma, rhabdomyosarcoma, poorly differentiated synovial sarcoma, Wilms Tumor, mesenchymal chondrosarcoma, and small cell carcinoma, but it is only rarely positive in Ewing sarcoma.

Other uses/miscellaneous: See hematolymphoid section for additional uses of CD56 in hematopoietic lesions.

Staining pattern: Membranous.

Clones: LEU-19; ERIC-1; 14-MAB735; 1B6; 24-MB2; 25-KD11; BC56C04; CD56; MAB 735; NCAM; NCC-LU-243; CD564; MOC-1; 123C3; NCL-CD56-1

Synaptophysin/chromogranin

Background: Synaptophysin is a major integral membrane protein of small synaptic vesicles which plays a role in regulating endocytosis during neuronal activity (Kwon & Chapman 2011) and is used as a highly sensitive marker for neuroendocrine differentiation. Chromogranins consist of a group of three types of proteins (A, B, and C) which make up a portion of the neurosecretory granules of neuroendocrine cells. One clone (LK2H10) to Chromogranin A, a 68 kDa protein, is the most widely used form of the antibody (Wilson & Lloyd 1984). Chromogranin has a higher specificity but lower sensitivity than synaptophysin. Chromogranin and synaptophysin are normally expressed in the neurosecretory granules of a variety of cells including Merkel cells in the skin.

Uses: Synaptophysin and chromogranin are used as markers of neuroendocrine differentiation. Cutaneous Merkel cell carcinomas are positive for synaptophysin, and the majority is also positive for chromogranin. Synaptophysin and chromogranin are positive in metastatic neuroendocrine tumors such as carcinoid and endocrine mucin-producing carcinoma, a rare eccrine tumor of the eyelid.

Staining pattern: Cytoplasmic.

Clones: SNP-88, SVP38; SY38; SYNAPTOPHYS; SP11; 27G12; MRQ-40

Other useful IHC markers in epithelial lesions

A summary of other commonly used IHC markers, many of which may be useful in the workup of systemic carcinomas, is summarized in **Table 6.4**.

Table 6.4 Other useful epithelial IHC markers					
Antibody	Clones	Background	Staining pattern	Positive	Other
CDX-2	7C7/D4; AMT28; CDx-2; EPR2764Y; CDX-2-88	Transcription factor important in GI tract development	N	Colorectal Mucinous Ovarian	
ER	6F11; EP1; ERB1; PPG5/10; SP1	Estrogen receptor	N	Breast Adnexal tumors	ER positivity virtually excludes a GI primary
GATA-3	GATA-3; HG3-31; L50-823; D13C9	Transcription factor highly expressed in breast epithelium	N	Breast Urothelial	Will stain primary cutaneous adnexal tumors
GCDFP	BRST-2; D6; GCDFP-15; 23A3	Proteins derived from analysis of fluid from gross cystic disease Gross cystic disease fluid protein	C	Breast Adnexal tumors	Negative staining in vulvar Paget's may indicate underlying malignancy
NKX3.1	NKX3.1	Androgen related gene specific to prostate	N	Prostate	
TTF-1	SC-13040; SPT-24; TTF-1; 8G7G3	Thyroid transcription factor	N	Thyroid Lung adenocarcinoma Lung neuroendocrine	
PAX-8	Pax-8; BC12	Transcription factor essential in development of kidneys, gyn organs, thyroid	N	Renal GYN tumors Thyroid	
P53	P53; 21N; AB6; CM1; DO1; MU195; PAB240; RSP53; DO7; SP5	Tumor suppressor gene	N	Maybe used in setting of dVIN – complete loss of p53 in dVIN; retained p53 in basilar keratinocytes in reactive processes	
Villin	I1D2C3; Villin; ID2C3; CWWB1	Actin binding cytoskeletal protein found in brush boarders	M	Colon Lung Stomach Pancreas Gall bladder	

C, cytoplasmic; dVIN, differentiated VIN; N, nuclear

Hematolymphoid IHC markers

IHC plays a large role in the evaluation of cutaneous lymphoproliferative infiltrates. IHC is used to differentiate reactive infiltrates from lymphomas, to sub-classify lymphomas, to obtain prognostic information, and to evaluate various cutaneous histiocytoses. The main IHC markers used for these purposes are highlighted below.

Work-up of B-cell proliferations

Bcl-2

Background: Bcl-2 is a 25 kDa regulator protein localized to the inner mitochondrial membrane involved in apoptosis, acting to either inhibit or promote cell death. Bcl-2 is normally expressed on mantle B-cells as well as the majority of T-cells. In nodal follicular lymphomas, there is often a t(14;18) chromosomal translocation which places the *BCL2* gene next to the immunoglobulin heavy chain locus leading to high levels of Bcl-2 and subsequent blocking of apoptosis.

Uses: Bcl-2 will stain B-cells of the mantle zone as well as T-lymphocytes. Bcl-2 is often positive in cutaneous marginal zone lymphomas (MZLs), but as these cases often have a reactive T-cell population, it is important to confirm that Bcl-2 is present on the B-cell population, and not just staining the background T-cells. Normal, reactive germinal centers (GCs) are Bcl-6+/Bcl-2-. Systemic follicular lymphomas have an abnormal Bcl-6+/Bcl-2+ GC profile (**Figure 6.8**). Cutaneous follicle center cell lymphomas (FCLs) often display a Bcl-6+/Bcl-2- phenotype. The literature varies on the percentage of primary cutaneous FCLs which express Bcl-2 in GCs, and in our experience a large number of cutaneous follicle center cell lymphomas do co-express Bcl-2; however, the presence of a Bcl-6+/Bcl-2+ phenotype should raise the possibility of a systemic nodal lymphoma secondarily involving the skin (Hoefnagel et al. 2003). In general, Bcl-2 expression on B-cells in the skin is of great concern for lymphoma.

Staining pattern: Membranous and cytoplasmic.

Clones: Bcl-2; 124; 124.3; ONCL2; BCL2/100/D5; C-2; E17

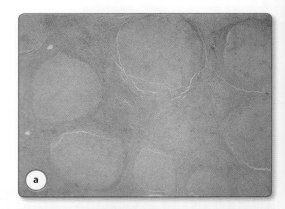

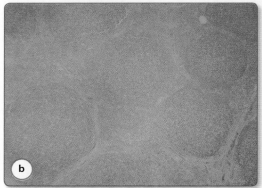

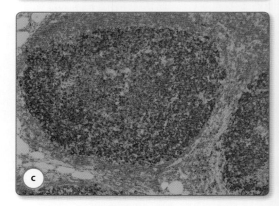

Figure 6.8 Bcl-2 and Bcl-6 in follicle center cell lymphoma. (a) Enlarged, abnormal germinal center (GC) formation in follicle center cell lymphoma (H&E, 100×). (b) Bcl-6 staining GC formation (BCL6, 100×) (c) Aberrant Bcl-2 expression in the Bcl-6 + germinal centers (BCL2, 100×).

Bcl-6

Background: Bcl-6 is a 95 kDa nuclear protein which has an important role in immune system regulation and is needed in germinal center differentiation and T-cell mediated immunity (Niu 2002).

Uses: Bcl-6 is expressed in both reactive and neoplastic germinal centers, and thus serves as an excellent marker of follicle centers. Thus, Bcl-6 is used in the diagnosis of cutaneous FCLs (see details above under uses of Bcl-2). In FCLs, Bcl-6 may also be expressed outside of germinal centers in inter-follicular areas, and this finding may be helpful in distinguishing follicular lymphomas from marginal zone lymphomas with secondary colonization of germinal centers (Dyhdalo et al. 2013; Dogan et al. 2000).

Along with CD10 and MUM-1/IRF, Bcl-6 is also used in the setting of the work up of cutaneous diffuse large B-cell lymphomas (DLBCL)(Berglund et al. 2005). These markers help to differentiate between DLBCL cases with a germinal center cell phenotype and cases with an activated B-cell phenotype (post germinal center cell) (**Figure 6.9**). Cutaneous DLBCL, leg type is an example of the activated B-cell phenotype. This distinction is important as the germinal center phenotype typically responds better to chemotherapy and DLBCL leg type behaves more aggressively.

In practice, some cases have weak or focal expression of Bcl-6, CD10 and/or MUM-1 and it may be difficult to accurately subtype the DLBCL. While Bcl-6 positivity is considered as >10% staining of the neoplastic cells, cases with diffuse Bcl-6 expression are considered more suggestive of a germinal center phenotype of cells.

Other: Bcl-6 is positive in Burkitt lymphoma, angioimmunoblastic T-cell lymphoma, and L&H cells of nodular lymphocyte predominant Hodgkin lymphoma. Bcl-6 may also stain squamous (including epidermal) and glandular epithelium.

Staining pattern: Nuclear.

Clones: GI191E/A8; PG-B6P; 3FR-1; N-3; P1F6; LN22; GL191E/A8; Bcl-6

CD10

Background: Also known as common acute lymphoblastic leukemia antigen (CALLA), CD10 is a 90–110 kDa cell membrane glycoprotein.

Uses: CD10 is a non-specific antibody as it stains a variety of epithelial, mesenchymal, and hematopoietic cells. In cutaneous lymphomas, in association with Bcl-6, CD10 is a marker of germinal center differentiation, and is therefore usually expressed in follicular lymphoma, more commonly in nodal follicular lymphoma involving the skin. As described above, it is used in conjunction with Bcl-6 and MUM-1 to classify DLBCL (**Figure 6.9**).

Other: Not lineage specific and stains a wide variety of epithelial cells, including bladder,

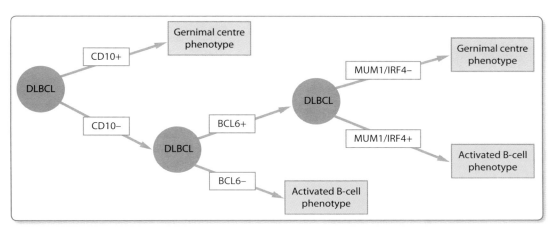

Figure 6.9 Diffuse large B-cell lymphoma (DLBCL) prognostic stratification flow chart.

kidney and liver. In the skin, it may be used to stain dermatofibromas (DF) and atypical fibrous xanthoma (AFX). CD10 may also be used to differentiate BCC from trichoepitheliomas (TEs), as BCC epithelium will stain for CD10 and its associated stroma is negative. In contrast, CD10 will stain the stroma of associated papillary mesenchymal bodies of TE, but not the tumor itself (Pham et al. 2006) (**Figure 6.10**). CD10 may be used to differentiate superficial BCC (CD10+) from actinic keratosis or squamous cell carcinoma (CD10-). CD10 is one of the first markers discovered for acute lymphoblastic leukemia.

Staining pattern: Membranous.

Clones: NCL-270; CD10; 56C6

CD20

Background: CD20 is a 33–37 kDa non-glycosylated phosphoprotein expressed on the vast majority of all normal and malignant B cells. It does not stain plasma cells. Of note, CD20 may be negative in lymphomas which have been treated with the anti-CD20 antibody rituximab.

Use: Used as a pan B-cell marker to evaluate both reactive processes, such as cutaneous lymphoid hyperplasia, as well as lymphomas.

Staining pattern: Membranous.

Clones: CD20; B1; FB1; L26

CD21

Background: CD21 is a 145 kDa membrane glycoprotein which functions as the complement receptor (CR2) for C3d as well as the receptor for Epstein-Barr virus (EBV) and Human Herpes Virus-8 (HHV-8). CD21 is a restricted B-cell antigen expressed on mature B cells and, like CD23, is also present on follicular dendritic cells (FDC).

Uses: As CD21 highlights the FDCs, it is very useful in clearly defining the architecture of germinal centers, and thus can be used to reveal abnormally expanded germinal centers in follicular lymphomas or germinal centers distorted by secondary colonization by lymphoma cells, as may occur within marginal zone lymphomas.

Other: Highlights expanded FDC network in angioimmunoblastic lymphomas. Stains tumors derived from follicular dendritic cells, such as follicular dendritic sarcomas. Although it is the receptor for EBV, it is not necessarily expressed in EBV+ lymphomas.

Staining pattern: Membranous.

Clones: CD21; IF8

CD23

Background: 45 kDa membrane glycoprotein and a low affinity IgE receptor on B-cells.

Uses: CD23 is useful in differentiating small lymphocytic lymphoma/leukemia (chronic lymphocytic lymphoma/leukemia, SLL/CLL) from other low grade B-cell lymphomas since SLL/CLL is CD23 positive, while other lymphomas, such as marginal or mantle zone lymphomas, are negative. CD23, like CD21, is also

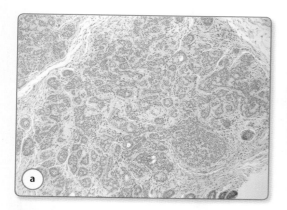
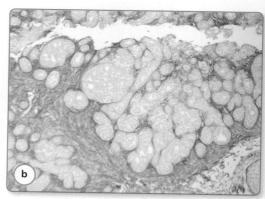

Figure 6.10 CD10 staining in trichoepithelioma. (a) Trichoepithelioma (TE) (H&E, 200×). (b) CD10 staining TE stroma (CD10, 200×).

expressed in follicular dendritic cells, and thus can be used to stain the follicular dendritic cell network and highlight expanded or abnormal follicle architecture in lymphomas. CD23 stains tumors of follicular dendritic cells and Reed-Sternberg cells of Hodgkin lymphoma.

Staining pattern: Membranous.

Clones: 1B12, BU38, MHM6, CD23, SP23

CD79a

Background: Like CD20, CD79a is a specific B-cell marker. CD79a is expressed on B-cells earlier than CD20, but also is retained longer during the maturation of B-cells and therefore will also stain plasma cells. CD79a also marks rituximab treated lymphomas.

Use: Similar to CD20 (see above)

Staining pattern: Membranous.

Clones: CD79a; 11D10; 11E3; HM47/A9; HM57; JCB117; MB-1; CD79A

CD138 (Syndecan-1)

Background: CD138/syndecan-1 is a cell membrane receptor and is expressed on the surface of mature epithelial cells and both normal and neoplastic plasma cells.

Uses: In hematolymphoid lesions, CD138 is a fairly good marker of plasma cells.

Other: CD138 must be interpreted in the appropriate context because it is non-specific and stains a variety of epithelial tumors, including breast, as well as non-epithelial tumors such as melanoma and synovial sarcomas (O'Connell et al. 2004).

Staining pattern: Membranous and cytoplasmic.

Clones: AM411-10M; B-B4; MI15; SYNDECAN; CD138; B-A38

Cyclin D1

Background: Cyclin D1 is a 34 kDa protein, and an important cell cycle regulator, and plays a crucial role in the G1/S transition phase of the cell cycle.

Use: Cyclin D1 stains mantle cell lymphoma, and is used to distinguish mantle cell lymphoma from other small B-cell lymphomas.

Other: May be expressed in various carcinomas, including breast, ovary, bladder, and squamous cell carcinoma.

Staining pattern: Nuclear.

Clones: A-12; AM29; D1GM; P2D11F11; PRAD1; SP4; DCS-6; CYCLIN D1; 5D4

Kappa (κ)/lambda (λ) light chains

Background: κ and λ immunoglobulin light chains comprise the small polypeptide subunit of an antibody. κ is located on chromosome 2 while λ is on chromosome 22. In tissues, the normal κ:λ ratio is roughly 2:1.

Uses: κ/λ stains are generally used in dermatopathology as a surrogate marker for clonality in a B-cell population. B cells can express either κ or λ light chains but not both, with the normal ratio of κ:λ B cells being approximately 2:1. Thus, a restricted population or marked predominance of κ or λ light chains is an indicator of a clonal population of B cells which would be supportive of a neoplastic process. In practice, κ/λ staining may be very helpful in the evaluation and discrimination of cutaneous low grade marginal zone lymphomas from reactive pseudolymphomas/cutaneous lymphoid hyperplasia.

Staining pattern: Cytoplasmic.

Clones: KAPPA; LAMBDA

Ki-67

Background: Ki-67 identifies a 395-kDa nuclear antigen expressed in all cells which are in not in the resting G0 phase of the cell cycle.

Use: Ki-67 is used as a marker of the proliferation index of cells. In lymphomas, Ki-67 has utility in differentiating lesions of cutaneous lymphoid hyperplasia with reactive germinal centers, which have high Ki-67 proliferative rate, from neoplastic germinal centers in FCL, which have a lower Ki-67 proliferation index.

Staining pattern: Nuclear.

Clones: KI88; MIB1; MMI; SP6; Ki-S5; KI-67; 30-9; IVAK-2; K2

MUM-1/IRF

Background: Multiple myeloma 1/interferon regulatory factor 4 (MUM-1/IRF) is a transcription factor involved in lymphocyte activation and plasma cell differentiation, and therefore is expressed in a variety of hematolymphoid tumors. In normal tissues, it is usually not expressed in areas with Bcl-6 since germinal center cells are

MUM1- BCL6+ CD10+, whereas post-germinal center cells are MUM1+ BCL6- CD10-.

Uses: As discussed under Bcl-6, MUM-1 is most often used in dermatopathology to evaluate DLBCL, and its presence indicates an aggressive activated B-cell phenotype as seen in DLBCL, leg type (**Figure 6.9**).

Other: MUM-1 is strongly positive in a variety of lymphomas, including multiple myeloma, natural killer cell lymphomas, and anaplastic large cell lymphomas (ALCL). MUM-1 may also be positive in melanoma.

Staining pattern: Nuclear.

Clones: M17; MUM1-IRF.4; MUM1; MUM1P

PAX-5

Background: Pax-5 encodes the 45 kDa B-cell specific transcription factor BSAP, and plays a crucial role in routing lymphoid progenitors to the B lymphocyte lineage (Cobaleda et al. 2007). Loss of Pax-5 also plays a crucial role in plasma cell development (Nera et al. 2006).

Uses: Similar to CD20 and CD79a, Pax-5 is used as a pan B-cell marker, and it generally stains similarly to CD20. PAX-5 may be especially useful in situations where CD20 may be negative, including classical Hodgkin lymphoma (cHL), B-lymphoblastic leukemia and B-cell lymphomas following rituximab therapy (Desouki et al. 2010). Unlike CD79a, Pax-5 is not expressed in plasma cells. Of note, PAX-5 is a nuclear stain, which facilitates interpretation of small biopsies.

Other: In the skin, PAX-5 has been shown to be expressed in the majority of merkel cell carcinomas.

Staining pattern: Nuclear.

Clones: PAX-5; PAX5 (BSAP); DAK-pax5; A-22

Zap-70

Background: Zap-70 is a 70 kDa tyrosine kinase involved in signal transduction pathways of both T and B cells (Au-Yeung et al. 2009).

Uses: Zap-70 is predominantly used as a prognostic marker in the setting of SLL/CLL. In CLL/SLL, the presence of an unmutated variable heavy-chain gene (IgV(H)) is an indicator of an aggressive clinical course. Zap-70 expression (considered significant if present in >20% of tumor cells) has been shown to act as a surrogate marker for the unmutated IGV(H) gene, and is thus predictive of a more aggressive clinical course (Crespo et al. 2003; Villamor 2005).

Zap-70 marks T cells in most tissues. Outside of CLL/SLL, Zap-70 is negative in most mature B-cell lymphomas.

Staining pattern: Cytoplasmic.

Clones: 2F3.2; ZAP-70-LR; ZAP-70; 1E7.2

Work-up of T-cell and NK-cell proliferations

Anaplastic lymphoma kinase (ALK)

Background: ALK is a receptor tyrosine kinase also known as CD246. It is involved in the characteristic t(2:5)(p23:q35) translocation involving the 2p23 ALK gene and the NPM 5q3 gene seen in a subset of anaplastic large cell lymphomas.

Uses: In the skin, ALK IHC is usually used in the evaluation of a CD30 lymphoproliferative process. The presence of ALK positivity in a CD30 positive disorder suggests a systemic ALCL secondarily involving the skin. ALK negativity does not, however, exclude a systemic ALCL involving the skin.

ALK may also be useful in the evaluation of spindle cell lesions in the skin as a subset of cutaneous inflammatory pseudotumors are ALK positive (El Shabrawi-Caelen et al. 2004).

Staining pattern: Cytoplasmic.

Clones: 5A4; ALKC; ALK; ALK1; D5F3; CD246

CD2

Background: Historically, human T lymphocytes were initially distinguished from B lymphocytes by their formation of spontaneous rosettes with sheep red blood cells, a phenomenon mediated by CD2. CD2 is a 50 kDa glycosylated transmembrane receptor molecule also known as LFA-3 (leukocyte function associated antigen-3), and is one of the earliest T-cell lineage restricted antigens to appear.

Uses: CD2 is used as a pan T-cell antigen, and will stain all normal T lymphocytes as well as the majority of T-cell lymphomas/leukemias. CD2 may be aberrantly lost in some T-cell lymphomas. It also stains NK cells.

Staining: Membranous and cytoplasmic.

Clones: MT910; 271; AB75; LFA-2; CD2; NCL-CD2-271

CD3

Background: The CD3 antigen consists of a complex group of at least four 20-28 kDa membrane glycoproteins, and is one of the earliest antigens expressed in T-cell differentiation.

Uses: Used as a pan T-cell specific marker due to presence on most normal resting and activated T lymphocytes. CD3 is often used along with other T-cell markers such as CD4, CD8, and CD7 in the evaluation of cutaneous T-cell lymphomas, including mycoses fungoides (MF).

Other: Polyclonal form of the antibody recognizes the epsilon chain of CD3, and may be positive in natural killer (NK) cell lymphomas; whereas the monoclonal form is usually negative in these lesions.

Staining pattern: Cytoplasmic and membranous.

Clones: A0452; CD3-M; CD3-P; PS1; F7238; SP7

CD4/CD8

Background: As CD4 and CD8 are often ordered together, they will be discussed under one heading.

CD4 is a 55 kDa glycoprotein found on T-helper cell subsets and acts as a co-receptor binding to MHC class II molecules. It is expressed on thymocytes, T-helper cells, monocytes, macrophages, and granulocytes. It also serves as the receptor for HIV on T-cells.

CD8 is a 34 kDa co-receptor involved in MHC class I antigen binding. It is expressed on T cytotoxic/suppressor lymphocytes and at low levels on NK cells.

Uses: CD4 and CD8 are generally mixed in reactive lymphoid populations as CD4 antibody will label T helper/inducer cells while CD8

highlights mature cytotoxic/suppressor cells. As the majority of peripheral T-cell lymphomas are derived from the helper T-cell subset, most of these neoplasms are CD 4+/CD 8-. Most cases of MF also display a CD4+/CD8- phenotype (**Figure 6.11**). In the evaluation of epidermotropic cells in MF, it is important to not over-interpret the presence of intra-epidermal Langerhans cells, as these cells are CD4+. Cases of juvenile MF are often CD8+CD4-(Whittam et al. 2000). Primary cutaneous epidermotropic cytotoxic T-cell lymphomas are aggressive lymphomas which also display a CD8+CD4- phenotype. As with other T-cell markers, CD4 and CD8 may be aberrantly deleted in neoplastic T-cell populations, and loss of both antigens is supportive of a diagnosis of lymphoma. **Table 6.5** summarizes the common CD4/CD8 staining patterns for common cutaneous T-cell lymphomas.

Staining pattern: Cytoplasmic.

Clones: CD4-1290; 1F6; 4B12; IF6; CD4; NCL-CD4-368; CD8-C8/144; C8/144B; CD8; M7103

CD5

Background: CD5 is a 67 kDa transmembrane glycoprotein involved in T and B-cell receptor signaling. It is a pan T-cell marker and is also present in a small subpopulation of B cells known as B-1 lymphocytes (Dono et al. 2004).

Uses: Along with CD3 and CD2, CD5 is used as a pan T-cell marker. The majority of T-cell malignancies are CD5+. Loss of expression in a T-cell process is evidence of malignancy. After CD7, it is the second most commonly lost antigen in MF. CD5 is negative in extranodal NK/T-cell lymphoma.

In B-cell lymphomas, CD5 is positive in both SLL/CLL and mantle cell lymphomas, and is useful in differentiating these entities from other B-cell lymphomas.

Table 6.5 Summary of CD4/CD8 expression in cutaneous lymphomas

Antigen	Conventional MF	Juvenile MF	Primary cutaneous epidermotropic T-cell lymphoma	γδ Lymphoma	ALCL	Subcutaneous panniculitis like T-cell lymphoma	Blastic plasmacytoid dendritic cell neoplasm
CD4	+	−	−	−	++/-	−	+
CD8	−	+	+	−	--/+	+	−

Other: Originally, immunoreactive only in fresh/ frozen tissue, but current clones such as Leu1 and 4C7 work on paraffin embedded formalin fixed tissue.

Staining pattern: Cytoplasmic.

Clones: 4C7; 54/B4; 54/F6; CD5; NCL-CD5; Leu-1

CD7

Background: CD7 antigen is a cell surface glycoprotein of 40 kDa expressed on the surface of immature and mature T cells and natural killer cells.

Uses: CD7 is specific for T-cell lineage and is positive in lymphoblastic leukemias/lymphomas. In peripheral T-cell lymphomas and MF, it is the most common pan T-cell antigen to be aberrantly lost (**Figure 6.11**).

Staining pattern: Cytoplasmic and membranous.

Clones: 272; CD7-272; CD7; NCL-CD7-272

CD30

Background: The first CD30 antibody to be identified and used was Ki-1, which only worked on frozen sections. Later, the BerH2 antibody was developed which can be used on formalin fixed paraffin sections. CD30 is a membrane-bound glycoprotein with a molecular mass of 105-120 kDa. CD30 is a lymphoid activation marker and can be induced on both B and T lymphocytes.

Uses: In the skin, CD30 is predominantly used in the assessment of lymphoproliferative disorders, and marks a variety of conditions under the broad category of CD30-positive lymphoproliferative disorders. CD30-lymphoproliferative processes include entities such as lymphomatoid papulosis, anaplastic large cell lymphoma (ALCL), transformed mycosis fungoides, and pseudolymphoma (**Figure 6.12**). Of note, CD30 is not evidence of malignancy and may be positive

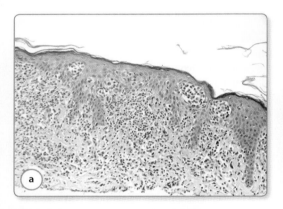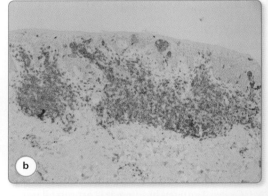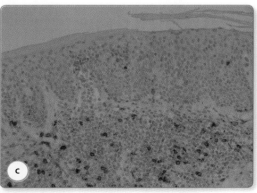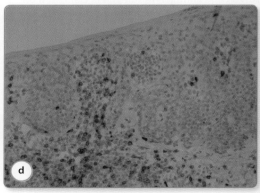

Figure 6.11 (a) Mycosis fungoides (MF) with Pautrier microabscess formation (H&E, 200×). (b) CD4+ atypical cells (CD4, 200×). (c) CD8 negative staining (CD8, 200X). (d) Loss of CD7 expression (CD7, 200×).

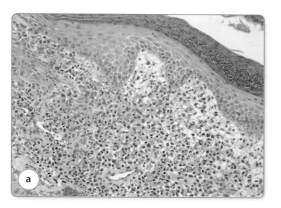

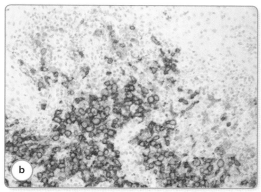

Figure 6.12 CD30 in lymphomatoid papulosis. (a) Large atypical cells in dermis of a case of lymphomatoid papulosis (H&E, 100×). (b) CD30 stain (CD30, 100×).

in a variety of reactive conditions including drug eruptions and arthropod assaults. CD30 is also positive in Epstein-Barr virus transformed B and T cells. It is positive in Reed-Sternberg cells of classical Hodgkin lymphoma.

Other: Histiocytes may express CD30 in various conditions including certain infections and in sarcoidosis. BER-H2 may label plasma cells. CD30 reactivity is impaired by mercury containing fixatives (Taylor & Cote 2006).

Staining pattern: Cytoplasmic and membranous.

Clones: CON6D/B9; BER-H2; KI-1; CD30; CON6D/B5; DT05 + BC98; 1G12

CD56

Background: CD56, also known as neural cell adhesion molecule (NCAM), was discovered as a cell surface molecule involved in inter-

cellular signaling during neural development (Rutishauser et al. 1988).

Uses: In the setting of hematolymphoid lesions, CD56 is expressed in NK/T- cell lymphomas, as well as $\gamma\delta$ lymphomas. Along with CD4, CD56 is positive in blastic plasmacytoid dendritic cell neoplasms (formerly known as blastic NK-lymphoma and CD4+/CD56+ hematodermic tumor). CD56 may also be expressed in acute myelogenous leukemia, acute lymphoblastic leukemia, and neoplastic plasma cells.

Staining pattern: Membranous.

Clones: LEU-19; ERIC-1; 14-MAB735; 1B6; 24-MB2; 5-KD11;BC56C04; CD56; MAB 735; NCAM;NCC-LU-243; CD564; MOC-1; 123C3; NCL-CD56-1B

Cytotoxic molecules (TIA-1, Granzyme B, Perforin)

Background: The cytotoxic molecules are found in cytoplasmic granules of natural killer cells and cytotoxic T cells. TIA-1 is present in both activated and inactivated cytotoxic cells, while granzyme and perforin are present only in activated cells.

Uses: Cytotoxic markers are positive in NK/T-cell lymphomas. 75% of ALCL are TIA-1 positive (Foss et al. 1996). They are also present in other lymphomas with cytotoxic phenotype including cytotoxic subsets of cutaneous T-cell lymphomas, intestinal T-cell lymphomas and large granular lymphocytic lymphomas. These markers may be positive in classical Hodgkin lymphoma.

Staining pattern: Granular, cytoplasmic.

Clones: TIA-1-NS/1-AG4; TIA-1; 2G9; Granzyme B- GRANZYME ; Perforin-P1-8; PE-41-PU; PERFORIN; 5B10

Histiocytic markers

CD1a

Background: CD1a is a membrane glycoprotein with a molecular weight of 49 kDa. It was initially found on human thymocytes and later on various T-cell populations and dendritic antigen presenting cells.

Uses: In dermatopathology, CD1a is a marker of Langerhans and Langerhans-like cells in the skin. Therefore, it is positive in Langerhans cell histiocytosis (LCH), congenital self-healing histiocytosis (a condition now considered a self-limited form of LCH), indeterminate cell histiocytosis and Langerhans sarcomas (**Figure 6.13b**). CD1a also stains immature cortical thymocytes and immature T-cell acute lymphoblastic lymphomas. It is negative in mature T-cell lymphomas including cutaneous T-cell lymphomas.

Other: CD1a may be helpful in the differentiation of cutaneous lymphoid hyperplasia (CLH)/ pseudolymphomas from cutaneous B-cell lymphomas, as CLH has been reported to have a high number of CD1a+ dendritic cells while B-cell lymphomas often lack such cells (Schmuth et al. 2001). It may also be helpful with CD4+ intra-epidermal infiltrates to distinguish Langerhans cells (CD4+/CD1a+) in allergic contact dermatitis (Langerhans cells) from mycosis fungoides T cells (CD4+/CD1a-).

Staining pattern: Membranous.

Clones: JPM30; NA1/34; O10; CD1A

CD68

Background: CD68 is a 110 kDa acidic, highly glycosylated lysosomal glycoprotein present in the cytoplasm of macrophages, monocytes, neutrophils and basophils. KP1 and PG-M1 are two commonly used monoclonal antibodies to CD68. KP1 labels monocytes and macrophages in all tissues as well as osteoclast giant cells, myeloid precursor cells, neutrophils and basophils. PG-M1 stains similarly to KP1; however, it is often negative in myeloid precursor cells and granulocytes.

Uses: Most commonly used as a marker of histiocytic differentiation and stains both reactive histiocytes as well as histiocytoses such as Rosai-Dorfman (R-D) and LCH. KP1 will also stain most acute myeloid leukemias, while PG-M1 will stain myelomonocytic leukemias. CD68 may also occasionally stain mast cells. As CD68 is associated with lysosomes, it is positive in entities with large numbers of lysosomes, including granular cell tumors and cellular neurothekeomas. PG-M1 has been reported to stain approximately 10% of melanomas (Leong et al. 1999).

Staining pattern: Cytoplasmic.

Clones: LN5; KP-1; PG-M1; CD68

CD163

Background: CD163 is a member of the scavenger receptor cystein-rich (SRCR) superfamily of receptors and is expressed on most

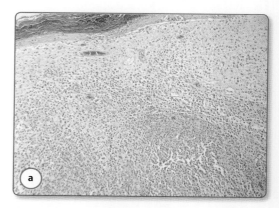

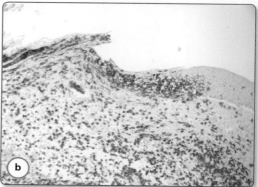

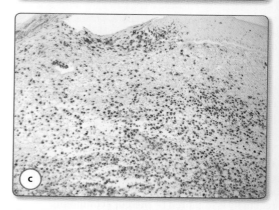

Figure 6.13 (a) Cutaneous Langerhans cell histiocytosis (H&E, 100×). (b) CD1a (CD1a, 100×). (c) Langerin (Langerin, 100×).

subpopulations of mature tissue macrophages (Fabriek et al. 2005).

Uses: Much like CD68, CD163 is primarily used as a marker of macrophages and histiocytic differentiation. CD163 stains macrophages in most normal tissues except for splenic histiocytes and lymph node tingible body macrophages (Lau et al. 2004).

CD163 is positive in reactive histiocytes; fibrous histioctyomas; chronic myelomonocytic leukemia; histiocytic sarcoma; sinus histiocytosis with massive lymphadenopathy (Rosai-Dorfman).

CD163 is negative in most cases of Langerhans cell histiocytosis; acute myeloid or myelomonocytic leukemias.

There are conflicting reports on CD163 staining in atypical fibrous xanthomas (AFX) (Pouryazdanparast et al. 2009; Sachdev et al. 2010).

Staining pattern: Membranous.

Clones: CD163; 10D6.

Langerin

Background: Langerin is a Birbeck granule associated type II transmembrane C-type lectin.

Uses: Used as a surrogate marker for the presence of Birbeck granules. Thus, like CD1a, langerin is used as a marker for Langerhans cells in the skin. Langerin is positive in LCH (**Figure 6.13 C**). It is sometimes negative in congenital self-healing histiocytosis. Langerin is negative in indeterminate cell histiocytosis, a lesion which has antigenic overlap with Langerhans cell histiocytosis and is CD1a+/S-100+ but lacks Birbeck granules.

Staining pattern: Membranous.

Clones: 12D6; Langerin

Other hematopoietic markers

CD25

Background: CD25 is a 55 kDa type I transmembrane glycoprotein and comprises the α chain of the IL-2 receptor. It is normally expressed on a subset of CD4+ regulatory T-cells as well as activated lymphocytes and monocytes.

Uses: Used in the evaluation of cutaneous mastocytosis. Reactive mast cells generally do not express CD25, while neoplastic mast cell populations may express CD25, and the presence of a CD25+ atypical immunophenotype is a minor diagnostic criteria for systemic mastocytosis (Horny 2009; Morgado et al. 2012). CD25 may sometimes be used in the evaluation of mycosis fungoides/Sezary syndrome as tumors with high expression (> 20% staining) of CD25

may respond to treatment with denileukin difitox therapy.

Staining pattern: Cytoplasmic and membranous.

Clones: 4C9; CD25; 2A3

CD45

Background: CD45 is the leukocyte common antigen (LCA), and is expressed on almost all bone marrow-derived cells. CD45 is a large molecule with multiple epitopes. As a result of post-translational change of the mRNA of the A, B and C exons, several isoforms are produced. CD45 antibodies are monoclonal antibodies, which react with all isoforms of CD45 proteins. The restricted CD45 (CD45R) antibody refers to those that recognize only a subset of CD45 proteins but not the entire class, and these CD45R antibodies can be further subdivided into CD45RA, CD45RB and CD45RO, depending on the isoform recognized by the antibody. CD45RA is located on naive T cells whereas CD45RO is a marker of memory T lymphocytes.

Uses: CD45 is used as a broad spectrum hematolymphoid marker and is thus used to prove hematolymphoid origin in undifferentiated tumors. The reactivity of anti-LCA antibodies is over 90% for most types of both B- and T-cell lymphomas. A potential pitfall in the workup of a poorly differentiated neoplasm may occur in the setting of ALCL, which may be CD45 negative. Therefore, in the skin, if CD45 is being used as a screening IHC in poorly differentiated lesions, CD30 should also be ordered so that lesions of ALCL are not missed. As ALCL may sometimes be CK positive, we have seen cases of CD45 negative ALCL called carcinomas when an accompanying CD30 stain was not performed. CD45RO is restricted to recognizing T-lymphocytes and is negative in B-cells, and may be positive in cases of ALCL which have lost other T-cell markers. CD45 is often negative in classic Hodgkin lymphoma.

Staining pattern: Membranous.

Clones: CD45- 1.22/4.14; 2D1; LCA; PD7; RP2/18; T29/33; CD45; PD7/26 CD45RO- UCHL-1; CD45RO; ACT-1; ICH1-L

CD117 (C-kit)

Background: 145 kDa tyrosine kinase growth factor receptor protein. Found on mast cells, various epithelial cells, melanocytes, and hematopoietic stem cells.

Uses: May be used as a marker for both reactive and neoplastic mast cell proliferations in the skin. CD117 is found on blasts in acute myelogenous leukemia.

Other: Mutations of CD117 occur in a variety of neoplasms including melanoma, mast cell disease, and gastrointestinal stromal tumors (GIST). In GISTs, the presence of CD117 expression often equates to mutations in exon 11 of the *KIT* gene, and these tumors are responsive to treatment with imatinib. Melanomas may have *KIT* mutations, with the highest mutation rates seen in acral and mucosal melanomas (Beadling et al. 2008). However, unlike in GIST tumors, IHC CD117 expression in melanoma does not correlate well with an underlying *KIT/CD117* mutation (Dai et al. 2013), and therefore is of limited use in predicting underlying mutation status and possible response to imatinib therapies.

Staining pattern: Membranous and cytoplasmic.

Clones: 104D2; 2E4; A4502; CMA-767; H300; CD117; YR145; Clone K45; 1A2.C5; C-KIT; T595; 9.7

CD123

Background: CD123 is the IL-3 alpha chain receptor and is found primarily on plasmacytoid dendritic cells (PDCs), but also may be expressed on monocytes, eosinophilic granulocytes, myeloid dendritic cells, and subsets of hematopoietic progenitor cells.

Uses: CD123 is positive in blastic plasmacytoid dendritic cell neoplasm (BPDCN), formerly known as blastic NK/T-cell lymphoma and CD4+/CD56+ dendritic cell neoplasm. BPDCN is a highly aggressive neoplasm which often presents with cutaneous lesions, and has a very poor prognosis (Julia et al. 2013). CD123 cells are increased in hypertrophic lesions of lupus, and may help differentiate cases of hypertrophic lupus from actinic keratosis and squamous carcinoma (Ko et al. 2011).

Staining pattern: Cytoplasmic.

Clones: CD123; 6H6; 9F5

Lysozyme

Background: Lysozyme is a 14.5 kDa mucolytic enzyme found in various secretions including saliva, tears, urine, serum, and gastrointestinal secretions (Leong et al. 1999). It is also present in granulocytes, macrophages and some epithelial cells.

Uses: Lysozyme is generally used as a marker of myeloid differentiation as well as a sensitive but non-specific histiocytic marker. It is often used in combination with myeloperoxidase as a myeloid differentiation marker when evaluating infiltrates for leukemia.

Lysozyme is also reported positive in Langerhans cell histiocytosis, follicular dendritic cell tumors, granular cell tumors, cellular neurothekeomas, malignant fibrous histiocytomas and other histiocytic tumor; apocrine glands and neoplasms.

Staining pattern: Cytoplasmic.

Clones: Lysozyme

Mast cell tryptase

Background: Mast cell tryptase (MCT) is a neutral serine protease and is a major component of mast cell granules.

Uses: Used as a fairly specific marker of mast cells for lesions of cutaneous mastocytosis (Irani et al. 1989). In subtle lesions of telangiectasia macularis perstans (TMEP), MCT may not only show increased numbers of mast cells, but also may highlight abnormally spindled mast cells, which are more indicative of a mastocytosis over a reactive process such as urticaria (**Figure 6.14**).

Staining: Granular, cytoplasmic.

Clones: AA1; TRYPTASE; G3

Myeloperoxidase

Background: Myeloperoxidase (MPO) is the major constituent of primary granules of both early and mature myeloid cells.

Use: Used as a specific marker for myeloid differentiation. MPO does not stain histiocytes, unlike other markers of myeloid differentiation such as lysozyme or CD68. It is positive in neutrophils. Like lysozyme, it is often used in the evaluation of leukemic-appearing infiltrates.

Staining pattern: Cytoplasmic.

Clones: MPO

Terminal deoxynucleotidyl transferase (TdT)

Background: Terminal deoxynucleotidyl transferase (TdT) is a 58 kDa DNA polymerase

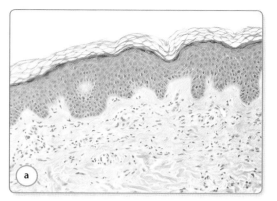

Figure 6.14 Mast cells in telangiectasia macularis eruptiva perstans (TMEP). (a) TMEP with subtle hypercellular dermis and telangiectasia (H&E, 100×). (b) Mast cell tryptase highlighting increased mast cells with spindled morphology (tryptase, 100×).

protein. TdT is normally present on precursor multipotent hematopoietic cells and immature B and T lymphocytes in the thymus and bone marrow. It is never present in normal peripheral T cells.

Uses: Mainly used as a marker for acute lymphoblastic lymphoma/leukemia of both B and T cell origin. Occasionally TdT is positive in myeloid leukemia. Of note, TdT is also positive in a large portion of merkel cell carcinomas (Buresh et al. 2008).

Staining pattern: Nuclear.

Clones: SEN 28; TDT; NCL-TdT-339

Melanocytic IHC markers

The use of IHC in melanocytic lesions plays an important role in the everyday practice of dermatopathology. Melanocytic markers may be used to detect the melanocytic nature of a tumor, to evaluate the number and growth pattern of melanocytes in junctional melanocytic lesions, to aid in the differentiation between benign and malignant melanocytic lesion, and finally, may be used as prognostic markers. The more commonly used markers are detailed below.

BAP-1

Background: BAP1 (BRCA1 associated protein 1) is a tumor suppressor protein which plays a key role in the function of the cell cycle. Wiesner et al. described *BAP1* mutations in two families who had characteristic melanocytic lesions with spitzoid features and an increased incidence of melanoma (Wiesner et al., 2012).

Uses: The BAP-1 antibody is used to evaluate for *BAP1*-mutated nevi, sometimes referred to as BAPomas or Wiesner nevi. These nevi have a characteristic histology generally consisting of large epithelioid, atypical appearing intradermal melanocytes with 'spitzoid' morphology (**Figure 6.15a**). There may often be bland, more conventional appearing nevus cells within the lesion as well. On IHC, the *BAP1* mutated cells demonstrate loss of nuclear BAP-1 staining (**Figure 6.15b**). Note that *BAP1* is a tumor suppressor gene and is mutated in many malignancies, including melanoma, and thus should be used in the appropriate context.

Staining pattern: Loss of nuclear BAP-1 staining.

Clones: C-4; BP1

HMB-45

Background: HMB-45 (human melanoma black 45) antigen is present on pre-melanosomes and is found on immature melanocytes, but not in resting adult melanocytes.

Uses: Used as a very specific but not sensitive marker for melanocytic differentiation. Stains activated melanocytes but not

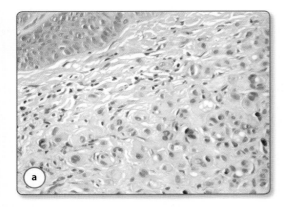

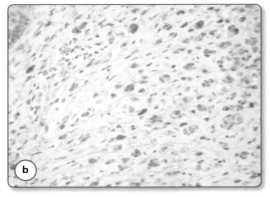

Figure 6.15 BAP-1-inactivated melanocytic tumor (BAPoma). (a) BAPoma with large epithelioid melanocytes with Spitzoid features (H&E 200×). (b) BAP1 IHC, negative staining in the large, lesional melanocytes (BAP1, 200×).

resting melanocytes. HMB-45 is positive in conventional melanomas, but negative in desmoplastic melanoma (DMM). In nevi, HMB-45 staining is present in junctional and superficial dermal melanocytes but is lost in the deeper maturing dermal melanocytes. This stratified loss of HMB-45 in the deep aspect of benign nevi may be helpful in the differential of atypical nevi versus melanoma, since melanomas mature poorly and thus retain deep HMB-45 expression. Similarly, HMB-45 may also be used to differentiate between nodal capsular nevi (HMB-45 -) and metastatic melanoma (HMB-45 +).

Also positive in: PEComa, clear cell sarcoma, lymphangiomyomatosis, melanotic schwannoma.

Staining pattern: Cytoplasmic, granular.

Clones: HMB-45

MART-1/Melan A

Background: MART-1 (melanoma antigen recognized by T cells 1) and Melan A (clone A103) are different clones which recognize the same antigen, a melanosome membrane protein.

Uses: It is a relatively specific marker for melanocytic differentiation, and stains all nevi, primary melanomas, and approximately 80% of metastatic melanomas. Unlike S-100, it is negative in nerves, Langerhans cells, and skin appendages. As it has much less background staining than S100, it is useful in evaluating the number and degree of junctional melanocytes in atypical pigmented lesions as well as for evaluation of lymph nodes for possible metastatic melanoma. Expression is lost in DMM. Shown to be more specific and sensitive than HMB-45 for melanoma (Jungbluth et al. 1998). MART-1 is useful in assessing number of melanocytes in junctional melanocytic proliferations. It may also be used in the assessment of vitiligo, which shows a complete loss of junctional melanocytes.

MART-1/Melan A may also stain adrenal cortical tumors (especially Melan A) and the PEComa family of tumors.

Staining pattern: Cytoplasmic.

Clones: MART-1; MELAN-A (A103); M2-7C10

MITF

Background: Microphthalmia-associated transcription factor (MITF) is a nuclear transcription protein involved in melanocyte regulation.

Uses: MITF was originally thought to be a very specific and sensitive nuclear marker for melanocytic differentiation. However, now it is known to be relatively non-specific as it also stains macrophages, fibroblasts, Schwann cells, smooth muscle cells, and mast cells. In our experience, it is also positive in a large portion of dermatofibrosarcoma protuberans. As it is a nuclear stain, some pathologists prefer to use MITF in junctional melanocytic proliferations to assess for intraepidermal melanocytes since the staining of dendritic cytoplasmic processes with MART-1 may lead to overestimation of junctional melanocytes. However, due to its low specificity, many pathologists now prefer to use Sox-10 for this purpose.

Staining pattern: Nuclear.

Clones: 34CA5; C5+D5; D5; MITF

S-100

Background: S-100 derived its name due to its 100% solubility in a saturated ammonium sulfate solution. S-100 is a protein dimer made up of α and β subunits and plays an important role in calcium regulation. S-100 has three isoforms: S-100ao (α-α), S-100a (α-β) and S-100b (β-β). Monoclonal antibodies specific to either the α or β subunits or polyclonal antibodies that recognize both subunits are available for use. In clinical practice, the polyclonal form which recognizes all three isoforms is the most widely used, allowing detection of a broader number of lesions than the monoclonal forms.

Uses: S-100 is widely used in dermatopathology as a screening stain as it is a highly sensitive, but not entirely specific, marker for both melanocytic and neural differentiation. S-100 will stain the majority of both benign nevi as well as melanomas. It has a classic strong, diffuse staining pattern in schwannomas (**Figure 6.16**). Neurofibromas are also S-100 +, but their staining may be more patchy. Malignant peripheral nerve sheath tumors (MPNST) may lose S-100 reactivity. S-100 will also stain Langerhans cells and dermal dendritic cells. Other lesions expressing S-100 include: granular cell tumors, myoepitheliomas, myoepithelial carcinomas, LCH, Rosai-Dorfman (R-D), cartilaginous tumors, adnexal eccrine tumors, slightly less than 50% of breast carcinomas, and adipocytes/lipoblasts. In the setting of cutaneous histiocytoses, S-100 positivity (as seen in LCH and R-D) is a clue to the presence of histiocytosis, since reactive histiocytes or granulomatous infiltrates secondary to infection are rarely S-100 positive. As S-100 often stains background dermal dendritic cells, it is important to not over interpret these cells in dermal lesions such as dermatofibromas. The polyclonal form of S-100 does not stain cellular neurothekeomas (CNT). However, the A6 isoform of S-100 will stain CNT as well as a variety of fibrohistiocytic lesions including atypical fibroxanthoma (AFX) and fibrous papules (Plaza et al. 2009; Fullen et al. 2001). S100A6 has also been reported to have different expression levels in Spitz nevi (strong, diffuse positivity) versus melanoma (30% positivity; patchy staining) (Ribé & McNutt 2003).

Staining pattern: Nuclear and cytoplasmic.

Clones: S-100 B; A6; 15E2E2; 4C4.9; S100-P; S-100; Z311

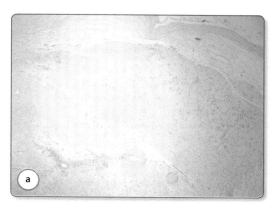

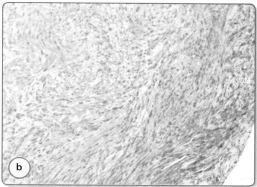

Figure 6.16 (a) S100 staining in schwannoma (H&E, 40×). (b) Diffuse strong S100 positivity, nuclear and cytoplasmic (S100, 40×).

SOX-10

Background: Sox-10 (sex determining region Y-box 10) is a nuclear transcription factor which plays an important role in melanocytic and schwannian differentiation.

Uses: Sox10 may be crudely thought of as having a similar application and staining profile as S-100, but as opposed to S-100 it is a nuclear stain. SOX-10 is very sensitive and relatively specific for melanocytic lesions. It is slightly more specific than S-100 as it does not stain Langerhans cells or dermal dendritic cells. Given its crisp nuclear staining, SOX-10 is useful in assessment of junctional melanocytic proliferations. It will also stain granular cell tumors, neural tumors, myoepitheliomas, some breast carcinomas, clear cell sarcoma, and a subset of MPNST.

Staining pattern: Nuclear.

Clones: Sox10; EP268; A-2

Tyrosinase

Background: Tyrosinase is a 75 kDa enzyme involved in the assimilation of tyrosine into melanin pigment.

Uses: Used as a general marker of melanocyte differentiation. Like HMB-45, expression may be diminished in mature melanocytes. Tyrosinase stains up to 1/3 of DMM. It is negative in PEComas. Tyrosinase is only used as a 2nd or 3rd tier melanocytic marker or in melanocytic cocktails.

Staining pattern: Cytoplasmic.

Clones: NCL-TYROS; T311; TYROSINASE

Other melanocytic lineage markers

Background: As with all fields new melanocytic markers are continually being developed. However, as these markers have not shown to be more beneficial than the above stains, they are not currently widely used in clinical practice, and they will be summarized in this section together.

PNL2: Antibody to somatostatin receptor which also strongly stains melanocytic lesions. PNL2 had a better sensitivity for melanoma than MART-1 and HMB-45 in one study (Busam et al. 2005). It is negative in DMM.

SM5-1: Recognizes a fibronectin variant expressed in melanoma, and is a very sensitive and specific marker of melanocytic lesions (Trefzer et al. 2000).

MAGE-1: Melanoma antigen encoding gene-1. Only positive in approximately 27% of melanomas, but is positive in some HMB-45 negative melanomas and 79% of DMM (Gajjar et al. 2004).

Melanocytic markers with prognostic or therapeutic significance

BRAF

Background: B-Raf is part of the Raf family of serine-threonine protein kinases. An activating mutation of the *BRAF* oncogene is the most common mutation in cutaneous melanoma, with *BRAF* mutations occurring in up to 60% of melanomas. >95% of these mutations occur at V600 with a specific valine to glutamic acid substitution (V600E mutation). As B-Raf

inhibitors have been developed to treat *BRAF* mutated melanomas, determination of a patient's *BRAF* mutation status is now necessary for treatment purposes. This assessment of treatment eligibility is conventionally performed by molecular PCR techniques.

Use: B-Raf IHC has been shown to be highly sensitive and specific in detecting the V600E and therefore is a useful screening tool which allows patients to be entered into treatment protocols in an expedited manner (Long et al. 2013). Because *BRAF* mutations are prevalent in benign nevi, identification of BRAF mutations is not useful for diagnostics.

Staining pattern: Cytoplasmic.

Clones: 26039; VE1

Elastin

Background: Elastin is a polymeric protein found in connective tissues and the dermis and imparts the property of elasticity to the skin.

Use: Up to 30% of melanomas have a background associated nevoidal component. As sometimes the melanoma is intimately admixed with the nevus, it may be difficult to accurately assess the Breslow depth of invasion in these cases. Elastin IHC may be useful in this setting to delineate between the nevus and melanoma. In this setting, the elastin immunostain is considered more useful than using elastin special stains. In nevi, elastin is preserved around the melanocytic nests and is often observed around individual melanocytes. In contrast, elastin staining is decreased within and around melanoma, and compressed elastin fibers are present at the base of the melanoma component (Kamino et al. 2009). Elastin may also be helpful in differentiating tumor regression from scar in melanoma, as regression has a well-defined compressed layer of elastin fibers at its base, while scarring fibrosis does not (Kamino et al. 2010).

Staining: Cytoplasmic.

Clones: ab2160; BA-4

Ki-67/MIB-1

Background: Ki-67 is a protein only expressed in the proliferative cell cycle, and is absent in the G0 resting phase.

Use: Ki-67 is used as a surrogate marker to assess the proliferative activity of lesions. Melanomas generally have a high dermal melanocytic proliferation index, while benign nevi are usually negative or only show rare superficial proliferative cells. As inflammatory cells have a high Ki-67 proliferation index, it is essential to not include them in the assessment of a tumor's proliferation index, as this would lead to a gross overestimation of the tumor proliferative rate. In order to alleviate this potential error, some labs use a dual MART-1/Ki-67 immunostain with MART-1 labeled with a red chromagen and Ki-67 staining the nucleus brown.

Other: The K2 clone may be used to mark lipoblasts (see 'Soft tissue markers' below)

Staining pattern: Nuclear.

Clones: KI88; MIB1; MMI; SP6; Ki-S5; KI-67; 30-9; IVAK-2; K2

PHH3

Background: Histone H3 is phosphorylated during the late G2 and M phases of a cell's mitotic cycle, leading to phosphohistone H3.

Uses: Anti-PHH3 ab labels mitotically active cells. Thus, it is used to facilitate mitotic counts, and to discriminate true mitotic cells from cells with bizarre or apoptotic nuclei. As the prophase portion of the mitotic cycle is not readily seen on routine H&E sections, PHH3 mitotic counts may be higher than H&E mitotic counts. Mitotic counts are extremely important, and the detection of a single mitosis in melanomas which are <1.0 mm in tumor thickness changes the AJCC tumor stage from T1a to T1b. An important caveat is to note that the current AJCC staging guidelines are based on H&E mitotic counts. Thus, PHH3 counts should not be used in isolation for mitotic counts in melanoma as PHH3 based cutoff levels for stage pT1b melanomas have not been determined. Nevertheless, PHH3 is remains useful in determining mitotic hotspots in melanomas and a combined PHH3/MART-1 immunostain may be helpful in confirming a dermal mitosis is indeed in a melanocyte and not an inflammatory cell. PHH3 may also be useful in soft tissue tumors for example during the evaluation of mitotic activity in smooth muscle lesions where mitotic activity is a major criterion used to differentiate cutaneous leiomyomas from superficial dermal cutaneous leiomyosarcomas.

Staining pattern: Nuclear.

Clones: PHH3; Ser10; RM

P16

Background: p16 is a cell cycle inhibitor encoded on 9p21. Comparative genomic hybridization and FISH studies have shown loss of p16 expression in spitzoid melanoma, a finding which correlates with loss of nuclear and sometimes cytoplasmic labelling of p16 on IHC.

Uses: Originally, p16 nuclear staining was reported to be lost in spitzoid melanomas and preserved in spitzoid nevi (Al Dhaybi et al. 2011); however, these findings have not been entirely confirmed on subsequent studies. May still be of use in helping differentiate between Spitz nevi and Spitzoid melanoma when combined with other IHC markers such as S100A6 (diminished staining in melanoma vs nevi, see above), HMB-45 to assess maturation, and Ki-67 to assess proliferation rates (Ferringer 2015).

Staining pattern: Nuclear and cytoplasmic.

Clones: sc1661; sc1661; 6H12; 6H12; DCS-50; DCS-50; F-12; F-12; G175-405; G175-405; ZJ11; ZJ11; JC8; JC8; 16P07; 16P07; P16; P16; P16_INK4A; P16_INK4A; 2D9A12; 2D9A12; E6H4; E6H4; 16P04; 16P04

Soft tissue markers

Soft tissue immunohistochemical markers play a major part in the dermatopathologist's ability to identify and diagnose a wide variety of mesenchymal tumors. Below is a list of some of the more widely used IHC markers.

Muscle markers

Caldesmon

Background: Caldesmon is a calmodulin binding protein which inhibits the ATPase activity of myosin, and is an essential component of smooth muscle contraction regulation.

Uses: Antibodies to caldesmon target the high molecular (93 kDa) form of the molecule. Caldesmon is a relatively specific marker for smooth muscle differentiation. However, it may be negative in a large portion of leiomyosarcomas (Hisaoka et al. 2001). It is also positive in myopericytomas and glomus tumors. It does not stain myofibroblasts.

Staining pattern: Cytoplasmic.

Clones: caldesmon

Calponin

Background: Calponin is a cytoskeleton associated protein involved in muscle contraction regulation.

Uses: Calponin is similar to SMA as it stains smooth muscle as well as myofibroblasts. It also stains myoepithelial cells.

Staining pattern: Cytoplasmic.

Clones: N3, 26A11, CALP, Calponin

Desmin

Background: Desmin is a 53 kDa cytoplasmic intermediate filament found in muscle cells.

Uses: Desmin is used as a marker of muscle differentiation and will stain both skeletal and smooth muscle. It does not stain myofibroblasts, and therefore is generally specific for true muscular differentiation. In our experience, desmin works better in staining skeletal muscle than smooth muscle tumors, and has been negative in some cutaneous leimyomas/superficial leiomyosarcomas. Along with EMA and CD68, it is positive in angiomatoid fibrous histiocytomas. Positivity may also be present in giant cell tumor of tendon sheath. Occasional expression present in melanomas and schwannoma.

Staining pattern: Cytoplasmic.

Clones: ZC18, DE-R-11, DE-U-10, DE5, DESMIN, M760, D33

Myogenin

Background: Myogenin is a 32 kDa intranuclear regulatory protein found in skeletal muscle cells.

Uses: Used as a specific marker for skeletal muscle differentiation.

Staining pattern: Nuclear.

Clones: F5D; MYF3; MYF4; MYOGENIN; LO26

Muscle specific actin (MSA; HHF35)

Background: MSA recognizes all four α-actin isoforms.

Uses: Similar to smooth muscle actin, muscle specific actin will stain myofibroblastic proliferations as well as true smooth muscle lesions. It will also stain skeletal muscle.

Staining pattern: Cytoplasmic.

Clones: HHF-35

Smooth muscle actin (SMA)

Background: Actins are a multifunctional protein which make up microfilaments and compose a large part of a cell's cytoskeleton. α-actins are present in muscle tissues and comprise the contractile apparatus of muscle fibers. SMA identifies the single α isoform present in smooth muscle cells and cells with myofibroblastic differentiation.

Uses: SMA highlights smooth muscle neoplasms such as cutaneous leiomyomas and leiomyosarcomas. It is important to note that SMA is not specific for true smooth muscle differentiation as it also marks cells with myofibroblastic differentiation. Therefore, it is positive in tumors with myofibroblastic differentiation including nodular fasciitis, some dermatofibromas, as well as early scar. SMA is positive in glomus tumors. It does not stain skeletal muscle. SMA can be expressed in painful variants of traumatic neuromas.

Staining pattern: Cytoplasmic. Myofibroblastic proliferations may display a characteristic 'tram track' pattern of distribution (**Figure 6.17**).

Clones: ASM-1, CGA7, HUC1-1, ACTIN-SM, 1A4, ASM/H12

Smooth muscle myosin (SMM)

Background: SMM is a cytoplasmic protein and a major constituent of the contractile apparatus in muscle cells.

Uses: Relatively sensitive and specific marker for smooth muscle derivation. SMM is also positive in myoepithelial cells. SMM is our preferred marker for smooth muscle neoplasms (**Figure 6.18**).

Staining pattern: Cytoplasmic.

Clones: HSM-V, ID8, SMMS-1, SM_MYOSIN_H

Vascular markers

CD31

Background: CD31 (platelet endothelial cell adhesion molecule-1/PECAM-1) is a 130 kDa glycoprotein normally expressed on endothelial cells as well as circulating hematopoietic cells including macrophages and plasma cells.

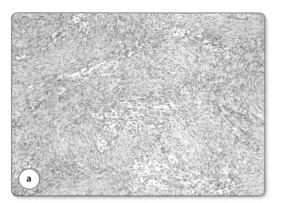

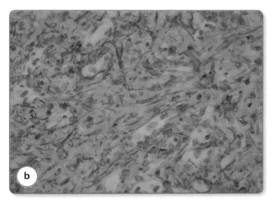

Figure 6.17 (a) SMA in nodular fasciitis (H&E, 200×). (b) SMA IHC with 'tram track' appearance (SMA, 200×).

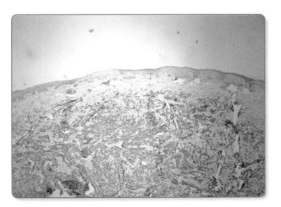

Figure 6.18 Smooth muscle myosin staining in a cutaneous leiomyoma (SMM, 40×).

Uses: A very sensitive and specific marker for endothelial cells, CD31 is positive in most vascular lesions including angiosarcomas. It is important to note that CD31 will stain histiocytes as well as plasma cells, and the authors have seen misdiagnosis of angiosarcoma based on CD31 staining of a histiocytic infiltrate. Intravascular macrophages have also been reported to have been misdiagnosed as vascular sarcomas (McKenney et al. 2001). CD31 will occasionally stain a subset of atypical fibrous xanthomas (AFX) which have a marked histiocytic component. The granular staining of histiocytes, as opposed to the smooth cytoplasmic staining of vascular lesions, should be a clue to this diagnosis.

Staining pattern: Vascular – membranous and cytoplasmic; histiocytes – granular.

Clones: CD31; JC/70; JC/70A; 1A10

CD34

Background: CD34 is a 110 kDa transmembrane glycoprotein thought to play a role in cell-cell adhesion. It is normally found on endothelial cells, dermal dendritic cells, hematopoietic stem cells, perivascular cells, and within the nerve sheath.

Uses: CD34 is an important immunostain used in the evaluation of soft tissue lesions. It is important to realize CD34 is non-specific, and present in a wide variety of lesions (**Table 6.6**). CD34 is prominently used in the differential diagnosis of dermatofibrosarcoma protuberans (DFSP), an aggressive cutaneous spindle cell neoplasm. DFSP is strongly and diffusely positive for CD34 (**Figure 6.19a,b**). Notably the cellular variant of dermatofibroma will have a zonal pattern of staining for CD34, with the outer tumor having strong CD34 positivity, while the central aspects of the lesion are negative. Diffuse neurofibromas (NF) may entrap subcutaneous adipose tissue and also be in the differential diagnosis of DFSP. We have seen cases of diffuse NF misdiagnosed as DFSP because NF may have strong expression of CD34. A helpful clue to NF is CD34 expression in these lesions often displays a so called 'fingerprint' type pattern of staining (**Figure 6.19c,d**). In this setting, an S-100 immunostain is essential to differentiate diffuse NF from DFSP, as NF is

Table 6.6 CD34 positive cutaneous lesions			
Fibrohistocytic	**Vascular**	**Neural**	**Other**
DFSP	Hemangiomas	Neurofibroma	Tricholemmoma
Cellular DF (zonal pattern with peripheral staining)	Kaposi sarcoma	Schwannomas- Antoni B areas	Spindle cell lipoma
Giant cell fibroblastoma	Angiosarcoma	Perineuriomas-non sclerosing type	Synovial sarcoma
Myxoinflammatory fibroblastic sarcoma	Epithelioid	Palisaded encapsulated neuroma	Blast cells in leukemia
	Hemangioendothelioma	Traumatic neuroma	+/- Melanomas
Solitary fibrous tumor			+/- Leiomyomas
Superficial acral fibromyxoma			+/- Glomus tumors
Nuchal fibroma sclerotic fibroma			+/- Myopericytoma
Pleomorphic fibroma			
Cellular digital fibroma			
Superficial angiomyxoma			

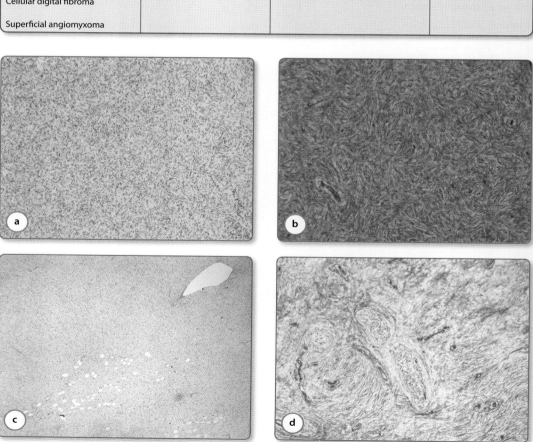

Figure 6.19 CD34 staining in DFSP and neurofibroma. (a) DFSP (H&E, 200×). (b) CD34 in DFSP (CD34, 200×). (c) Diffuse neurofibroma (NF) (H&E, 200×). (d) CD34 in NF with 'fingerprint' sign (CD34, 200×).

strongly S-100+ while DFSP is S-100-. CD34 can also be used as a vascular marker as it stains the majority of endothelial neoplasms.

Staining pattern: Cytoplasmic.

Clones: 1309; 8G12; CD34; HPCA; HPCA-1; IOM34; MY10; NU-4A1; TUK4; clone 581; QBEND10; BI-3C5; NCL-L-END; 43A1; MEC 14.7

Claudin-5

Background: The claudin family is a group of integral transmembrane proteins which are important components of intercellular tight junctions. Claudin-5 expression is normally limited to endothelial cells and glomeruli.

Uses: Claudin-5 is a relatively sensitive endothelial marker; however, it is not a specific marker and also positive in various carcinomas and synovial sarcoma.

Staining pattern: Membranous.

Clones: 4C3C2; Claudin-5

D2-40 (Podoplanin)

Background: D2-40 is a 40 kDa transmembrane sialoglycoprotein normally expressed on lymphatic endothelial cells.

Uses: D2-40 stains dermal lymphatics and may be used as marker of lymphatic derivation, and as such stains cutaneous lymphangiomas. However, while it was originally thought to be relatively specific marker for lymphatic tumors, it is now known to be relatively non-specific and stains a variety of cutaneous lesions including Kaposi sarcoma, some hemangiomas and angiosarcomas, synovial sarcoma, leiomyosarcomas, DF, DFSP, solitary fibrous tumors, and spindle cell melanomas (Kalof & Cooper 2009). D2-40 is useful in finding lymphatic invasion in tumors, including melanomas, which may be missed on routine H&E sections (Rose et al. 2011). D2-40 may also be useful in conjunction with p63 and CK15 in the differential diagnosis of primary adnexal carcinomas vs metastatic adenocarcinomas (**Table 6.3**). These markers have a much higher rate of positivity in primary adnexal tumors, and therefore, positivity in all three markers is a strong sign indicating a primary cutaneous adnexal tumor (Mahalingam et al. 2010).

Staining pattern: Cytoplasmic.

Clones: D2-40; D2-40 clone

ERG and Fli-1

Background: ERG (ETS Related Gene) and Fli-1 are nuclear proteins and members of the ETS transcription family. ERG is normally expressed on endothelial cells and is also involved in various oncogenic gene fusions including variants of prostate carcinoma, acute myelogenous leukemias (AML), and Ewing's sarcoma (EWS).

Uses: Both markers stain the vast majority of endothelial derived neoplasms including hemangiomas, hemangioendotheliomas, angiosarcoma and Kaposi sarcoma (**Figure 6.20**). As Fli-1 is less specific than ERG, we prefer to use ERG. Of note, in one study, ERG stained over 30% of epithelioid sarcomas, so it may not be the best immunostain to differentiate between epithelioid angiosarcoma and epithelioid sarcoma (Miettinen et al. 2013). Due to its presence as a

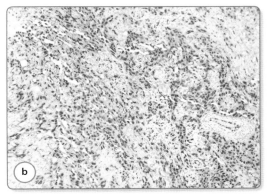

Figure 6.20 ERG. (a) Angiosarcoma (H&E, 200×). (b) ERG IHC, nuclear positivity (ERG, 200×).

gene fusion product, it will also stain a subset of prostate carcinomas, as well as EWS and blastic acute myeloid leukemias.

Staining pattern: Nuclear.

Clones: ERG; EPR3864; 9FY1

Glut-1

Background: Glut-1 is a glucose transporter found in erythrocytes and upregulated in many tumor types.

Uses: Glut-1 is often used in the evaluation of pediatric vascular tumors, and its expression is seen in juvenile capillary hemangiomas, but not in other pediatric vascular tumors such as malformations. It also marks perineural tumors such as perineuriomas. Red blood cells can serve as positive internal control in tissues. Glut-1 will often be positive in areas of necrosis.

Staining pattern: Membranous.

Clones: SPM498; GLUT1

vWF (Von Willebrand Factor; Factor VIII related antigen)

Background: vWF is the largest soluble human plasma protein. It is found in plasma where it serves as a carrier protein for Factor VIII. It is also present in the Weibel Pallade bodies of endothelial cells, in the alpha-granules of megakaryocytes and platelets, and the subendothelial matrix of vessel walls.

Uses: vWF was the first used IHC marker of endothelial differentiation. However, its current use is limited as it is the least sensitive marker for vascular tumors. Also, as vWF is a plasma protein, it has high degree of background staining in areas of tumor necrosis and hemorrhage. Therefore, vWF has generally been replaced by more specific vascular markers such as CD31 and ERG.

Staining pattern: Cytoplasmic.

Clones: F8/86; FVIIIRAG; 36B11

Other soft tissue markers

Beta-catenin

Background: Fibromatoses are known to harbor APC or beta-catenin gene mutations. Beta-catenin immunostaining for the protein product can be a valuable adjunct for separating fibromatoses from a number of other, morphologically similar spindle cell lesions.

Uses: Although nuclear beta-catenin staining is not specific for the diagnosis of fibromatosis, it is especially useful in separating fibromatoses from other lesions which demonstrate morphologic overlap with fibromatoses such as low grade fibromyxoid sarcoma, leiomyosarcomas, myofibromas, scars, and nodular fasciitis all of which typically lack nuclear beta-catenin (Bhattacharya et al. 2005). It is important to realize that other spindle cell lesions such as, malignant melanoma, synovial sarcoma, solitary fibrous tumor, and metaplastic carcinoma of the breast can demonstrate nuclear staining. In addition, keloid scars may occasionally express beta-catenin. We have seen rare cases of sarcomatoid carcinoma with nuclear expression of beta-catenin. As with most immunostains, beta-catenin is best utilized in the context of a panel of immunostains.

Staining pattern: Nuclear and cytoplasmic (though only nuclear staining is significant).

Clones: 5H10, E-5, 17C2, RB-9035Po, CLONE 14, B-catenin, 6B3, 15B8, B-CATEN-MEM

Calretinin

Background: 31 kDa calcium binding protein and member of the same protein family as S-100. Normally found in central and peripheral nervous system as well as mesothelial cells.

Uses: Calretinin may be used to differentiate schwannomas, which are diffusely calretinin positive, from neurofibromas which are negative (Fine et al. 2004). Calretinin is also positive in granular cell tumor, cellular neurothekeoma, synovial sarcoma, desmoid fibromatosis, and mesothelioma.

Staining pattern: Cytoplasmic.

Clones: 5A5; AB149; CAL 3F5; DC8; DAK-CALRET; CALRETININ; 2 E7; SP13

Cathepsin K

Background: Cathepsin K is a cysteine protease which plays an important role in osteoclast function where its expression is regulated by MITF.

Uses: Stains melanocytic lesions including clear cell sarcoma (melanoma of soft parts), and is also a sensitive and specific markers of the PEComa (perivascular epithelioid cell neoplasm) family of tumors which include angiomyolipoma, clear cell sugar tumor of lung, lymphangioleiomyomatosis, lymphangiomyoma, cutaneous clear cell myomelanocytic tumor, clear cell myomelanocytic tumors of the falciform ligament, and a host of similar tumors which can arise in virtually any organ (Rao et al. 2013).

Other: Cathepsin K also is immunoreactive in a significant proportion of translocation associated renal cell carcinomas, osteoclasts and osteoclastic giant cells. In our own practice we have observed immunoreactivity for cathepsin K in endothelial cells within some tumors, histiocytes, pleomorphic sarcomas, synovial sarcoma, and gastrointestinal stromal tumors (weak staining). We have also seem cathepsin K reactivity in pleomorphic undifferentiated sarcomas,

Staining pattern: Cytoplasmic.

Clones: 3F9 (Cathepsin K)

CD99

Background: 32 kDa transmembrane glycoprotein encoded by MIC2 gene.

Uses: Best known for its use in the evaluation of small round blue cell tumors and the Ewing Family of Tumors (EFT). Sensitive marker for EFT as it stains over 90% of EFT. However, it is not specific for EFT as it also stains lymphoblastic lymphomas, as well as a subset of rhabdomyosarcomas. Also positive in: synovial sarcoma, superficial acral fibromyxomas, solitary fibrous tumors, leiomyosarcoma, undifferentiated pleomorphic sarcoma/malignant fibrous histiocytoma (MFH).

Staining pattern: Membranous.

Clones: CD99, HBA71, M3601, MIC2, P30/32MIC2, CD99-MEMB; 12E7; O13;H036-1.1

CDK4

Background: CDK4 stands for cyclin dependent kinase 4, a catalytic subunit of the protein kinase complex important for cell cycle G1 phase progression. Mutations in the *CDK4* gene can be associated with tumorigenesis of a variety of cancers.

Uses: CDK4 staining is characteristic of well differentiated liposarcoma/atypical lipomatous tumor and dedifferentiated liposarcoma. Osteosarcomas can also demonstrate CDK4 staining and it can be seen in a minority of other types of soft tissue tumors such as

pleomorphic undifferentiated sarcoma (MFH), leiomyosarcoma, and liposarcoma. In our experience, we have also seen a sarcomatoid carcinoma demonstrate positive staining. We use the same criteria to interpret CDK4 immunostaining as MDM2 (see below).

Staining pattern: Nuclear and cytoplasmic.

Clones: C-22, DC5-31

Claudin-1

Background: The claudin family is a group of integral transmembrane proteins which are important components of intercellular tight junctions. Claudin-1 is limited to perineural cells.

Uses: Positive in the majority of perineuriomas. Claudin-1 is negative in other spindle cell lesions within the differential diagnosis of perineuriomas including schwannomas, fibromatosis, DFSP, solitary fibrous tumors, and sclerotic fibromas.

Staining pattern: Membranous.

Clones: CLAUDIN-1; JAY.8

Factor XIIIa

Background: Factor XIIIa (A subunit) is part of the blood coagulation cascade which crosslinks fibrin.

Uses: Factor XIIIa is present in many cell types including monocytes/macrophages, dendritic cells of the skin and other sites, chondrocytes, and osteocytes (Sandell et al. 2015). Factor XIIIa is most commonly used in the differential diagnosis of dermatofibroma (DF, fibrous histiocytoma) vs. DFSP, with DF showing many positive background macrophages and DFSP showing only a few positive background macrophages.

Staining pattern: Cytoplasmic.

Clones: FXIIIA, EP3372, AC-1A1, SP196, E980.1

H3K27me3

Background: Polycomb group proteins are a family of proteins involved in chromatin remodeling and subsequent epigenetic silencing of genes. PRC2 (Polycomb repressive complex 2) trimethylates histone H3 on lysine 27 (H3K27me3).

Use: Malignant peripheral nerve sheath tumors (MPNST) often have PRC2 mutations and subsequent loss of H3K27me3 nuclear staining. H3K27me3 is lost in 2/3 of all MPNSTs and is lost in >90% of high grade MPNSTs (Prieto-granada et al. 2015)CDKN2A, and polycomb repressive complex 2 component genes (Embryonic Ectoderm Development [EED] and Suppressor of Zeste 12 [SUZ12] It has thus far proven to be a fairly specific and sensitive marker for MPNST and is useful in distinguishing MPNST from its mimics including spindle cell melanoma.

Staining pattern: Nuclear.

Clone: H3k27me3; trimethyl K27; Lys27

Inhibin

Background: 32 kDa peptide hormone normally produced by ovarian granulosa cells. Its name derives from the fact it selectively inhibits the secretion of follicle stimulating hormone from the pituitary gland.

Uses: In the skin, inhibin is positive in granular cell tumors. It also stains adrenocortical tumors, ovarian tumors, and sex cord stromal tumors.

Staining pattern: Cytoplasmic.

Clones: Inhibin; alpha subunit

INI-1/SMARCB1(BAF47)

Background: SMARCB1 is a ubiquitously expressed nuclear protein which is a component of the SWItch/Sucrose Non-Fermentable complex. The SWI/SNF complex functions as a tumor suppressor in many human malignancies and specifically loss of SMARCB1 expression at the protein level (as assessed by IHC) can be a very sensitive and specific way to diagnose a number of tumors associated with its loss (Margol & Judkins 2014) (Agaimy 2014).

Uses: Loss of nuclear staining of INI-1 is significant, and is seen only in a specific set of neoplasms. Tumors which characteristically show loss of INI-1 include epithelioid sarcoma, epithelioid malignant peripheral nerve sheath tumors (MPNST), atypical teratoid/rhabdoid tumors of the central nervous system, myoepithelial carcinomas, renal rhabdoid tumors, and renal medullary carcinomas. In addition, sinonasal carcinomas and a proportion of collecting duct carcinomas of the kidney can demonstrate loss of this marker. Interestingly, ossifying fibromyxoid tumor can demonstrate a mosaic pattern of staining in which a proportion of the neoplastic cells demonstrate INI-1 loss.

Staining pattern: Nuclear (loss of nuclear staining is considered significant).

Clones: MRQ-27, 3E10

Ki-67 (K2 Clone)

Background: Ki-67 identifies a 395 kDa nuclear antigen expressed in all cells in non-G0 phases of the cell cycle and therefore is positive in all proliferating cells.

Uses: As mentioned in the melanocytic section, Ki-67 is used as a proliferation marker and can be used in the setting of almost any neoplastic process in order to assess the proliferation rate of the lesion. In addition to being a nuclear marker of proliferation activity, the K2 clone of Ki-67 specifically stains the cytoplasm of fat cells. As such it can be used as a marker for lipoblasts (**Figure 6.21**) helping to differentiate true lipoblasts from pseudolipoblasts which may be seen in myxoinflammatory fibroblastic sarcoma or areas of fat necrosis with 'lipoblast-like' cells.

Staining pattern: Nuclear (proliferation index) and cytoplasmic (in lipoblasts).

Clones: K2

MDM2

Background: MDM2 is an oncogene that plays a role in controlling the cell cycle by binding to TP53 and preventing its degradation. As such it is thought to be involved in the pathogenesis of a number of neoplasms including atypical lipomatous tumor, well differentiated liposarcoma, and dedifferentiated liposarcoma (Weaver et al. 2009).

Uses: In the appropriate morphologic context, the detection of MDM2 amplification (either by FISH or by protein expression manifested

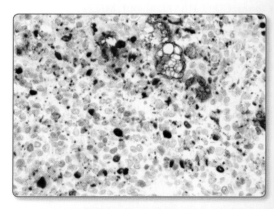

Figure 6.21 Ki-67 K2 clone cytoplasmic staining of lipoblasts (Ki-67 K2, 100×).

by nuclear IHC staining) provides strong evidence for the diagnosis of atypical lipomatous tumor/well differentiated liposarcoma or dedifferentiated liposarcoma. However, other tumors can demonstrate nuclear staining with this marker including a subset of angiomyolipomas, low grade osteosarcomas (MDM2 can also be very useful in the differential diagnosis of fibrous dysplasia vs. low grade osteosarcoma), and inflammatory myofibroblastic tumors. We have also seen significant MDM2 expression in some cases of sarcomatoid carcinoma. The interpretation of MDM2 immunostaining can be challenging as scattered positive cells can be rather non-specific, and as a result, performing FISH for MDM2 amplification in appropriate cases is warranted. The criteria we use in our lab for positive staining is one positive tumor nucleus per high power field (Binh et al. 2005). In our own practice, we have seen cytoplasmic staining of a proportion of the neoplastic cells in most cases of myxofibrosarcoma.

Staining pattern: Nuclear (strong and diffuse).

Clones: HDM2, MDM-2, IF2, SMP14, 1B10

MUC-4

Background: Differential gene expression profiling has recently identified the MUC-4 (mucin-4) gene as upregulated in cases of low grade fibromyxoid sarcoma with a corresponding overexpression of MUC-4 at the protein level.

Uses: A sensitive and specific marker of low grade fibromyxoid sarcoma (Doyle et al. 2011). As low grade fibromyxoid sarcomas are EMA positive bland appearing spindle cell tumors, they may be easily misdiagnosed as perineuriomas, and MUC-4 can be used in this setting to differentiate between these entities as perineuriomas are MUC-4 negative. MUC-4 also stains sclerosing epithelioid fibrosarcoma (Doyle et al. 2012). In our laboratory we typically follow-up suspected cases of low grade fibromyxoid sarcoma, which are MUC-4 positive, with FISH to demonstrate the FUS rearrangement characteristic of these tumors.

Staining pattern: Cytoplasmic.

Clones: 8G7, 5B12

Neurofilament

Background: Neurofilament proteins (NFP) are the largest of the intermediate filaments,

composed of three subunits of 68, 150, and 200 kDa respectively. Constitute a major component of the cytoskeletal framework of neurons and axons.

Uses: Stains axonal processes. As such, will show diffuse axons in neurofibroma (NF) and palisaded encapsulated neuromas. Schwannomas were originally described as lacking axons or only displaying peripheral axons under the capsule. However, many sporadic schwannomas have been shown to contain diffuse intra-tumoral axons, and therefore the presence or absence of NFP+ axons should not be used to discriminate between NF and schwannoma (Nascimento & Fletcher, 2007). NFP has a characteristic dot like perinuclear pattern in merkel cell carcinoma. NFP is also expressed in neuroblastoma, ganglioglioma, and paraganglioma.

Staining pattern: Cytoplasmic.

Clones: NEFH; NEFL; NEFM; NFP; TA-51; SMI33; TPNFP-1A3;NFP; SMI31; SM132; 2F11; FNP-7

NKI/C3 (CD63)

Background: NKI/C3 is also known as melanoma associated antigen, a glycoprotein located in the cytoplasm inside vacuoles and strongly expressed in cells with a large number of melanosomes. While the antibody which recognizes this antigen was originally described as a melanoma marker, it is rather non-specific with reactivity being seen in a variety of other tumors including fibrohistiocytic tumors, granular cell tumors, and neurothekeomas.

Uses: NKI/C3 is typically used in the diagnosis of cellular neurothekeomas, though this immunostain is non-specific. In addition to melanomas, cellular neurothekeomas, and various fibrohistiocytic tumors, NKI/C3 can stain schwannomas, neurofibromas, granular cell tumors, neuroendocrine neoplasms, and PEComas. We have also seen NKI/C3 staining in mast cells, spindle cell squamous carcinoma, and DFSP (Sachdev & Sundram 2006).

Other: NKI/C3 is a marker of lysosomes, so it tends to demonstrate positive staining in essentially any lesion that shows granular cell change.

Staining pattern: Cytoplasmic.

Clones: NKI/C3, CD63

NY-ESO-1

Background: NY-ESO-1 stands for New York

squamous carcinoma 1, which is a cancer-testis antigen that was identified in the serum of a patient with esophageal squamous carcinoma. Cancer-testis antigens are typically only expressed in adult testicular germ cells with atypical expression in a number of malignancies. They may also be used as a target of immunotherapy, as they are highly immunogenic and expressed in a number of malignancies including a variety of carcinomas, melanomas, and sarcomas.

Uses: In the appropriate context NY-ESO-1 has shown itself to be a relatively sensitive and specific marker of synovial sarcoma and myxoid/round cell liposarcoma (especially in distinguishing myxoid/round cell liposarcoma from other soft tissue lesions with myxoid or adipocytic features). In addition, NY-ESO-1 has shown immunoreactivity in a number of undifferentiated Ewings-like sarcoma with CIC-DUX4 rearrangements. This may prove to be of great utility as these tumors show a very non-specific immunophenotype without a clear line of differentiation.

Staining pattern: Nuclear and cytoplasmic. Positive staining is defined as moderate to strong staining in 50% or more of neoplastic cells (Endo et al. 2014).

Clones: E978

P75NTR

Background: p75NTR is a 75 kDa nerve growth factor receptor normally expressed on axons, Schwann cells, perineural cells, fibroblasts, outer root sheath, and myoepithelial cells.

Use: Stains 80% of malignant peripheral nerve sheath tumors (MPNST). P75NTR is positive in NF, schwannoma, and granular cell tumors. Also stains desmoplastic/spindled melanoma and synovial sarcoma. May have some utility in differentiating desmoplastic trichoepithelioma (strong P75+) from sclerosing/morpheaform basal cell carcinoma (P75-) (Krahl & Sellheyer 2010).

Staining pattern: Nuclear.

Clone: MS-394-P1; NGFR5; P75NGFR; P75NTR

Procollagen-1

Background: Procollagen is the soluble precursor of collagen produced by fibrocytes.

Uses: Procollagen is generally used as a marker of fibrohistiocytic differentiation. It is positive in AFX; however, it is not a specific marker and has been reported to be positive in carcinomas and melanomas. Therefore, it must be used as part of a panel including more lineage specific immunostains to be useful.

Staining pattern: Cytoplasmic.

Clones: PC1

Rb Protein

Background: Retinoblastoma (Rb) is an important tumor suppressor protein which plays an important role in cell cycle progression. Disruptions to the Rb protein allow tumor cells a proliferative advantage which can result in a number of human cancers. In addition, Rb is involved in the differentiation of a number of tissue types including adipocytic tissue.

Uses: In the context of soft tissue pathology, loss of immunohistochemical staining for Rb is seen in a host of related soft tissue neoplasms which include spindle cell lipoma, pleomorphic lipoma, mammary type myofibroblastoma, and cellular angiofibroma.

Staining pattern: Loss of nuclear staining is significant. Deficient expression of Rb is defined as nuclear staining in less than 10% of neoplastic cells (Chen et al. 2012).

Clones: 13A10, PRB, 1F8, 3C8, 3H9, G3-245, PRB1, RB-1, RB-WL 1, RB1, RB, 84-B3-1

SATB2

Background: Special AT-rich sequence-binding protein 2 (SATB2) is a nuclear matrix protein which plays a role in osteoblast development.

Uses: While SATB2 was first shown to be a specific marker of colorectal origin among carcinomas, it has also been shown to be a sensitive and specific marker of osteoblastic differentiation in various bone and soft tissue tumors.

Other: Previously we used antibodies against **osteocalcin** and **osteonectin** to assess osteoblastic differentiation, however osteocalcin is no longer easily available, is difficult to optimize for clinical practice, and suffers from relatively low sensitivity and specificity (Conner & Hornick 2013). It is important to note that SATB2 does not distinguish neoplastic from non-neoplastic osteoblastic cells.

Staining pattern: Nuclear.

Clones: SATB2

STAT6

Background: The NAB2-STAT6 fusion gene has been detected in up to 100% of solitary fibrous tumors (SFT), and thus far has not been identified in other types of tumors. The fusion gene results in an aberrant concentration of the STAT6 fusion protein in the nucleus, which can be detected using the IHC stain (Yoshida et al. 2014).

Uses: STAT6 is a very sensitive and specific marker in the diagnosis of SFT, and distinguishes it from other morphologically similar soft tissue tumors such as myofibroblastoma, spindle cell lipoma, various nerve sheath tumors, synovial sarcoma, dermatofibrosarcoma protuberans, and cellular fibrous histiocytoma (**Figure 6.22**).

Staining pattern: Nuclear.

Clones: sc-621

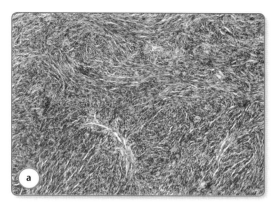

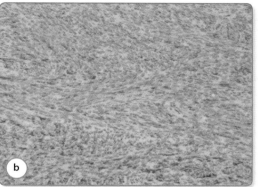

Figure 6.22 (a) STAT6 staining in solitart fibrous tumor (SFT) (H&E, 200×). (b) STAT6 nuclear stain (STAT6, 200×).

TFE-3

Background: TFE3 is a transcription factor which contains a nuclear localization signal that maps to a portion of TFE3 retained within all known TFE3 fusion proteins. TFE3 is ubiquitously expressed in humans and presumed to regulate many genes, most of which remain to be identified. Native TFE3 protein is usually not detected by IHC. The mechanism of TFE3 nuclear overexpression in tumors associated with such rearrangements is unknown, but may be a result of overexpression of the TFE3 fusion protein relative to native TFE3, impaired degradation of the fusion protein, increased antigenicity as a result of the fusion, or upregulation of native TFE-3 (Argani et al. 2003).

Uses: Typically used in the diagnosis of alveolar soft part sarcoma and translocation associated renal cell carcinomas (PPRC-TFE3, ASPL-TFE3, PSF-TFE3). Also stains a subset of PEComas (Argani et al. 2010). Granular cell tumors can also express TFE-3 by IHC without evidence of the corresponding gene rearrangement (Schoolmeester & Lastra 2015). In our practice, we have found TFE-3 a technically difficult antibody to use and have discontinued its use in favor FISH testing.

Staining pattern: Nuclear.

Clones: MRQ37, EPR11591, P-16

TLE-1

Background: DNA microarray expression profiling has shown a major association of the Wnt signaling pathway with synovial sarcoma. TLE-1 represents a prominent gene related to the Wnt pathway, and has been found to be a good discriminator of synovial sarcoma in multiple studies. TLE-1 overexpression may also represent a potential therapeutic target (Terry et al. 2007).

Uses: TLE-1 is used in the diagnosis of synovial sarcoma. The criteria for positive staining is described as greater than 50% of cells showing nuclear staining at low power (40X), 3+, or 10-50% showing intense staining on low power or 50% well above background at 100X, 2+. Other spindle cell tumors can demonstrate positive staining including up to 40% of schwannomas and 20% of solitary fibrous tumors, so it is important that results be interpreted in the context of a panel of immunostains (Terry et al. 2007). In our practice we typically follow-up positive TLE-1 immunostains with FISH studies for SYT rearrangement if synovial sarcoma is suspected.

Staining pattern: Nuclear.

Clones: TLE-1 (p)

Vimentin

Background: Vimentin (58 kDa) is one of the most widely distributed intermediate filaments, and is present in most mesenchymal cells.

Uses: Vimentin was originally used as a marker of mesenchymal differentiation; however, vimentin expression is also present in a variety of carcinomas. As such, vimentin is not generally useful as a specific tumor marker, and thus is of limited practical use. In the setting of a poorly differentiated tumor which may be negative on an initial wide battery of immunostains, vimentin may be useful in proving the tumor is immunoreactive.

Staining pattern: Cytoplasmic.

Clones: RPN1102; V10; V9; VIM-3B4; 43BE8; 3B4; SRL33

WT-1

Background: Wilms tumor protein (WT-1) is encoded by the WT1 gene on chromosome 11p. The WT-1 gene normally plays a role in the development of the urogenital system and mesothelial formation in embryonic development. WT-1 protein can be detected by IHC in most mesotheliomas, ovarian serous carcinomas, and Wilms tumors.

Uses: WT-1's relevance in soft tissue lies mainly in its immunoreactivity in desmoplastic small round cell tumor, a rare tumor typically arising in the abdomen and pelvis of children and young adults (although many other locations can be involved) . The tumor is classically associated with a t(11;22)(p13;q11.2 or q12), EWS-WT1 translocation producing a chimeric protein detected by the C-19 clone of the WT-1 antibody or with the use of FISH techniques (Zhang et al. 2003).

Staining pattern: Nuclear staining is considered significant.

Clones: 6F-H2, C-19, WT1

Infectious immunohistochemistry

In dermatopathology cultures, special stains (including Brown-Brenn, PAS, GMS, Fite, AFB),

molecular techniques, and in situ hybridization are the predominant methods used for the evaluation of infections. However, IHC does play a significant role in infections, especially in viral infections, when there are a paucity of organisms, or when organisms are difficult to culture. The more widely used IHC stains employed by dermatopathologists are detailed below.

Anti-BCG

Background: Anti-BCG is the antibacillus Calmette–Guérin polyclonal antibody directed against *Mycobacterium bovis*.

Use: Early on, anti-BCG was used as a screening tool due to its cross-reactivity with virtually all bacteria, fungi, and mycobacteria. In essence it served a similar function to the combined use of Brown–Brenn, PAS and Fite special stains (A M Molina–Ruiz et al. 2015). However, the current form of anti-BCG has been over purified, and is no longer recommended as a screening marker, but rather should be restricted to mycobacterial pathogens.

Staining pattern: Intact organisms.

Clone: B124

Bartonella species

Background: The genus *Bartonella* consists of small, gram-negative intracellular bacilli which are often difficult to culture. Of the 19 species of *Bartonella*, the most commonly encountered by dermatopathologists is *Bartonella henselae* which is the predominant pathogen in cat scratch disease and bacillary angiomatosis. Bacillary angiomatosis may also be secondary to *B. quintana* infection.

Use: As in syphilis, *Bartonella* species were originally identified using Warthin–Starry stains. IHC has been shown to be effective in highlighting organisms in bacillary angiomatosis as well as differentiating cat scratch disease from other etiologies of suppurative lymphadenitis.

Staining pattern: Intact bacteria.

Clones: HAS10; anti-*B. quintana*

Cytomegalovirus (CMV)

Background: CMV belongs to the β subgroup of the Herpesviridae family. CMV infections are more common in immunocompromised patients and may present with a variety of cutaneous manifestations including ulcers, papular lesions, vesicles or verrucoid lesions. CMV typically presents in endothelial cells of dermal blood vessels and presents with large nuclei surrounded by a clear halo (owl's eye inclusion).

Uses: CMV infection in the skin may be difficult to detect, often presenting with only a few infected cells and with background obscuring inflammation. Thus, CMV IHC allows for greater sensitivity of detection of CMV infection and is on par with culture and ISH methods (Molina–Ruiz et al. 2015).

Staining pattern: Early stage infections = nuclear; later stage infections = nuclear and cytoplasmic.

Clones: CCH2; DDG9

Epstein–Barr virus (EBV)

Background: EBV is a DNA γ-herpes virus also known as HHV4. The DNA core is surrounded by a nucleocapsid and envelope. EBV was the first described oncovirus, and is associated with a variety of lymphoproliferative disorders (including Burkitt lymphoma, classic Hodgkin lymphoma, post-transplant lymphoproliferative disorders, extra nodal NK/T-cell lymphoma, angioimmunoblastic T-cell lymphoma), and nasopharyngeal lymphoepithelial carcinomas.

Uses: IHC antibodies which recognize latent membrane protein 1(LMP 1) are available to detect EBV but have a very low detection sensitivity in comparison to Epstein-Barr-encoded RNAs (EBER) in situ hybridization (ISH). Thus, EBER ISH is generally preferred over the IHC method (see Chapter 13).

Staining pattern: Cytoplasmic and membranous.

Clones: CS1-4; LMP-1

Herpes simplex virus (HSV1/HSV2) and varicella zoster virus (VZV)

Background: Herpes simplex virus I and 2 (HSV-1 and HSV-2) and varicella zoster virus (VZV) are members of the Herpesviridae family of viruses which are relatively common causes of cutaneous infections.

Uses: HSV and VZV infections often show characteristic histologic changes with classic multinucleated keratinocytes with nuclear molding and margination of nuclear chromatin (**Figure 6.23a**). However, in early infections, these

classic findings may not be apparent and IHC to HSV 1/2 and VZV is extremely useful in detecting these early infections. The polyclonal nature of the antibodies to HSV-1 and HSV-2 are unable to distinguish between HSV-1 and HSV-2 infections. It can however distinguish between HSV-1/HSV-2 and VZV infections, which may have epidemiologic and therapeutic significance.

Staining pattern: Nuclear (accentuated in the periphery of nuclei which correlates with the areas of margination) and cytoplasmic (**Figure 6.23b**).

Clones: HSV-1/HSV-2 polyclonal, DAKO

Human herpesvirus 8 (HHV-8)

Background: HHV-8 was discovered in 1994 when it was isolated from lesions of Kaposi sarcoma (KS) and was originally termed KS-associated herpesvirus. In addition to KS, HHV-8 is the causative agent in primary effusion lymphoma and Castleman's disease.

Use: HHV-8 virus is present in all phases of KS from early patch stage lesions to the nodular phase. Thus, HHV-8 IHC is primarily used to diagnose and distinguish lesions of KS from other vascular lesions. It is highly specific and sensitive and present in virtually all cases of KS. Other entities which may mimic KS on H&E sections (such as angiosarcomas, hobnail hemangiomas, spindle cell hemangioma, and kaposiform hemangioendothelioma) are negative for HHV-8.

Staining pattern: Nuclear, often in a stippled pattern (**Figure 6.24**).

Clones: HHV8;LNA1;13B10;BB10

Rickettsial infections

Background: Rickettsia are obligate intracellular bacteria often transferred by the bite of an arthropod such as a tick. *Rickettsia rickettsii* is the causative agent of Rocky Mountain spotted fever (RMSF).

Use: Anti-rickettsial IHC may be used in cases of RMSF to detect organisms most often present in endothelial cells or histiocytes. Antimicrobial treatment of RMSF greatly diminishes the ability to find organisms in tissue.

Staining pattern: Intact bacteria.

Clone: Not commercially available

Treponema pallidum

Background: *T. pallidum* is a spirochete and the causative agent of syphilis. Its subspecies are also

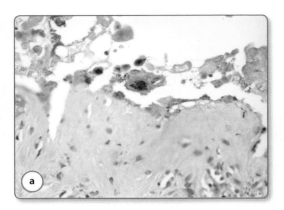 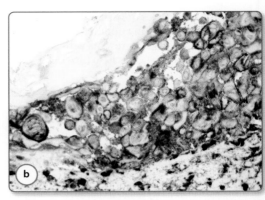

Figure 6.23 Varicella zoster virus (VZV) detection. (a) VZV infection (H&E, 200×). (b) VZV IHC (VZV, 200×).

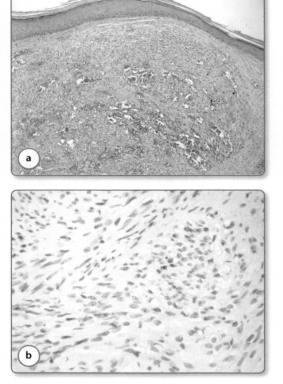 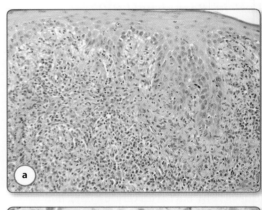

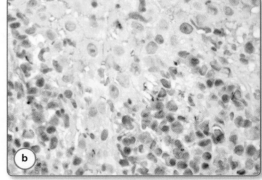

Figure 6.24 (a) HHV-8 in Kaposi sarcoma (H&E, 100×). (b) HHV-8 with fine stippled nuclear positivity (HHV-8, 400×).

Figure 6.25 (a) Syphilis detection (H&E, 100×). (b) IHC (*Treponema pallidum*, 400×).

the causative agent for endemic syphilis/bejal (*Treponema endemicum*), yaws (*T. pertenue*), and pinta (*T. carateum*).

Use: *T. pallidum* was historically detected in tissue by silver stains such as Warthin-Starry (WS) stain, but this stain has such a high degree of background staining that some pathologists resort to giving it the unfortunate moniker of the 'worthless and sorry' stain. While the WS stain is more useful than this moniker would indicate, it is true that IHC techniques have greatly improved the sensitivity of finding spirochetes in tissue. It is important to note that *T. pallidum* IHC is not specific for syphilis and will cross react with the other subspecies of *T. pallidum* as well as *Borrelia*. It may also cross react with *Treponema*–positive bacteria that may be present in water baths contaminating histologic sections (Molina-Ruiz et al. 2015).

Staining pattern: Intact spirochete (**Figure 6.25**).

Clones: anti-T.pallidum, polyclonal

Other infectious IHC stains

Several other IHC stains are available to the dermatopathologist but are generally not in widespread clinical use. Some of these markers include *Borrelia burgdorferi* (Lyme disease), Merkel cell polyomavirus, trichodysplasia polyomavirus, rabies virus, *Cryptococcus*, histoplasmosis, coccidoides, leishmaniasis, *Candida albicans*, and *Aspergillus* spp. A monoclonal antibody against ORF (ecthyma contagiosum) has been developed but is not currently available for commercial use (Molina-Ruiz et al. 2015).

References

Agaimy A. The Expanding Family of SMARCB1 (INI1-deficient Neoplasia: Implications of Phenotypic , Biological , and Molecular Heterogeneity, 2014

Alvarez-Cañas MC, et al. Perianal basal cell carcinoma: a comparative histologic, immunohistochemical, and flow cytometric study with basaloid carcinoma of the anus. American Journal of Dermatopathology 1996; 18:371–379.

Ansai SI, et al. Ber-EP4 is a useful marker for follicular germinative cell differentiation of cutaneous epithelial neoplasms. J Dermatol 2012; 39:688–692.

Argani P, et al. A distinctive subset of PEComas harbors TFE3 gene fusions. American Journal of Surgical Pathology, 2010.

Argani P, et al. Aberrant nuclear immunoreactivity for TFE3 in neoplasms with TFE3 gene fusions: a sensitive and specific immunohistochemical assay. Am J Surg Pathol, 2003.

Asioli S, et al. p63 expression as a new prognostic marker in Merkel cell carcinoma. Cancer 2007; 110:640–647.

Au-Yeung BB, et al. The structure, regulation, and function of ZAP-70. Immunological Reviews 2009; 228:41–57.

Bayer-Garner IB, Givens V, Smoller B. Immunohistochemical staining for androgen receptors: a sensitive marker of sebaceous differentiation. American Journal of Dermatopathology 1999; 21:426–431.

Beadling C, et al. KIT gene mutations and copy number in melanoma subtypes. Clinical Cancer Research 2008; 14:6821–6828.

Beer TW, Shepherd P, Theaker JM. Ber EP4 and epithelial membrane antigen aid distinction of basal cell, squamous cell and basosquamous carcinomas of the skin. Histopathology 2000; 37:218–223.

Berglund, M. et al. 2005. Evaluation of immunophenotype in diffuse large B-cell lymphoma and its impact on prognosis. Modern Pathology 2005; 18:1113–1120.

Bhattacharya B. et al. Nuclear beta-catenin expression distinguishes deep fibromatosis from other benign and malignant fibroblastic and myofibroblastic lesions. The American journal of surgical pathology, 2005.

Binh MBN, et al. MDM2 and CDK4 immunostainings are useful adjuncts in diagnosing well-differentiated and dedifferentiated liposarcoma subtypes: a comparative analysis of 559 soft tissue neoplasms with genetic data. The American Journal of Surgical Pathology, 2005.

Buresh CJ, Oliai BR, Miller RT. Reactivity with TdT in merkel cell carcinoma: A potential diagnostic pitfall. American Journal of Clinical Pathology 2008; 129:894–898.

Busam KJ, et al. Immunohistochemical analysis of novel monoclonal antibody PNL2 and comparison with other melanocyte differentiation markers. The American Journal of Surgical Pathology 2005; 3:400–406.

Chen BJ, et al. Loss of retinoblastoma protein expression in spindle cell/leomorphic lipomas and cytogenetically-related tumors. The American Journal of Surgical Pathology, 2012.

Cobaleda C, et al. Pax5: the guardian of B cell identity and function. Nature immunology, 2007; 8:463–470.

Conner JR, Hornick JL. SATB2 is a novel marker of osteoblastic differentiation in bone and soft tissue tumours. Histopathology, 2013.

Crespo M, et al. ZAP-70 expression as a surrogate for immunoglobulin-variable-region mutations in chronic lymphocytic leukemia. The New England journal of medicine, 2003; 348:1764–1775.

Dai B, et al. Analysis of KIT expression and gene mutation in human acral melanoma: With a comparison between primary tumors and corresponding metastases/recurrences. Human Pathology 2013; 8:1472–1478.

Desouki MM, et al. PAX-5: A valuable immunohistochemical marker in the differential diagnosis of lymphoid neoplasms. Clinical Medicine and Research, 2010; 8:84–88.

Al Dhaybi R, et al. P16 Expression: A marker of differentiation between childhood malignant melanomas and Spitz nevi. Journal of the American Academy of Dermatology 2011; 65:357–363.

Dogan, A, et al. CD10 and BCL-6 expression in paraffin sections of normal lymphoid tissue and B-cell lymphomas. The American Journal of Surgical Pathology 2000; 24:846–852.

Dono M, Cerruti G, Zupo S, The CD5+ B-cell. International Journal of Biochemistry and Cell Biology 2004; 36:2105–2111.

Doyle LA, et al. MUC4 is a highly sensitive and specific marker for low-grade fibromyxoid sarcoma. The American Journal of Surgical Pathology, 2011.

Doyle LA, et al. MUC4 Is a Sensitive and Extremely Useful Marker for Sclerosing Epithelioid Fibrosarcoma. The American Journal of Surgical Pathology, 2012.

Dyhdalo KS, et al. Immunoarchitectural patterns of germinal center antigens including LMO2 assist in the differential diagnosis of marginal zone lymphoma vs follicular lymphoma. American Journal of Clinical Pathology 2013; 140:149–154.

Endo M, et al. NY-ESO-1 (CTAG1B) expression in mesenchymal tumors. Modern Pathology.

Fabriek BO, Dijkstra CD, van den Berg TK. The macrophage scavenger receptor CD163. Immunobiology 2014; 210:153–160.

Ferringer T. Immunohistochemistry in dermatopathology. Archives of Pathology and Laboratory Medicine 2015; 139:83–105.

Fine SW, McClain, SA & Li M. Immunohistochemical staining for calretinin is useful for differentiating schwannomas from neurofibromas. American Journal of Clinical Pathology 2004; 122:552–559.

Foss HD, et al. Anaplastic large-cell lymphomas of T-cell and null-cell phenotype express cytotoxic molecules. Blood 1996; 88:4005–4011.

Franke WW, et al. Diversity of cytokeratins. Differentiation specific expression of cytokeratin polypeptides in epithelial cells and tissues. Journal of Molecular Biology 1981; 153:933–959.

Fullen DR, et al. S100A6 expression in fibrohistiocytic lesions. Journal of Cutaneous Pathology 2001; 28:229–234.

Gleason BC, et al. Utility of p63 in the differential diagnosis of atypical fibroxanthoma and spindle cell squamous cell carcinoma. Journal of Cutaneous Pathology 2009; 36:543–547.

Henderson S, et al. p40 Is More Specific Than p63 for the distinction of atypical fibroxanthoma from other cutaneous spindle cell malignancies. The American Journal of Surgical Pathology 2014; 38:1102–10.

Hisaoka M. et al. Specific but variable expression of h-caldesmon in leiomyosarcomas: an immunohistochemical reassessment of a novel myogenic marker. Applied immunohistochemistry & molecular morphology: AIMM / official publication of the Society for Applied Immunohistochemistry 2001; 9:302–308.

Hoefnagel JJ, et al. Bcl-2, Bcl-6 and CD10 expression in cutaneous B-cell lymphoma: Further support for a follicle centre cell origin and differential diagnostic significance. British Journal of Dermatology 2003; 149:1183–1191.

Horny HP. Mastocytosis: An unusual clonal disorder of bone marrow-derived hematopoietic progenitor cells. American Journal of Clinical Pathology 2009; 438–447.

Irani AM, et al. Detection of MCT and MCTC types of human mast cells by immunohistochemistry using new monoclonal anti-tryptase and anti-chymase antibodies. The Journal of Histochemistry and Cytochemistry 1989; 37:1509–1515.

Ivan D, et al. Use of p63 expression in distinguishing primary and metastatic cutaneous adnexal neoplasms from metastatic adenocarcinoma to skin. Journal of Cutaneous Pathology 2007; 34:474–480.

Izikson L, Bhan A, Zembowicz A. Androgen receptor expression helps to differentiate basal cell carcinoma from benign trichoblastic tumors. The American Journal of Dermatopathology 2005; 27:91–95.

Julia F, et al. Blastic plasmacytoid dendritic cell neoplasm: Clinical features in 90 patients. Br J Dermatol 2013; 169:579–586.

Jungbluth AA, et al. A103: An anti-melan-a monoclonal antibody for the detection of malignant melanoma in paraffin-embedded tissues. The American Journal of Surgical Pathology 1998; 22:595–602.

Kalof AN, Cooper K, D2-40 immunohistochemistry--so far! Advances in anatomic pathology, 2009; 16:62–64.

Ko CJ, et al. Hypertrophic lupus erythematosus: The diagnostic utility of CD123 staining. Journal of Cutaneous Pathology 2011; 38:889–892.

Krahl D, Sellheyer K. P75 Neurotrophin receptor differentiates between morphoeic basal cell carcinoma and desmoplastic trichoepithelioma: Insights into the histogenesis of adnexal tumours based on embryology and hair follicle biology. British Journal of Dermatology 2010; 163:138–145.

Kwon SE, Chapman ER. Synaptophysin regulates the kinetics of synaptic vesicle endocytosis in central neurons. Neuron 2011; 70:847–854.

Lau SK, Chu PG, Weiss LM. CD163: A specific marker of macrophages in paraffin-embedded tissue samples. American Journal of Clinical Pathology 2004; 122:794–801.

Leong AS-Y, Cooper K, Leon FJW-M. Manual of Diagnostic Antibodies for Immunohistology 1st ed., London: Oxford University Press, 1999.

Long GV et al. Immunohistochemistry is highly sensitive and specific for the detection of V600E BRAF mutation in melanoma. The American Journal of Surgical Pathology 2013; 37:61-65.

Mahalingam M, et al. The diagnostic utility of immunohistochemistry in distinguishing primary skin adnexal carcinomas from metastatic adenocarcinoma to skin: an immunohistochemical reappraisal using cytokeratin 15, nestin, p63, D2-40, and calretinin. Modern Pathology 2010; 23:713-719.

Margol AS, Judkins AR. Pathology and diagnosis of SMARCB1-deficient tumors. Cancer Genetics, 2014.

McKenney JK, Weiss SW, Folpe AL. CD31 expression in intratumoral macrophages: a potential diagnostic pitfall. The American Journal of Surgical Pathology 2001; 25:1167–1173.

Miettinen M, et al. ERG expression in epithelioid sarcoma: a diagnostic pitfall. Am J Surg Pathol 2013; 37:1580–1585.

Molina-Ruiz, AM, et al. Immunohistochemistry in the Diagnosis of Cutaneous Bacterial Infections. American Journal of Dermatopathology 2015; 37:179–196.

Molina-Ruiz AM, et al. Immunohistochemistry in the Diagnosis of Cutaneous Viral Infections—Part I. Cutaneous Viral Infections by Herpesviruses and Papillomaviruses. Am J Dermatopathol 2015; 37:1–14.

Morgado JMT et al. Immunophenotyping in systemic mastocytosis diagnosis: 'CD25 positive' alone is more informative than the 'CD25 and/or CD2' WHO criterion. Modern Pathology 2012; 25:516-521.

Gajjar NA, Cochran AJ, Binder SW. Is MAGE-1 expression in metastatic malignant melanomas really helpful? American Journal of Surgical Pathology 2004; 28:883–888.

Nera KP, et al. Loss of Pax5 promotes plasma cell differentiation. Immunity 2006; 24:283-293.

Niu H. The proto-oncogene BCL-6 in normal and malignant B cell development. Hematological Oncology 2002; 20:155-166.

O'Connell FP, Pinkus, JL, Pinkus, GS. CD138 (Syndecan-1), a Plasma Cell Marker: Immunohistochemical Profile in Hematopoietic and Nonhematopoietic Neoplasms. American Journal of Clinical Pathology 2004; 121:254–263.

Orta L, et al. Towards identification of hereditary DNA mismatch repair deficiency: sebaceous neoplasm warrants routine immunohistochemical screening regardless of patient's age or other clinical characteristics. The American Journal of Surgical Pathology 2009; 33:934–44.

Ostler DA, et al. Adipophilin expression in sebaceous tumors and other cutaneous lesions with clear cell histology: an immunohistochemical study of 117 cases. Modern Pathology 2010; 23:567–573.

Ozawa M, et al. Ber-EP4 antigen is a marker for a cell population related to the secondary hair germ. Experimental Dermatology 2004; 13:401–405.

Pham TTN, et al. CD10 expression in trichoepithelioma and basal cell carcinoma. Journal of Cutaneous Pathology 2006; 33:123–128.

Pinkus GS, Kurtin PJ. Epithelial membrane antigen--a diagnostic discriminant in surgical pathology: immunohistochemical profile in epithelial, mesenchymal, and hematopoietic neoplasms using paraffin sections and monoclonal antibodies. Human Pathology 1985; 16:929-940.

Plaza JA, et al. Immunohistochemical expression of S100A6 in cellular neurothekeoma: clinicopathologic and immunohistochemical analysis of 31 cases. The American Journal of Dermatopathology 2009; 31:419–22.

Pouryazdanparast P, et al. Diagnostic value of CD163 in cutaneous spindle cell lesions. Journal of Cutaneous Pathology 2009; 36:859-864.

Prieto-Granada CN, et al. Loss of H3K27me3 expression Is a highly sensitive marker for sporadic and radiation-induced MPNST. Am J Surg Pathol 2016; 40:479–489.

Rao Q, et al. Cathepsin K expression in a wide spectrum of perivascular epithelioid cell neoplasms (PEComas): A clinicopathological study emphasizing extrarenal PEComas. Histopathology 2013; 62:642-650.

Ribé A, McNutt NS. S100A6 protein expression is different in Spitz nevi and melanomas. Modern Pathology 2003; 5:505-11.

Rose AE, et al. Clinical relevance of detection of lymphovascular invasion in primary melanoma using Endothelial Markers D2-40 and CD34. The American Journal of Surgical Pathology 2011; 35:1441-1449.

Rutishauser U, et al. The neural cell adhesion molecule (NCAM) as a regulator of cell-cell interactions. Science 1988; 240:53–57.

Sachdev R, et al. CD163 expression is present in cutaneous histiocytomas but not in atypical fibroxanthomas. American Journal of Clinical Pathology 2010; 133:915-921.

Sachdev R, Sundram UN. Frequent positive staining with NKI/C3 in normal and neoplastic tissues limits its usefulness in the diagnosis of cellular neurothekeoma. American Journal of Clinical Pathology 2006; 126:554–563.

Sandell RF, Carter JM Folpe AL. Solitary (juvenile) xanthogranuloma: a comprehensive immunohistochemical study emphasizing recently developed markers of histiocytic lineage. Human Pathology 2015; 46:1390–1397.

Schmuth M, et al. Reduced number of CD1a+ cells in cutaneous B-cell lymphoma. American Journal of Clinical Pathology 2001; 116:72–78.

Schoolmeester JK, Lastra RR. Granular cell tumors overexpress TFE3 without corollary gene rearrangement. Human Pathology 2015; 46:1242–1243.

Sellheyer K, Krahl D. Ber-EP4 enhances the differential diagnostic accuracy of cytokeratin 7 in pagetoid cutaneous neoplasms. Journal of Cutaneous Pathology 2008; 35:366–372.

El Shabrawi-Caelen L. et al. Cutaneous inflammatory pseudotumor--a spectrum of various diseases? Journal of Cutaneous Pathology 2004; 31:605-611.

Smith KJ, et al. Neuroendocrine (Merkel cell) carcinoma with an intraepidermal component. The American Journal of Dermatopathology 1993; 15:528–533.

Swanson PE, et al. Eccrine sweat gland carcinoma: an histologic and immunohistochemical study of 32 cases. JCutan Pathol 1987; 14:65-86.

Taylor C, Cote R. Immunomicroscopy: A diagnostic tool for the Surgical Pathologist 3rd ed. M. Houston, ed., Saunders Elsevier, 2006.

Terry J, et al. TLE1 as a diagnostic immunohistochemical marker for synovial sarcoma emerging from gene expression profiling studies. The American Journal of Surgical Pathology 2007; 31:240-246.

Trefzer U, et al. SM5-1: a new monoclonal antibody which is highly sensitive and specific for melanocytic lesions. Archives of Dermatological Research 2000 292;12:583-9.

Villamor N. ZAP-70 staining in chronic lymphocytic leukemia. Current Protocols in Cytometry 2005; 6:6-19.

Weaver J, et al. Detection of MDM2 gene amplification or protein expression distinguishes sclerosing mesenteritis and retroperitoneal fibrosis from inflammatory well-differentiated liposarcoma. Modern Pathology 2009; 22:66–70.

Whittam LR, et al. CD8-positive juvenile onset mycosis fungoides: An immunohistochemical and genotypic analysis of six cases. British Journal of Dermatology 2000; 143:1199-1204.

Wilson BS, Lloyd RV. Detection of chromogranin in neuroendocrine cells with a monoclonal antibody. The American Journal of Pathology 1984; 115:458–468.

Yoshida A, et al. STAT6 Immunohistochemistry is helpful in the diagnosis of solitary fibrous tumors. The American Journal of Surgical Pathology, 2014.

Zhang PJ, et al. Immunophenotype of desmoplastic small round cell tumors as detected in cases with EWS-WT1 gene fusion product. Modern Pathology 2003; 16:229–235.

Marc R. Lewin

IHC panel for pagetoid proliferations (Table 7.1)

Many different entities may present as pagetoid proliferations within the epidermis. As these entities have similar histologic appearances, IHC plays a crucial role in the diagnosis of these lesions. Squamous cell carcinoma in situ (SCCIS)/ Bowen's disease may present as a pagetoid proliferation, and generally can be distinguished from extramammary Paget's disease (EMPD) by its strong CK5 reactivity. It is important to note that while CK7 is generally negative in SCC in situ, it can be positive in a significant subset of tumors. Ber-EP4 is also useful in the setting of pagetoid proliferations as it is positive in EMPD and Merkel cell carcinoma, but negative in most other pagetoid proliferations.

Sclerosing epithelial neoplasms (Table 7.2)

Sclerosing epithelial tumors often present a diagnostic challenge to the dermatopathologist. Since mBCC and MAC are aggressive carcinomas, it is vital to differentiate these entities from the indolent DTE. As these lesions are often located on the face, the biopsies may be relatively superficial leaving the pathologist with only a small portion of the lesion to evaluate. Given

Table 7.1 IHC panel for pagetoid proliferations

	CK5	P63	CK7	CK20	Ber-EP4	CEA	CDX-2	GCDFP	Androgen receptor	Mart-1
Primary mammary Pagets and EMPD	-	-	+	-	+	+	-	+	-	-
SCCIS, Bowens	+	+	-/+	-	-	-	-	-	-	-
Metastatic colorectal	-	-	+/-	+	-	+	+	-	-	-
Metastatic urothelial	+	+	+	+	-	+	-	-	-	-
Melanoma	-	-	-	-	-	-	-	-	-	+
Merkel	+	+	-	+	+	-	-	-	-	-
Sebaceous carcinoma	+	+	-	-	-	-	-	-	+	-

Table 7.2 Sclerosing epithelial neoplasms

Lesion	CK7	CK20	Bcl-2	P63	CD10	P75	CK15
mBCC	-/+	-	+, strong, diffuse	++	+ tumor/-stroma	-	+
MAC	+	-	-	-	-	-	-
DTE	-	+ merkel cells	Peripheral cells only	++	-tumor/+in stroma	+	+

DTE, desmoplastic trichoepithelioma; MAC, microcystic adnexal carcinoma; mBCC, morpheaform basal cell carcinoma this fact, and as these lesions have similar histologic features, distinction may be difficult on H&E sections alone. By using the different IHC expression profile of these tumors, an immunopanel made up of markers including CK7, CK20, bcl-2, p63, CD10, and CK15 forms a relatively reliable way to differentiate between these entities.

Small round blue cell tumors (Table 7.3)

This table lists a variety of entities which may present as cutaneous small round blue cell tumors. The IHC stains listed can be used as screening tools to differentiate between these entities.

Table 7.3 Small round blue cell tumors	
Tumor	IHC
Lymphoma	CD45 B-cell lymphoma – CD20 T-cell lymphoma – CD3 Lymphoblastic lymphoma – TdT
Merkel cell carcinoma	CK20; TdT-; CK7-
Metastatic small cell carcinoma	CK7+/CK20-
Melanoma	Mart-1; Sox10; S-100
Ewing sarcoma/PNET	NSE; CD99; Fli1
Rhabdomyosarcoma	Myogenin; MyoD

Basal cell carcinoma (BCC) vs sebaceous carcinoma (SebCa) (Table 7.4)

Basal cell carcinomas (BCCs) and sebaceous carcinoma (SebCa) may both present as cutaneous basaloid lesions. In addition, BCC may also have a component of sebaceous differentiation, which can make distinguishing between these entities difficult. The use of a panel approach to this differential diagnosis is

Table 7.4 Basal cell carcinoma (BCC) vs sebaceous carcinoma (SebCa)		
Stain	BCC	SebCa
Androgen receptor (AR)	- / focal (<5%)	++
CAM 5.2	-	++
Ber-EP4	+	-

extremely helpful in distinguishing these entities. A caveat is AR may stain some BCCs, but in general, it is present focally in BCC compared to the strong, diffuse positivity seen in SebCa.

B-cell lymphoma (Table 7.5)

Figure 7.1 shows a simplified flow chart with key IHC breakpoints in the evaluation of a cutaneous predominantly CD20 + B-cell process. The first break point is based on the presence or absence of high grade histologic features such as marked atypia, pleomorphism, and necrosis. When these changes are present, the lymphoma is a DLBCL, and further IHC including MUM-1 and Bcl-6 stains is performed to assess whether the lymphoma has an activated B-cell phenotype or a germinal center cell phenotype. If high grade cytology is not observed, additional IHC stains are performed in order to evaluate the lesion. Of note, while mantle cell lymphoma (MCL) is an intermediate to high grade lymphoma, it often has a bland, monotonous cytologic appearance, and therefore is placed in the low grade cytology for the purposes of this flow chart. This flow chart is in no means all encompassing, and there is often considerable histologic and immunophenotypic overlap between lesions of exuberant CLH/pseudolymphomas and low grade B-cell lymphomas. For example, marginal zone lymphoma (MZL) may present with no distinct IHC abnormalities. Bcl-6+/Bcl-2- GC formation may be observed in reactive GCs as well as neoplastic GC of cutaneous follicle center lymphoma. In the latter

Table 7.5 IHC panel	
Stain	Use
CD20/CD79a	Pan-B cell markers
Bcl-6	Highlights GC; used to subclassify DLBCL
Bcl-2	Over expressed in MZL; aberrantly expressed in Bcl-6 + GC in FCL; also stains T-cells
CD10	Marker of GC differentiation
CD23	+ in CLL/SLL; + in MCL highlights dendritic cell network and architecture of GCs
CD21	Defines GC architecture
k/l stains	Evaluate for restricted clonal populations in MZL
MUM-1	Indicator of activated B phenotype in DLBCL

DLBCL, diffuse large B-cell lymphoma; FCL, follicle center lymphoma; GC, Germinal Center; MZL, marginal zone lymphoma

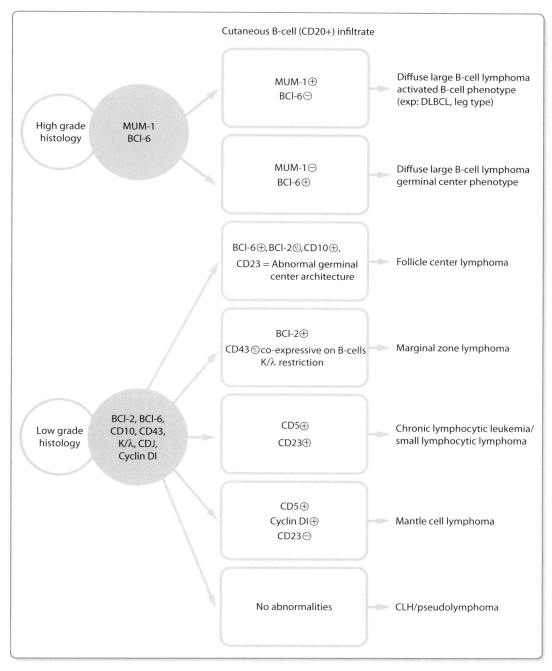

Figure 7.1 Key IHC breakpoints of a cutaneous predominantly CD20+ B-cell process.

setting, IHC markers such as CD21 or CD23 may be of value to highlight an abnormal GC architecture. Ki-67 may also be of use as it is actually decreased in neoplastic GCs compared to their reactive counterparts. In some instances, a diagnosis of lymphoma can only be rendered after sequential sampling over time, and often with the use of ancillary studies such as IgH gene rearrangement studies or flow cytometric analysis.

Mycosis fungoides (MF) panel (Table 7.6)

The most common immunoprofile of MF cells is CD3+, CD4+, CD8-, CD7- . Of note, MF in juvenile patients often presents with a CD8+/CD4- phenotype. In assessing IHC in a suspected case of MF, it is essential to evaluate the correct population of cells. Cases of MF may present with an exuberant reactive dermal infiltrate, and it is critical to limit the assessment of an atypical immunoprofile to the cells of interest, namely the atypical epidermotropic lymphocytes or the lymphocytes tagging the dermal-epidermal

junction. Also, intraepidermal Langerhans cells are CD4+, and can be misinterpreted as Pautrier microabscesses; however, true MF cells are CD3+/CD1a -, while Langerhan cells are CD3-/CD1a +.

Panel for poorly differentiated dermal spindle cell tumors (Table 7.7)

In the skin, one is often faced with the challenge of evaluating a very poorly differentiated dermal spindle cell neoplasm. In this setting, it is essential to use a panel-based approach to the IHC assessment of a tumor. For example, if one does not perform a complete IHC panel, the presence of strong CK positivity may lead to the erroneous diagnosis of a sarcomatoid squamous cell carcinoma. However, CK positivity may also be seen in cases of epithelioid angiosarcomas, ALCL, and even LMS. Procollagen-1 is strongly positive in AFX; however, it may also stain a broad range of other tumors including carcinomas and melanomas. Therefore, it is only useful in the setting of a complete IHC panel including more lineage specific IHC markers. Another potential pitfall is in the use of CD31. CD31 is an excellent vascular marker, but one must also be aware that it will stain histiocytes and therefore will sometimes stain a subset of AFXs with prominent histiocytic differentiation. Our preferred panel includes IHC markers that cover most lines of differentiation including epithelial (CK5); vascular (CD31/ERG); smooth muscle (SMM); neural (S-100); melanocytic (S-100, Mart-1); hematopoietic (CD45 or CD30 for ALCL); and fibrohistiocytic (Procollagen-1;CD10; CD68).

This use of a complete IHC panel on these undifferentiated lesions greatly diminishes the chance of a misdiagnosis.

Table 7.6 Mycosis fungoides (MF) panel

Stain	Use
CD3	Pan T-cell marker
CD4	Most MF cases are CD4+/CD8-; will stain histiocytes including LCs
CD8	Most MF are CD8-; + in juvenile and hypopigmented MF
CD7	Lost in a large portion of MF
CD30	May be + in transformed MF; + in LYP, ALCL
CD2/CD5	May be lost in subset of MF

ALCL, anaplastic large cell lymphoma; LC, Langerhans cells; LYP, lymphomatoid papulosis

Table 7.7 Panel for poorly differentiated dermal spindle cell tumors

Entity	CK5	P63 or p40	ERG or CD31/CD34	SMM	S100	CD30	Procollagen-1
Poorly differentiated SCC	+	+	-	-	-	-	-/+
Melanoma	-	-	-	-	++	-	-/+
Angiosarcoma	-/+	-	+++	-	-	-	-
ALCL	-/+	-	-	-	-	+++	-/+
AFX	-	-	-/+	-	-	-	++++
LMS	-+	-	-	+++	-	-	-

AFX, atypical fibroxanthoma; ALCL, anaplastic large cell lymphoma; LMS, leiomyosarcoma; SCC, squamous cell carcinoma

Section 4

Point of care testing

Chapter 8   Dermatological point of care tests

Dermatological point of care tests

Travis Vandergriff

The first step in successfully treating a patient with a dermatological condition is to secure the correct diagnosis. In many cases, the diagnosis can be made confidently based on clinical findings. When the clinical differential diagnosis includes entities with divergent prognoses or treatments, then additional diagnostic maneuvers are typically warranted. Point-of-care (POC) tests represent one such set of diagnostic techniques that can be used to quickly and accurately secure a diagnosis at the patient's bedside. This chapter will explore POC tests applicable to the practice of dermatology. Emphasis will be given to potassium hydroxide preparations, mineral oil preparations, Tzanck smears for cytodiagnosis, and frozen section analysis of skin samples.

All testing performed on samples from human patients are subject to regulations passed by the United States Congress in 1988 known as Clinical Laboratory Improvement Amendments (CLIA). CLIA is a complex set of regulatory statutes which are meant to ensure accuracy, reliability, and timeliness of patient test resulting. CLIA regulations apply to all health care settings, including physician in-office testing. All laboratories and physician offices performing laboratory tests are required to enroll in the CLIA program. Each individual test is assigned a level of complexity which determines the type of CLIA certification required for the laboratory. Most of the POC tests performed by dermatologists fall into the 'moderate complexity' category, including its subcategory of 'provider performed microscopy procedures'. Mohs micrographic surgery and other frozen section analyses of skin fall under the 'high complexity' designation and are subject to more stringent CLIA requirements. Complete and current CLIA requirements can be found online (cms.gov/clia).

Potassium hydroxide preparation

Preparation of skin scrapings with potassium hydroxide (KOH) is the preferred POC method for diagnosing superficial cutaneous mycoses. Fungal infections of the skin are generally divided into three categories:

1. Superficial
2. Subcutaneous
3. Deep

All three categories of mycoses are amenable to diagnosis by KOH preparation, but the technique is most commonly applied to diagnose superficial mycoses.

Superficial mycoses affect only the hair, nails, and epidermal stratum corneum. Fungal agents known to cause superficial mycosis include dermatophytes and non-dermatophytes. Approximately 40 species of dermatophytes are recognized and fall within three genera (*Epidermophyton*, *Trichophyton*, and *Microsporum*). Non-dermatophyte causes of superficial mycosis are uncommonly implicated and include yeasts (e.g. *Candida* spp.) and molds [1].

When a superficial mycosis is suspected clinically, keratin-containing material (i.e. epidermal scale, nail debris, or hair shafts) can be examined for fungal elements by KOH preparation. Performance of a KOH preparation requires a 15 blade scalpel, a glass slide with coverslip, KOH solution, and a source of a gentle flame to warm the material (e.g. matches or a lighter).

To reduce the risk of sampling error, the test material must be chosen and obtained carefully. For suspected fungal infections of the skin, scale should be scraped from the edge of an annular lesion with a 15 blade scalpel held perpendicular to the skin surface. Scale is dislodged directly onto the glass slide which is held beneath the scraping site [2]. When onychomycosis is suspected, subungual debris is similarly obtained with a 15 blade scalpel and dislodged directly onto a microscopic slide. For suspected tinea capitis, hair shafts may be plucked from the scalp with forceps, then laid carefully onto the glass slide. Regardless of the source of the keratin material, one principle holds true: copious material should be obtained in order to maximize the chances of finding fungal elements when present.

Once the keratin material has been transferred to the glass slide, the KOH solution is added. One or two drops of 10–20% KOH solution are added directly to the slide. A coverslip is then placed over the material in solution. As a relatively potent base, the KOH solution dissolves keratinaceous debris such as corneocytes, onychocytes, and hair shafts, while sparing the chitin-enriched fungal elements [3]. The clearing of keratin debris can be accelerated by gently warming the specimen with a flame or by adding dimethyl sulphoxide (DMSO) to the solution. Specimens prepared by KOH technique are labile and should be examined microscopically within hours of their preparation.

When examining KOH preparations microscopically, the condenser should be moved down and the diaphragm position relatively closed. By creating contrast, low lighting improves the ability to discern fungal hyphae and to distinguish them from keratin debris [2, 3]. The characteristic finding in KOH preparation of dermatophytosis is the presence of long, branching septate hyphae (**Figure 8.1**). In hair samples, the hyphae and their spores can be seen within hair shafts (endothrix) or surrounding hair shafts (ectothrix). Importantly, specific dermatophyte species cannot be ascertained on KOH preparation. A fungal culture would be required for that determination. *Candida* spp. will reveal clustered pseudomycelia or pseudohyphae which lack septation. Round to oval yeast forms will be admixed. Other yeasts may also be identified on KOH. *Malassezia furfur*, the causative agent of tinea versicolor, appears as short hyphae with numerous round yeast, the so-called 'spaghetti and meatballs' appearance.

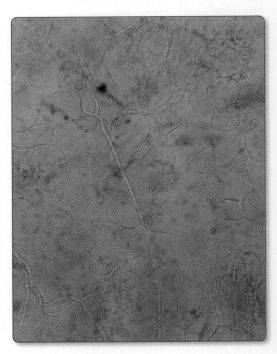

Figure 8.1 Potassium hydroxide preparation for fungal assessment. Branching, septate hyphae are seen to cross epithelial cells (KOH preparation, 400×).

Artifacts may be confused with fungal elements and lead to false-positive findings. Clothing fibers are typically larger in caliber than are fungal hyphae (**Figure 8.2**). They also have an irregular or twisted form, whereas hyphae have parallel edges [3]. Fibers lack septations. When fibers are dyed, their unnatural colors make them easily recognizable as foreign. Human hair shafts are also larger caliber and lack septation. When epithelial cells (corneocytes, onychocytes, etc.) are clustered, their cell membranes may align to form a confluent contour resembling hyphae. A cotton tip applicator can be used to gently press on the coverslip in this area to disperse the cells; the presence of fungal hyphae would then be easily recognizable.

KOH appears to be more sensitive than fungal culture for the identification of superficial mycoses [4, 5]. The sensitivity of the test depends somewhat on operator experience, but reports indicate that the sensitivity of KOH preparation for diagnosing dermatophytosis ranges from 75%

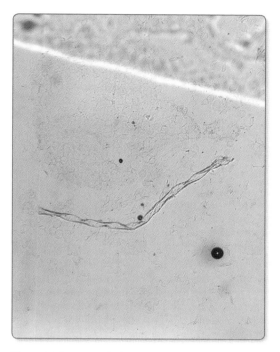

Figure 8.2 Potassium hydroxide preparation for fungal assessment, mimickers. Clothing fibers may resemble hyphae but they are larger and typically have twisted forms (KOH preparation, 200×).

to over 90%. A modest increase in sensitivity can be achieved if a chitin-avid stain such as chlorazol black E is added to the KOH solution [5, 6]. Other fungal stains have been reported to increase the sensitivity of KOH preparation and include both calcofluor white and acridine orange [3, 6]. Because both of these stains require fluorescent microscopy, their practical utility is limited.

Mineral oil preparation

Human ectoparasites are arthropods that burrow into or attach onto the human integument and extract nutrients from the human host. In some cases, ectoparasites may be facultative and cause no discernible disease. However, they commonly cause human disease by virtue of host inflammatory reactions or as vectors of microbial pathogens. Human ectoparasites include mites, lice, scabies, fleas, ticks, and maggots.

Some ectoparasites, including ticks and maggots, are macroscopic and are generally recognizable without microscopy. Mites and lice range in size and may be too small to discern without microscopy or magnification. When an ectoparasite-associated disease is suspected clinically, skin scraping or hair fragments can be viewed microscopically by way of mineral oil preparation to aid in identification of the parasite. Mineral oil preparation techniques for diagnosis of scabies, lice, and mite infestations will be presented herein.

The necessary supplies for performing a mineral oil preparation include a 15 blade scalpel, a glass slide with coverslip, mineral oil, a rubbing alcohol pad, and perhaps an ink pen.

Diagnosis of scabies

Scabies is an ectoparasite disease caused by the scabietic mite *Sarcoptes scabiei var hominis*, an obligate human parasite which burrows into the host skin. The host inflammatory reaction to the burrowed mites leads to an intensely pruritic eruption. The disease is most prevalent in conditions of overcrowding, homelessness, and in some institutional settings including hospitals and nursing homes [7].

Patients with scabies typically present with intense pruritus that is characteristically worse at night. Excoriated papules may be widespread but predominate in the axillary folds, around the umbilicus and nipples, on the genitals, on the wrists, and in the interdigital spaces. The pathognomonic clinical sign is the burrow: a linear or serpiginous track measuring 1–10 mm in length [7]. A burrow represents the migratory route created by a mite within the stratum corneum. Burrows are most readily apparent around the wrists and in the interdigital spaces, and identification of a burrow is an important first step in choosing areas for diagnostic skin scrapings.

The diagnosis of scabies can be confirmed by identifying the mite, its eggs, or its feces (scybala) on microscopic examination of skin scrapings (**Figure 8.3**). Because the mite burden in most hosts is usually quite low (10–12 mites), identification of the mite requires careful consideration and execution of skin scrapings. The highest-yield anatomic sites for finding burrows and other lesions suitable for scraping include the anterior axillary folds, the ventral aspect of the wrists, the periumbilical area, and

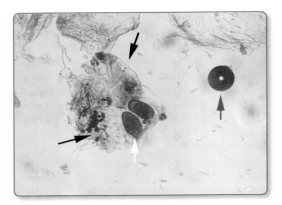

Figure 8.3 Mineral oil preparation for diagnosis of scabies. Scabies mite (black arrow), eggs (white arrow), and scybala (blue arrow) are seen (mineral oil preparation, 400×). An air bubble under the coverslip (red arrow) may be confused with eggs but is distinguished by its opacity and its circular rather than ovoid shape. Courtesy of Jake Turrentine MD.

the interdigital spaces. Suspected burrows can be highlighted by the 'burrow ink test' [8]. An inexpensive ballpoint inkpen with blue or black ink is used to thoroughly cover a suspected burrow. A rubbing alcohol pad is then used to wipe away the ink from the skin. If a burrow is present, the ink will track down and through its tunnel and will not wipe away. The burrow is then marked by the color of the ink and is a high-yield site for scraping.

The scraping technique is simple. A drop of mineral oil is placed onto the skin over a burrow or suspect papule, and another drop of mineral oil is placed onto the glass slide. The burrow or papule is scraped down its entire length with a 15 blade scalpel held perpendicular to the skin surface. A 3 mm disposable curette may be substituted for the scalpel blade [9]. The debris collected on the blade or curette is then transferred to the slide, and a coverslip is placed. Microscopic examination of the slide is done on scanning magnification. A diagnosis of scabies can be confirmed when a mite, egg or fecal pellet (scybala) is seen. The female mite measures 0.3–0.4 mm in length, with male mites measuring half that size [7, 10]. Mites have eight short legs with hair-like projections, a round undivided abdomen and cephalothorax, and a small but identifiable head [7]. Eggs are usually ovoid and transparent, but small mites are sometimes identifiable

encased within egg shells. Fecal pellets are dark brown or golden round to ovoid structures. The sensitivity of skin scrapings for diagnosing scabies is operator dependent and has been reported to be low (46% in one study by Walter, et al) [11]. Therefore, failure to identify scabietic elements on a scraping does not exclude the diagnosis.

Diagnosis of pediculosis

Pediculosis is the human infestation by lice. Three types of lice predominate: the head louse (*Pediculus humanus capitus*), the body louse (*Pediculus humanus humanus*), and the crab louse (*Pthirus pubis*). Infestation by lice can be confirmed when the louse or its ova (which are encased in chitinous shells called nits) are identified microscopically [12].

Pediculosis capitis is infestation of the human scalp by *Pediculus humanus capitus*. Children are affected preferentially, and girls more often than boys [12]. Infestation may be asymptomatic or manifest as scalp pruritus leading to excoriations. Adult lice may be seen crawling near the scalp. A fine-toothed louse comb can be used to extract the lice. Louse ova are housed in chitinous shells called nits which are securely adherent to hair shafts. Nits predominate on the proximal aspect of the hair shaft and are mostly found within 1 to 2 mm of the scalp [12]. Nits extend upwardly at an acute angle away from the shaft (**Figure 8.4**). Because they are firmly cemented to the hair shaft, nits are not freely mobile along the shaft.

The head louse measures 1–2 mm in length and can be seen without microscopy [12]. Nits are also visible without microscopy. However, microscopic examination of the louse or its nits allows for recognition of unique and identifying anatomic characteristics. Suspected lice or nits can be plucked from the scalp and placed onto a microscope slide prepared with a drop of mineral oil. The head louse has an elongate body with six clawed legs, short antennae, and small anteriorly situated mouthparts (**Figure 8.5**) [12].

Body lice infestation, or pediculosis corporis, is seen preferentially in settings of overcrowding, poverty, homelessness, or war. Infestation may be asymptomatic but typically leads to pruritus. Papules, excoriations, and lichenification may be seen clinically. Body lice are also potential vectors of serious bacterial

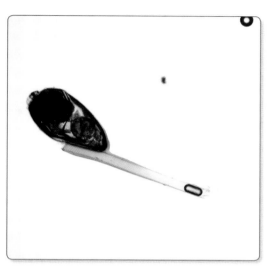

Figure 8.4 Mineral oil preparation for diagnosis of pediculosis, nits. Head louse nit (mineral oil preparation, 200×).

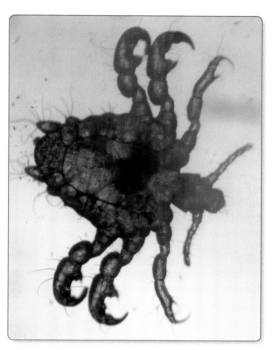

Figure 8.6 Mineral oil preparation for diagnosis of pediculosis, pubic louse. Pubic louse (mineral oil preparation, 200×). Courtesy of Jake Turrentine MD.

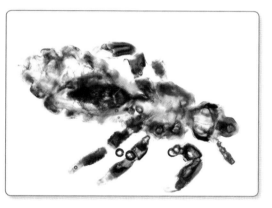

Figure 8.5 Mineral oil preparation for diagnosis of pediculosis, head louse. Head louse (mineral oil preparation, 200×).

diseases including epidemic typhus, trench fever, and relapsing fever.

The body louse and its nits are found in the seams of clothing, rather than directly attached to the patient's skin. Clothing seams around the waist are the highest-yield areas [12]. The body louse measures 2–4 mm in length but is otherwise morphologically similar to the head louse.

The crab louse preferentially attaches to pubic hair but is sometimes found on the chest, thighs, buttocks, and eyelashes. Similar to head lice and body lice, the infestation may be asymptomatic or patients may present with pruritus. When crab lice bite their human hosts for a blood meal, the bite marks leave characteristic red-blue macules known as maculae ceruleae [12]. The pubic louse measures approximately 1 mm in length. Unlike the head and body lice, the pubic louse's body is round rather than elongate. The pubic louse has six legs, but the anterior-most set of legs is small and vestigial in appearance (**Figure 8.6**) [12]. Nits of the pubic louse resemble those of the head louse.

Diagnosis of demodicosis

Demodex mites are a normal part of the human skin microbiome and are found within hair follicles. The mites were first identified in 1841 and later classified into two separate species

(*Demodex folliculorum* and *Demodex brevis*) in 1963 [13]. *Demodex folliculorum* is the larger of the two species and is mostly found in clusters in the pilosebaceous unit of the face [14]. *Demodex brevis* is the smaller of the two mite species and is typically found as single units in follicles on the trunk [14]. As a normal constituent of the skin microbiome, demodex mites are routinely found in the follicle in the absence of any clinical disease. However, an abnormal inflammatory response to the mites can occur, usually in the setting of increased mite numbers. This inflammatory response leads to clinical disease and usually presents as a pustular eruption resembling acne or folliculitis. An important corollary is that clinical correlation is essential for diagnosing demodex folliculitis, and the diagnosis should only be made in the proper clinical context. Simply identifying the mite on a skin scraping is insufficient for the diagnosis.

Demodex folliculorum is an oblong microscopic mite with eight short legs which are situated anterior to a long tail. Identification of the mite by point of care testing can be accomplished via a variety of techniques. The simplest method is direct microscopic examination of expressible folliculosebaceous contents. A standardized technique has been published whereby an area of 1 cm² of lesional skin is squeezed between the thumb and index finger, and the blunt end of a scalpel blade is used to collect secretions and pustular contents by scraping the skin surface [15]. The collected material can then be transferred to a microscope slide and covered with a coverslip. Direct microscopic examination is used to search for and quantify demodex mites. Another technique for collecting mites is called standardized skin surface biopsy, first described in 1971 [16]. A 1 cm² area is marked with a pen onto a glass microscope slide, and then a cyanoacrylic adhesive drop is placed into the marked square. The slide is then placed on the patient's lesional skin, with the adhesive surface in direct contact with the skin. After the adhesive dries, which may take about one minute, the slide is gently dislodged and a drop of mineral oil is placed onto the adhesive surface. After covering with a coverslip, microscopic examination is performed and mites are counted.

Because demodex mites are a normal constituent of the skin microbiome, simply identifying a mite on microscopy does not diagnose a disease state. However, abnormally increased numbers of mites support a diagnosis of demodex-related inflammatory disease of the pilosebaceous unit in the proper clinical context. A threshold value of at least 5 mites per cm² has been proposed and remains the most widely applied criterion [17].

Tzanck preparation (cytodiagnosis)

In 1947, the technique of point-of-care cutaneous cytodiagnosis was introduced by French Physician Arnault Tzanck [18]. In addition to his efforts in pioneering the use of blood transfusions, Tzanck described a simple technique whereby blistering diseases could be differentiated by microscopic visualization of blister contents and scrapings. The practice of cutaneous cytodiagnosis is now widely and eponymously known as the Tzanck smear or Tzanck preparation.

In addition to cytodiagnosis for distinguishing blistering diseases, Tzanck also described the application of the technique for the bedside diagnosis of cutaneous neoplasia. This application will not be addressed here, since the Tzanck preparation is almost exclusively used in practice today for differentiating inflammatory diseases.

Within the spectrum of inflammatory skin disease, those presenting with vesicles, bullae, or pustules are most suitable for cytodiagnosis. Microscopic examination of the blister contents and the surrounding epithelial cells can be used to rapidly identify diagnoses. The first and most important step in performing a Tzanck preparation for a blistering skin disease is to select the best lesion for examination. Intact vesicles or pustules early in their stage of evolution (1–2 days) are most likely to yield diagnostic findings. Older vesicles or pustules may have crusting, impetiginization, ulceration, or excoriation, features which can obscure diagnostic findings.

Once a suitable vesicle or pustule is identified, the lesion is sterilized by gently cleaning with isopropyl alcohol or chlorhexidine. A 15-blade scalpel is used to incise the roof of the vesicle or pustule. The roof, if flaccid, can be reflected with the blade. Contents of the vesicle or pustule are scraped with the scalpel blade and transferred to a clean and dry glass slide. Importantly, the deep side of the blister roof as well as the blister base are also scraped with the scalpel blade and their yield is also transferred to the glass slide. The goal is to collect both inflammatory cells and epithelial cells for examination. Blister fluid will contain inflammatory cells and acantholytic epithelial cells, but the roof and base must be scraped to collect adherent epithelial cells.

Once the scraped material has been transferred to the glass slide, the material is allowed to air dry. A stain is then applied directly to the slide. The rapidly applied Giemsa stain is the most commonly applied stain in practice [19]. Essentially, the slide is exposed to the Giemsa stain for 30–40 seconds, then rinsed with tap water and again allowed to air dry [18, 20]. A coverslip is then placed. Numerous other stains have been employed and described in the literature, including: Wright stain [21], Diff-Quik [22], May-Grunwald-Giemsa [23], and Papanicolaou [18].

Diagnosis of herpes virus infections

By far, the most common setting for clinical use of the Tzanck smear is when an infection with either herpes simplex virus (HSV) or varicella zoster virus (VZV) is suspected. The cytological features of HSV (both types 1 and 2) and VZV are essentially identical, and distinguishing between the two would require clinical correlation and/or ancillary tests such as viral culture, PCR analysis, direct fluorescent antigen testing, or biopsy with immunohistochemical analysis.

Herpes virus causes characteristic cytopathic effects in epithelial cells (keratinocytes, follicular epithelium, and mucosal squamous epithelial cells) that can be readily identified on specimens prepared by the Tzanck technique (**Figure 8.7**). Namely, multinucleated syncytial giant cells are formed by fusion of epithelial cells. These cells may be acantholytic within blister fluid or adherent to the blister roof or base. The nuclear shapes of infected epithelial cells are no longer uniformly round or ovoid, but they become polygonal or crescentic as they are compressed together and mold to one another's form. Chromatin is peripherally marginated within

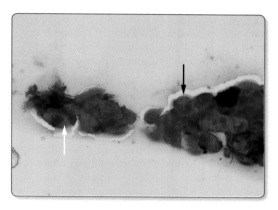

Figure 8.7 Tzanck preparation for herpes virus cytopathic effect assessment. A multinucleate keratinocyte is seen, with nuclear molding and margination of chromatin (white arrow), as well as a Cowdry A body (black arrow) (Tzanck preparation, 400× original magnification).

individual nuclei, imparting a hyperchromatic rim appearance. Additionally, infected cells may have glassy intranuclear inclusions called Cowdry A bodies.

The cardinal cytopathic effects of herpes virus infection can be remembered with the mnemonic of '3 Ms':

- **Multinucleation**
- **Molding**
- **Margination**

Diagnosis of pustular dermatoses

A pustule is a papule or papulovesicle which contains an accumulation of inflammatory cells. Microscopic examination of pustular inflammatory contents can narrow the differential diagnosis of pustular eruptions considerably.

Pustular contents can be harvested by unroofing the surface of a pustule with a 15 blade and then gently scraping the purulent material from the center and base of the pustule. The contents are transferred to a glass slide and allowed to air dry before application of a suitable stain, such as Giemsa's reagent. A coverslip is placed, and microscopic examination can be performed. The most important observation to make is the identification of the predominate inflammatory cell type. Most pustules will be formed by either neutrophils or eosinophils. Neutrophils can be recognized by their multi-lobed nucleus (typically three to five lobes) and vaguely granular cytoplasm. Eosinophils are recognizable by virtue of a bilobed nucleus with oblong or elliptical lobes, and a distinctly granular cytoplasm.

A particularly salient application of this technique is for distinguishing pustular eruptions in the neonate [19, 24]. Numerous eosinophils in pustular contents correspond to a diagnosis of erythema toxicum neonatorum. Occasionally, pustular eruptions of incontinentia pigmenti may also contain copious eosinophils. When neutrophils are identified as the predominate cell type, the diagnosis could be acropustulosis of infancy, transient neonatal pustular melanosis, or bullous impetigo [19]. Bullous impetigo may be distinguished by the additional finding of bacterial colonies and dyskeratotic acantholytic cells within the pustule smears [25].

Frozen section technique

Application to Mohs micrographic surgery

Formalin fixation followed by paraffin embedding is the standard histological technique for creating archival tissue from surgical pathology specimens. This technique has emerged as the standard histological processing technique but the time required for processing poses a limitation in some scenarios. When a short turn-around time is required (e.g. intraoperative diagnosis, etc.), frozen section technique may be used to rapidly prepare surgical pathology specimens for microscopic interpretation. In dermatology, this technique finds its widest application in the field of Mohs micrographic surgery.

A description of a rapid, reliable frozen section technique was first published in 1895 when the technique was developed by surgeons at The Johns Hopkins Hospital [26]. In the late 1800s and early 1900s, pathological diagnosis of surgical specimens was mostly made by surgeons intraoperatively based on gross findings and sometimes on microscopic findings [26]. The frozen section technique began to gain traction in the 1920s and in modern times represents an indispensible component of surgical management of disease.

In dermatology, the frozen section technique has been applied most prolifically in Mohs micrographic surgery, a form of microscopically controlled surgery first developed by Dr. Frederic Mohs beginning in the 1930s. The technique he developed now represents the standard of care treatment for many forms of skin cancer.

Mohs was a surgeon who spent his entire career in practice at the University of Wisconsin. Early in his career, he was an assistant to the chairman of the Department of Zoology and spent considerable time researching treatments for cancer. During an experiment, he made the unanticipated observation that injection of 20% zinc chloride leads to tissue necrosis as well as in situ fixation, allowing for identification of structural features on microscopy [27, 28]. From this observation, Mohs deduced that in situ tissue fixation along with microscopic examination could allow for microscopically controlled excision of cancerous tissue from patients. However, each stage of the excision could take 1 day or more because of time required for fixation [28]. In 1953, Mohs began to use frozen section technique for tissue processing in order to reduce the time needed for fixation. By 1974, the frozen tissue technique had become widely accepted for use in microscopically controlled excision [28]. Currently, frozen section technique is the standard for preparation of tissue sections using the Mohs micrographic surgery (MMS) method.

Entire texts have been written on histological preparations for MMS, and an exhaustive description of the technique is beyond the scope of this chapter. Rather, a summary of the technique will be presented with emphasis on the properties which lead to extremely high cure rates for many forms of skin cancer.

MMS is able to achieve extremely high cure rates for treatment of skin cancer largely because Mohs surgeons are able to assess 100% of operative margins of resection. This is in contrast to the traditional serial vertical sections ('bread-loaf') technique in which less than 1 percent of margins are assessed histologically. In the Mohs technique, the tumor is first debulked by curettage or sharp excision. Then a narrow margin (typically 2–3 mm) is defined around the debulked area. This margin is circumferentially excised on the oblique, at a 45° inwardly-directed angle to the skin [29, 30]. The excision is continued under the debulked surface (usually within the subcutis) in a plane parallel to the skin. Importantly, the excised specimen is marked with colored inks to denote orientation which will be critical later for mapping of positive margins.

Grossing in of the fresh tissue is done with the primary goal of converting a three-dimensional specimen into a two-dimensional histological preparation [29]. First, water must be removed from the specimen in order to prepare quality tissue sections. Frozen water crystals in tissue impede processing and create histological artifact [29]. Dehydration of tissue can be achieved by pressing the tissue between mesh gauzes [29]. Specimens are mounted onto cryostat chucks with a few drops of embedding media [29, 30]. The chuck inserts into a rapidly freezing metal bar within the cryostat, and a heat extractor rapidly freezes the tissue [29]. Horizontal sections measuring 5–7 µM in thickness are then cut with a microtome, capturing the outermost periphery (including epidermis, dermis, and subcutis) of the resected specimen [30]. These sections are analogous to en face sections but they capture 100% of peripheral and deep margins in a single plane. Sections are transferred to glass slides and fixed with acid formalin. Fixed specimens are then stained. Hematoxylin and eosin are widely used, but toluidine blue and safranin O are acceptable alternatives [29]. Excess stains are removed by clearing agents such as xylene, d-limonene, or alkanes [29].

The technique also allows for immunohistochemical staining of frozen tissue sections. Various immunohistochemical stains have been applied, most commonly melanocytic markers such as Melan-A for treating melanoma in situ, as well as cytokeratin stains for keratinocytic tumors and to assess perineural invasion.

Lastly, sections are covered with glass coverslips and are ready for microscopic interpretation. Slides are reviewed by the Mohs surgeon. When residual tumor is identified within sections, the map is referenced and orientation of the margins is recognized by color-coding of inked margins. Positive margins are then selectively re-excised using the same technique.

Once the tumor has been successfully removed, attention can be turned to repairing the defect.

MMS offers high cure rates for surgical treatment of skin cancer, and the processing and interpretation of resected tissue can be done rapidly and reliably because of the application of frozen section processing technique.

Distinguishing exfoliative dermatitis

Frozen section analysis may be used to rapidly distinguish between two important causes of abrupt-onset exfoliative dermatitis, namely toxic epidermal necrolysis (or its severity variant, Stevens–Johnson syndrome) and staphylococcal scalded skin syndrome. Toxic epidermal necrolysis (TEN) and Stevens–Johnson syndrome (SJS) are both syndromes of acute apoptosis of keratinocytes, most often caused by drug hypersensitivity. The management of TEN or SJS requires identification and withdrawal of the offending agent, as well as supportive care. Staphylococcal scalded skin syndrome (SSSS) is an exfoliative dermatitis caused by bacteremic staphylococcal infection. The bacteria elaborate an exotoxin which cleaves desmoglein 1, an important intercellular adhesion molecule for keratinocytes, leading to widespread superficial intraepidermal blistering. The management of SSSS requires antibiotic treatment. Because of the differences in managing TEN/SJS or SSSS, rapid distinction between the two diagnosis may be important.

The pan-epidermal apoptosis characteristic of TEN or SJS can be readily identified on frozen section, as can the intraepidermal cleavage of SSSS, allowing for their distinction. The analysis is done by scissor excision of a small sheet of exfoliative scale from blistered (lesional) skin [31,32]. This sample is snap-frozen, sectioned on the cryostat, and then transferred to a glass slide. Hematoxylin and eosin staining is performed per routine, and a coverslip is placed. In SSSS, frozen section will reveal an exfoliative sheet formed by an orthokeratotic stratum corneum, beneath which a few adherent or acantholytic keratinocytes will be seen. In contrast, frozen section analysis of TEN/SJS blister roofs will reveal an epidermis with full-thickness necrosis (**Figure 8.8**).

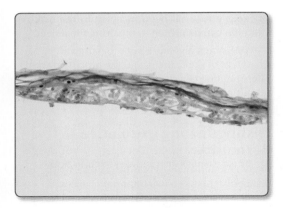

Figure 8.8 Frozen section for toxic epidermal necrolysis assessment. Section of exfoliative blister roof reveals full thickness epidermal necrosis beneath an orthokeratotic cornified layer in toxic epidermal necrolysis (hematoxylin and eosin, 400×).

Conclusion

POC tests allow dermatologists to make rapid, reliable diagnoses at the bedside, bypassing standard processing and H&E evaluation. The ability to quickly diagnose skin diseases by way of POC tests can improve patient care by leading to faster, more effective treatment interventions. While many of the POC tests used by dermatologists in current practice take their origin from observations made decades ago, they offer reproducible and reliable diagnostic tools that maintain relevance in modern clinical practice.

References

1. Kemna ME, Elewski BE. A U.S. epidemiologic survey of superficial fungal diseases. J Am Acad Dermatol 1996; 35:539–542.
2. Brodell RT, Helms SE, Snelson ME. Office dermatologic testing: the KOH preparation. Am Fam Physician 1991; 43:2061–2065.
3. Ruocco E, Baroni A, Donnarumma G, Ruocco V. Diagnostic procedures in dermatology. Clin Dermatol 2011; 29:548–556.
4. Levitt JO, Levitt BH, Akhavan A, Yanofsky H. The sensitivity and specificity of potassium hydroxide smear and fungal culture relative to clinical assessment in the evaluation of tinea pedis: a pooled analysis. Dermatol Res Pract 2010; 2010:764–843.
5. Lilly KK, Koshnick RL, Grill JP, Khalil ZM, Nelson DB, Warshaw EM. Cost-effectiveness of diagnostic tests for toenail onychomycosis: a repeated-measure, single-blinded, cross-sectional evaluation of 7 diagnostic tests. J Am Acad Dermatol 2006; 55:620–626.
6. Panasiti V, Borroni RG, Devirgiliis V, et al. Comparison of diagnostic methods in the diagnosis of dermatomycoses and onychomycoses. Mycoses 2006; 49:26–29.
7. Hicks MI, Elston DM. Scabies. Dermatol Ther 2009; 22:279–292.
8. Woodley D, Saurat JH. The Burrow Ink Test and the scabies mite. J Am Acad Dermatol 1981; 4:715–722.
9. Jacks SK, Lewis EA, Witman PM. The curette prep: a modification of the traditional scabies preparation. Pediatr Dermatol 2012; 29:544–545.
10. Brodell RT, Helms SE. Office dermatologic testing: the scabies preparation. Am Fam Physician. 1991; 44:505–508.
11. Walter B, Heukelbach J, Fengler G, Worth C, Hengge U, Feldmeier H. Comparison of dermoscopy, skin scraping, and the adhesive tape test for the diagnosis of scabies in a resource-poor setting. Arch Dermatol 2011; 147:468–473.
12. Ko CJ, Elston DM. Pediculosis. J Am Acad Dermatol 2004; 50:1–12.
13. Aylesworth R, Vance JC. Demodex folliculorum and Demodex brevis in cutaneous biopsies. J Am Acad Dermatol 1982; 7:583–589.
14. Elston CA, Elston DM. Demodex mites. Clin Dermatol 2014; 32:739–743.
15. Aşkin U, Seçkin D. Comparison of the two techniques for measurement of the density of Demodex folliculorum: standardized skin surface biopsy and direct microscopic examination. Br J Dermatol. 2010; 162:1124–1126.
16. Marks R, Dawber RP. Skin surface biopsy: an improved technique for the examination of the horny layer. Br J Dermatol 1971; 84:117–123.
17. Forton F, Seys B. Density of Demodex folliculorum in rosacea: a case-control study using standardized skin-surface biopsy. Br J Dermatol 1993; 128:650–659.
18. Barr RJ. Cutaneous cytology. J Am Acad Dermatol 1984; 10:163–180.
19. Kelly B, Shimoni T. Reintroducing the Tzanck smear. Am J Clin Dermatol 2009;10:141–152.
20. Spiller WF, Spiller RF. Giemsa stain for Tzanck smear. J Am Acad Dermatol 1983; 9:464.

21. Grossman MC, Silvers DN. The Tzanck smear: can dermatologists accurately interpret it? J Am Acad Dermatol 1992; 27:403–405.

22. O'Keefe EJ, Burke WA, Steinbaugh JR. Diff-Quik stain for Tzanck smears. J Am Acad Dermatol 1985; 13:148–149.

23. Eryılmaz A, Durdu M, Baba M, Yıldırım FE. Diagnostic reliability of the Tzanck smear in dermatologic diseases. Int J Dermatol 2014; 53:178–186.

24. Van Praag MC, Van Rooij RW, Folkers E, Spritzer R, Menke HE, Oranje AP. Diagnosis and treatment of pustular disorders in the neonate. Pediatr Dermatol 1997; 14:131–143.

25. Durdu M, Baba M, Seçkin D. The value of Tzanck smear test in diagnosis of erosive, vesicular, bullous, and pustular skin lesions. J Am Acad Dermatol 2008; 59:958–964.

26. Juan Rosai, ed. Guiding the Surgeon's Hand: The History of American Surgical Pathology. Washington, D.C.: Armed Forces Institute of Pathology, 1997, pp14–20.

27. Mohs FE. Frederic E. Mohs, M.D. J Am Acad Dermatol 1983; 9:806–814.

28. Trost LB, Bailin PL. History of Mohs surgery. Dermatol Clin 2011; 29:135–139.

29. Davis DA, Pellowski DM, William Hanke C. Preparation of frozen sections. Dermatol Surg 2004; 30:1479–1485.

30. Shriner DL, McCoy DK, Goldberg DJ, Wagner RF Jr. Mohs micrographic surgery. J Am Acad Dermatol 1998; 39:79–97.

31. Amon RB, Dimond RL. Toxic epidermal necrolysis. Rapid differentiation between staphylococcal- and drug-induced disease. Arch Dermatol 1975; 111:1433–1437.

32. Honig PJ, Gaisin A, Buck BE. Frozen section differentiation of drug-induced and staphylococcal-induced toxic epidermal necrolysis. J Pediatr 1978; 92:504–505.

Section 5

Immunofluorescence

9

Principles of immunofluorescence

Robert M. Law

As discussed in Chapters 5 and 6, selective antibody detection of human antigens via the use of immunohistochemical techniques has revolutionized diagnostic dermatopathology beginning in the 1960s. It is interesting to note that fluorescent antibody detection predated this revolution by several decades (Coons 1941). Dr Albert Coons (1912–1978) was an American immunologist and pathologist whose group at Harvard Medical School perfected techniques and optical filter protocols that allow for antigen detection on tissue sections and smears (**Figure 9.1**). Initially, this procedure was used in his laboratory to detect *Pneumococcus* in tissue sections with a high degree of specificity. This technique has since been adopted in several diagnostic subspecialties, including renal pathology as well as dermatopathology, where detection of deposited autoantibodies at target sites is essential. In 1964, Beutner described the use of indirect immunofluorescence to detect circulating antibodies in the sera of pemphigus vulgaris patients (Beutner, 1964), and Jordon subsequently reported deposition of human immune globulin at the basement membrane zone in bullous pemphigoid (Jordon, 1967) using direct immunofluorescence protocols.

The basement membrane zone

One of the target sites for autoantibody deposition is located immediately subjacent to the epithelial cell layer, and provides a substrate for cell attachment. The basement membrane zone (BMZ) is a complex region consisting of numerous interacting adhesion proteins (Woodley 2001). Within the skin, these proteins are produced by both epidermal keratinocytes as well as dermal fibroblasts. Ultrastructurally, the BMZ is subdivided into distinct subregions, each of which harbor antigens which interact with others both within subregions and between adjacent ones (**Figure 9.2** and **Table 9.1**). Based on transmission electron microscopy, there are four of these major subregions:

- Basilar keratinocyte/hemidesmosome/plasma membrane
- Lamina lucida (an electron lucent region, perhaps an artefact of dehydration (Goldberg 1986)
- An electron dense lamina densa
- The sublamina densa region within the dermal papillae

Cytoskeleton and hemidesmosome region

Assembly of the BMZ begins with keratin 5 and keratin 14 intermediate filaments within the cytoskeleton of the basilar keratinocyte. These filaments attach to the plaque-like regions known

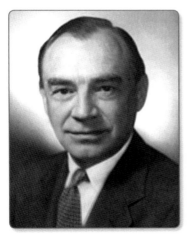

Figure 9.1 Albert H. Coons, MD (photo by Bachrach).

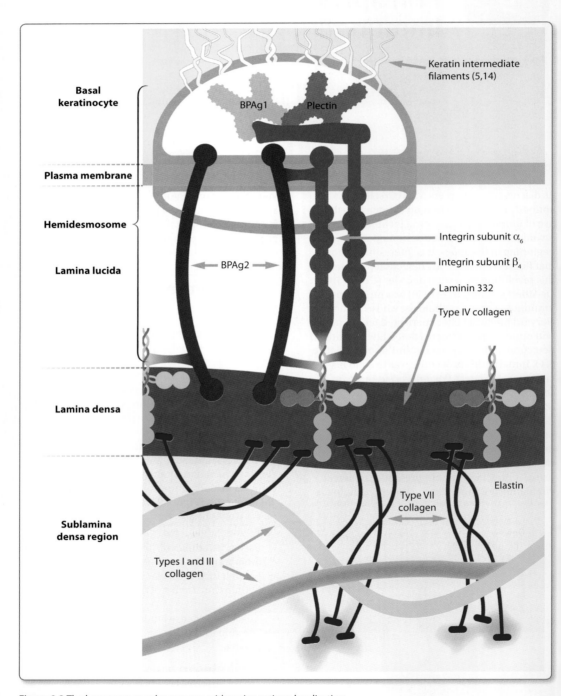

Figure 9.2 The basement membrane zone with major antigen localization.

Table 9.1 Antigen localization within the basement membrane zone (BMZ)

Ultrastructural compartment	Major antigen(s)
Basilar keratinocyte	Intermediate filaments (keratins 5 and 14)
Hemidesmosome region	Bullous pemphigoid antigen 1 (BPAG1, 230 kDa) Bullous pemphigoid antigen 2 (BPAG2, 180 kDa) Plectin β4-integrin, α6-integrin
Lamina densa	Laminin 332 Proteoglycans Type IV collagen
Sublamina densa	Type VII collagen Elastin Types I/III collagen

as hemidesmosomes. A 500 kDa protein known as plectin binds these filaments via its carboxy terminus, while its amino terminus binds such proteins as β4-integrin, bullous pemphigoid antigen 2 (BPAG2, 180kDa), as well as actin (Wiche, 1998). Bullous pemphigoid antigen 1 (BPAG1) also resides within the hemidesmosome, and is a 230 kDa protein with a globular carboxy terminus whose amino acid makeup encourages association of keratins 5 and 14. The opposing amino terminus in turn attaches to the cytoplasmic portion of BPAG2 as well as β4-integrin. BPAG2 is a transmembrane protein that then provides a linkage across the lamina lucida via association with α6-integrin and into the subjacent lamina densa through laminin 332 (Masunaga 1997).

Lamina densa and sublamina densa

The laminins are heterotrimeric proteins with varying isoform compositions of α, β, and γ subunits, each subunit variant reflected in the corresponding nomenclature. Laminins 332 (α 3β3γ2), 311, and 511 comprise the majority of isoforms found within epidermal basement membrane zones (Aumailley 1999). These heterotrimeric laminins associate with a 150kDa protein known as nidogen, which in turn binds tightly to type IV collagen. Type IV collagen is comprised of three α-chains, which

exhibit a triple-helical structure common to the family of collagen proteins. Throughout and within adjoining ultrastructural regions, acidic proteoglycans percolate, intercalate, and strengthen the scaffolding of the entire basement membrane zone. Within the sublamina densa, anchoring fibrils of type VII collagen associate with dermal collagen I, while the anchoring plaques of type VII collagen provide attachment to the overlying type IV collagen-rich lamina densa (Chen 1997). Defects in the gene encoding type VII collagen (*COL7A1*) or aberrant mRNA processing are described in both dominant and recessive forms of dystrophic epidermolysis bullosa (EB) (Christiano 1996).

Intercellular keratinocyte adhesion

While the complex interactions within the BMZ provide a firm attachment for basilar keratinocytes to the dermis, equally important is providing cell-to-cell adhesion within the multilayered epidermis itself. This is accomplished by two types of cell-cell interactions, one at the adherens (quick but weak) junction and the other at the desmosome (slow but strong). Similar to the hemidesmosome region, actin and keratin filaments provide the root of attachment between neighboring cells. The desmosome is a 'spot-weld' between cells, where keratins 1 and 10 sweep into plaque regions containing several members of the plakin family of proteins. Desmoplakin has an affinity for intermediate filaments as well as for other members of its family such as plakoglobin and plakophilin (Green 2000). Adjacent association with transmembrane proteins such as desmogleins 1 and 3 as well as desmocollin provide the direct intercellular linkage at the desmosome (**Figure 9.3**). Adherens junctions are similarly arranged, with cadherins associating with one another in the intercellular space.

Direct immunofluorescence

In many dermatologic scenarios, supplementary clinical techniques and procedures must be performed and integrated into the diagnostic

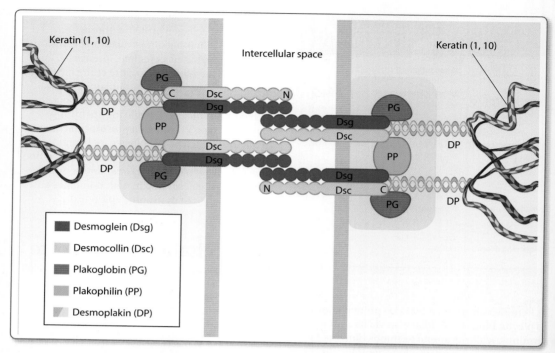

Figure 9.3 Intercellular space (desmosome) with major antigen localization.

equation. One such methodology is direct immunofluorescence (DIF), particularly when interpreted in conjunction with routine H&E histologic sections. DIF is a laboratory technique which requires special training, personnel, and equipment to interpret correctly. Specimens submitted for DIF consist of either a punch or shave biopsy of skin, placed not in formalin as for H&E processing, but rather submitted in a special transport media known as Zeus' fixative or Michel media. In contrast to formalin, these solutions do not irreversibly crosslink proteins within the sample, but provide a static but reversible 'preservative' milieu during the biopsy's short transit time to the laboratory. Unlike immunohistochemical techniques performed on formalin-fixed, paraffin embedded (FFPE) tissue, harsh methods of antigen retrieval (microwaving, protease treatment, etc.) are not necessary, and accordingly, a greater degree of detection sensitivity is afforded.

Upon receipt, the laboratory rinses away the transport media and begins the direct immunofluorescence procedure (**Figure 9.4**).

The biopsy is frozen in mounting media on a cryostat, paying careful attention to orientation. This can be particularly challenging with mucosal or conjunctival specimens. Tissue sections are taken at 5 µM thickness and mounted on a number of glass slides, one slide per target antibody probed. These sections are then incubated with commercially available, fluorescein isothiocyanate (FITC)-conjugated goat antibodies directed against human immunoglobulins, complement fractions, and fibrinogen. FITC is a photolabile molecule, and some degree of photoprotection should be ensured during subsequent steps to minimize photobleaching and signal degradation. Following incubation with the FITC-conjugated antibodies, the slides are rinsed to remove excess antibody, coverslipped, and visualized on a fluorescence-equipped microscope. Fluorochromes like FITC have a low quantum yield when excited, and therefore high levels of excitation are required for the human eye to detect the characteristic green color of FITC. The specialized fluorescence microscopes

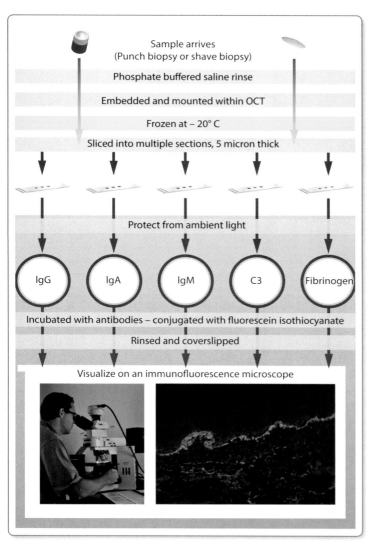

Figure 9.4 Direct immunofluorescence procedure protocol. A patient's biopsy, transported in Michels media is rinsed free of salts in phosphate buffered saline. The rinsed biopsy is mounted in optimum cutting temperature (OCT) compound and frozen on a cryostat at -20°C. Multiple 5 µM tissue sections are cut and mounted on slides. Protected from light, these slides are incubated with goat anti-human antibodies which are directed to either IgG, IgA, IgM, C3, or fibrinogen, and conjugated with fluorescein isothiocyanate (FITC). Following incubation, the slides are rinsed to remove nonspecific binding, and visualized on a fluorescence equipped microscope in a darkroom.

use a high intensity mercury or xenon arc lamp encased in quartz under high pressure. These lamps are used in conjunction with specialized excitation and emission cube filters which selectively pass specific wavelengths depending on the fluorochrome used. For FITC, the excitation wavelength is 467–498 nm and the emission wavelength is 513–566 nm. Using this procedure, a high degree of sensitivity is achieved, allowing for visualization of deposited autoantibodies within human skin (**Figure 9.5**).

Indirect immunofluorescence and special substrates

Although direct immunofluorescence probing of the patient's tissue has a very high (~90%) reported rate of sensitivity in diseases like bullous pemphigoid (Sardy 2013), ancillary testing of the patient's serum may also be useful in certain instances. Unlike DIF, indirect immunofluorescence (IIF) aims to detect

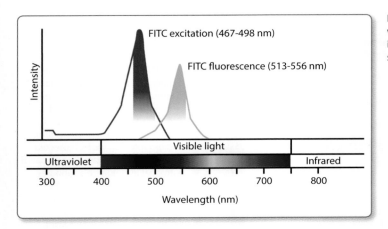

Figure 9.5 Excitation and emission wavelengths for fluorescein isothiocyanate (FITC). Visible light spectrum shown for comparison.

circulating autoantibodies utilizing the patient's serum rather than a tissue biopsy. It may be useful when biopsy is impractical or not feasible, or in instances of clinicopathologic discrepancy following initial DIF examination. IIF begins with a blood draw, and uses the patient's spun-down serum as the primary antibody step (**Figure 9.6**). The serum is incubated on special substrates, which can either be purchased or prepared by the technician themselves. Salt-split human skin, monkey esophagus, rat bladder, and guinea pig lip are all examples of such substrates, each utilized for a selected clinical scenario (**Table 9.2**). The most commonly utilized is salt-split human skin, which can be prepared by treatment of surplus human skin (foreskin, for example) in 1.0 M NaCl. This treatment induces a cleft between the lamina lucida and allows for distinction of subepidermal disease processes based on the resultant signal localization (**Figure 9.7**). Following incubation with the patient's serum, the special substrate is rinsed, and the two-step procedure continues with addition of commercially available FITC-conjugated antibodies, the remaining steps identical to those in DIF.

diseases such as epidermolysis bullosa variants are the prototypical scenario where this process is performed by the laboratory (**Table 9.3**). Immunomapping begins with biopsy of a freshly induced blister, typically induced by rotating a pencil eraser on intact skin. Old blisters must be avoided, as any degree of re-epithelialization will obscure the cleavage plane on immunomapping. The biopsy is submitted to the laboratory in immunofluorescence transport media (Zeus' or Michel), often accompanied by a second biopsy in glutaraldehyde for electron microscopy. It is rinsed, and multiple 5 µM frozen sections are cut, depending on the number of antibodies to be used in the panel. Initially, a panel consisting of anti-BP180, collagen IV, laminin 332, and collagen VII are used, possibly followed by more esoteric ones (**Figure 9.8**). Secondary detection and visualization is similar to that used in IIF. Diagnosis of the inherited mechanobullous diseases is often aided by the use of electron microscopy (Chapter 12) and mutational analysis for keratin 5 (*KRT5*) and keratin14 (*KRT14*) mutations via molecular sequencing techniques (Chapter 7).

Immunomapping

While DIF and IIF aim to detect deposited autoantibodies directed against specific antigens, immunomapping is a technique used to localize blister cleavage planes secondary to structurally defective proteins within the BMZ region. The inherited mechanobullous

Optimum specimen submission

As mentioned earlier, tissue biopsies are not submitted in formalin fixative for performing DIF, but rather in specialized transport media (Zeus' or Michel media). Both of these fluids are saturated salt (typically ammonium sulfate)

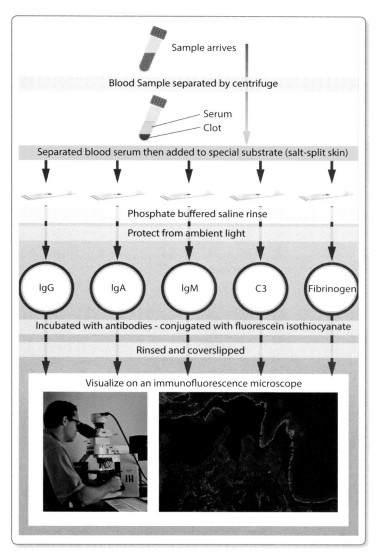

Figure 9.6 Indirect immunofluorescence procedure protocol. In contrast to direct immunofluorescence, indirect IF begins with the patient's serum, typically spun down in a red-top tube. The serum is used as a primary antibody incubation step on special substrates. Subsequent rinsing and secondary antibody probing is identical to that done for direct immunofluorescence (DIF).

Table 9.2 Use of special substrates in indirect immunofluorescence (IIF)

Substrate	Immunobullous disease
Monkey esophagus	Pemphigus vulgaris
Salt-split human skin	Bullous pemphigoid, epidermolysis bullosa acquisita (EBA), bullous lupus, cicatricial pemphigoid
Guinea pig esophagus	Pemphigus foliaceus
Rat bladder epithelium	Paraneoplastic pemphigus

solutions containing proteinase inhibitors as well as pH buffers. Cold saline may also be used, but only if transport time to the laboratory is in the order of hours, not days. There are occasions where the sample is initially and inadvertently exposed to formalin, raising questions as to the viability of subsequent testing. Reports indicate that transient exposure to formalin (2 minutes) results in loss of detectable signal in pemphigus, while signal retention is still possible in the setting

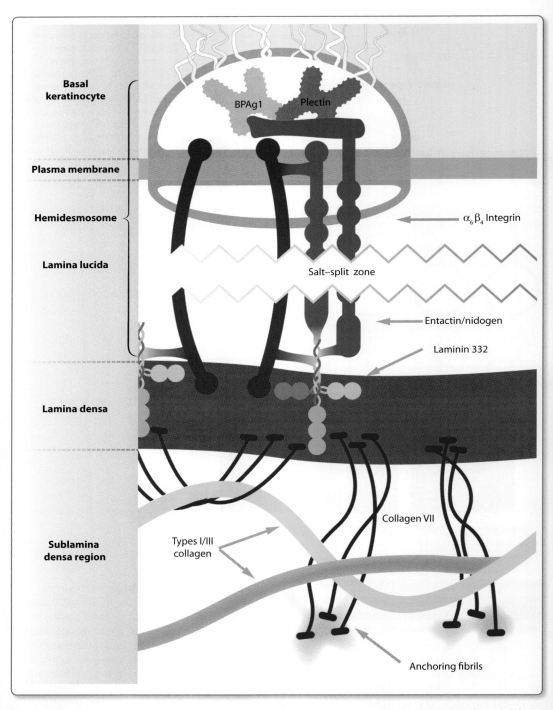

Figure 9.7 Human salt-split skin cleavage plane. Incubation of human tissue in 1.0 M NaCl induces an artifactual cleft between the lamina lucida and lamina densa, with antigen localization shown above.

Table 9.3 Mechanobullous diseases and representative defective proteins

Disease	Protein and gene
Epidermolysis bullosa simplex (EB-simplex)	Keratin 5 (*KRT5*) and keratin 14 (*KRT14*)
EB-simplex with muscular dystrophy	Plectin (*PLEC1*)
Recessive EB-simplex	BP230 (*DST*)
Junctional EB, non-Herlitz	BPAG2 (*COL17A1*) Laminin 332, various subunits (LAM) β4-integrin (*ITGB4*)
Junctional EB with pyloric atresia	β4-integrin (*ITGB4*) α6-integrin (*ITGA6*)
Junctional EB, Herlitz	Laminin 332, various subunits (LAM)
Dominant dystrophic EB Recessive dystrophic EB	Type VII collagen (*COL7A1*)

pemphigoid patients via immunoperoxidase detection and conventional light microscopy (Chandler 2009) and (Pfaltz 2010).

Biopsy location

Optimally, two biopsies are taken from the patient, one for formalin fixation and routine H&E histology, the other for direct immunofluorescence studies. A 3 mm or 4 mm punch biopsy is recommended, however, a 'scoop-shave' biopsy of small, fresh blisters is also acceptable in the setting of immunobullous disorders. Perilesional samples should be adjacent to a blister site to include the erythematous base predominantly, with a smaller peripheral 'bite' of the edge of the blister to provide an additional opportunity to assess cleavage plane. One should never biopsy an older blister or erosion, which may exhibit re-epithelialization. Other clinical scenarios will dictate biopsy location, as illustrated in **Table 9.4**.

Biopsy timing

Just as important as where the biopsy is taken anatomically is when the biopsy is taken during the disease course. Particularly in the superficial blistering diseases, sample acquisition prior to any secondary ulceration or re-epithelialization is important. In suspected vasculitis, an early stage (within 48 hours, if possible) lesion would be ideal to avoid clearance of deposited immunoreactants within vessels. On the other hand, in the connective tissue diseases such as lupus erythematosus, deposition of the classic granular band of immunoreactants takes some time, and biopsies of early lesions (less than 4–6 weeks old) may yield false negative results.

of pemphigoid and dermatitis herpetiformis after longer exposure (10 minutes) (Arbesman, 2011). Of note, this same study describes the appearance of a spurious anti-nuclear antibody (ANA) signal with formalin exposure. Therefore, it is important to communicate this accidental exposure to the laboratory to prevent unnecessary workups for a connective tissue disease.

Often, clinicians will inquire about performing immunofluorescence on formalin fixed tissue to circumvent a second biopsy. While DIF remains the gold-standard in evaluation of immunobullous diseases at this time, reports in a small series of patients have yielded promising results in detecting C3d and C4d in formalin-fixed, paraffin embedded tissue of bullous

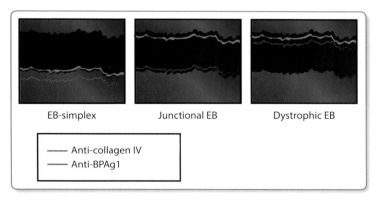

EB-simplex   Junctional EB   Dystrophic EB

—— Anti-collagen IV
—— Anti-BPAg1

Figure 9.8 Example of immunomapping displaying antigen localization in selected immunobullous diseases. In EB-simplex, the cleavage plane is within the basilar keratinocyte, so both collagen IV and BPAg1 will localize to the dermis in a fresh blister. In contrast, in dystrophic EB, type VII collagen is defective, driving both signals up to the epidermis in a fresh blister.

Table 9.4 Optimal biopsy location for direct immunofluorescence	
Disease	Optimal biopsy location
Pemphigus vulgaris	Perilesional
Pemphigus foliaceus	Perilesional
IgA pemphigus	Perilesional
Paraneoplastic pemphigus	Perilesional
Bullous pemphigoid	Perilesional
Cicatricial pemphigoid (MMP)	Perilesional skin, mucosa, or conjunctiva
Herpes gestationis	Perilesional
Epidermolysis bullosa acquisita	Perilesional
Dermatitis herpetiformis	Lesional or normal skin from disease-prone area
Lichen planus	Inflamed, but non-ulcerated mucosa or skin
Discoid lupus erythematosus	Lesional skin
Systemic lupus erythematosus	Lesional skin
Bullous lupus erythematosus	Perilesional skin
Vasculitis	Early lesion, above waist preferably
Linear IgA dermatitis	Perilesional skin
Porphyria/pseudoporphyria cutanea tarda	Perilesional

Often, patients present to the dermatologist having undergone a therapeutic course of systemic corticosteroid treatment without a confirmed positive immunofluorescence result. In this scenario, such therapy does not necessarily negate potential direct immunofluorescence results, and should not dissuade the clinician from pursuing a biopsy for DIF. Deposited immunoglobulins must undergo several half-lives (21 days for IgG) to clear completely, and short courses of steroids (less than a month) will not likely affect DIF test results.

Clinicopathologic discrepancies

False negatives

When met with a negative DIF in the setting of high clinical suspicion, it is important to consider potential causes of a false negative result. Expired transport media, biopsy of an older stage lesion or outdated laboratory reagents are all potential sources. From the laboratorians' side, daily performance of positive controls will verify correct procedures and antibody titers. However, other scenarios may contribute to a false negative result. Some commercially available anti human IgG conjugates have limited reactivity to the IgG4 subclass, and a predominant expression of this IgG4 in a patient with bullous pemphigoid may be responsible for a false-negative result (Buschman 2002). In these cases, either indirect immunofluorescence examination of serum or a sandwich double antibody (SDAI) method may be required. In SDAI, additional mouse monoclonal antibodies are used to detect specific subclasses in addition to the goat anti-human IgG primary antibody.

In addition, reports also indicate a higher rate of false-negatives in biopsies from the lower extremities. Weigand demonstrated a false negative rate of 33% in a cohort of bullous pemphigoid patients whose direct immunofluorescence biopsies were taken from the lower extremity (Weigand 1985).

False positives

False positives are typically operator dependent causes, often over-interpretation of autofluorescence. In human tissue, normal components may exhibit some degree of autofluorescence in the same spectrum as fluorescein isothiocyanate (FITC). Elastin and collagen excite at 440–480 nm and emit at 470–520 nm, overlapping FITC. When viewed in cross section, enough autofluorescent elastic fibers may mimic a granular pattern, particularly on the scalp. Other macromolecules with overlapping autofluorescence spectra include lipofuscins as well as nicotinamide adenine dinucleotide and its derivatives (NAD and NADPH). Use of tight band-pass filters rather than broad ones will help minimize autofluorescence.

One anatomic location where the interpreter should proceed with caution is the lower extremity in the setting of suspected vasculitis. In patients with chronic stasis/edema, non-specific deposition of C3 and fibrinogen can be seen in the absence of other immunoreactants such as IgG, IgM, and C3. A corresponding H&E slide helps demonstrate lack of vascular injury and avoid a false-positive DIF.

Ancillary serologic testing

Overall, direct immunofluorescence examination of skin biopsies exhibits a high degree of sensitivity (>90%), particularly in diseases such as bullous pemphigoid. In contrast, indirect immunofluorescence on special substrates tends to be slightly less sensitive (75%) (Sardy 2013). There are currently commercially available enzyme-linked immunosorbent assays (ELISA) which can detect antibodies with specific target antigens within serum, such as anti BP180 or BP230, anti Desmoglein 1 and Desmoglein 3, as well as the NC1 domain of collagen VII for epidermolysis bullosa acquisita. In addition to their specificity, these are rapid tests which also afford an additional opportunity to monitor antibody titers, and their sensitivity approaches that of direct immunofluorescence (87% pooled sensitivity) (Tampoia 2012).

References

Arbesman JG. Can direct immunofluorescence testing still be accurate if performed on biopsy specimens after brief inadvertent immersion in formalin? J Am Acad Dermatol 2011; 65:106–111.

Aumailley MRP. Laminins of the dermoepidermal junction. Matrix Biol 1999; 18:19–28.

Beutner EA. Demonstration of skin antibodies in sera of pemphigus vulgaris patients by indirect immunofluorescence staining. Exp Biol Med 1964; 117:505–510.

Buschman KS. A predominant IgG4 subclass may be responsible for false-negative direct immunofluorescence in bullous pemphigoid. J Cutan Pathol 2002; 29:282–286.

Chandler WZ. C4d immunohistochemical stain is a sensitive method to confirm immunoreactant deposition in formalin fixed paraffin embedded tissue in bullous pemphigoid. J Cutan Pathol 2009; 36:655–659.

Chen MM. Interactions of the amino-terminal noncollagenous (NC1) domain of type VII collagen with extracellular matrix components. A potential role in epidermal-dermal adherence in human skin. J Biol Chem 1997; 272:14516–22.

Christiano AM et al. Molecular diagnosis of inherited skin diseases: the paradigm of dystrophic epidermolysis bullosa. Adv Dermatol 1996; 11:199–213.

Coons AH et al. Immunological properties on an antibody containing a fluorescent group. Proc Soc Exp Biol Med 1941; 47:200–202.

Goldberg ME et al. Is the lamnia lucida of the basement membrane a fixation artifact? Eur J Cell Biol 1986; 42:365–368.

Green KJ et al. Are desmosomes more than tethers for intermediate filaments? Nat Rev Mol Cell Biol 2000; 1:208–16.

Jordon RB. Basement zone antibodies in bullous pemphigoid. JAMA 1967; 200:751–756.

Masunaga T et al. The extracellular domain of BPAG2 localizes to anchoring filaments and its carboxyl terminus extends to the lamina densa of normal human epidermal basement membrane. J Invest Dermatol 1997; 109:200–206.

Pfaltz KM. C3d immunohistochemistry on formalin-fixed tissue is a valuable tool in the diagnosis of bullous pemphigoid of the skin. J Cutan Pathol 2010; 37:654–658.

Sardy MK. Comparative study of direct and indirect immunofluorescence and of bullous pemphigoid 180 and 230 ELISA for diagnosis of bullous pemphigoid. J Am Acad Dermatol 2013; 69:748–753.

Tampoia MG. Diagnostic accuracy of ELISA to detect anti-skin autoantibodies in autoimmune blistering skin diseases: a systematic review and meta-analysis. Autoimmun Rev 2012; 12:121–126.

Weigand D. Effect on anatomic region on immunofluorescence diagnosis of bullous pemphigoid. J Am Acad Dermatol 1985; 12:274–278.

Wiche G. Role of plectin in cytoskeleton organization and dynamics. J Cell Sci 1998; 111:2477–86.

Woodley DT et al. The Basement Membrane Zone. New York: Parthenon, 2001.

10

Immunofluorescence: applications in dermatopathology

Robert M. Law

The practicing dermatopathologist must incorporate a broad armamentarium of both routine (H&E) and ancillary laboratory methods to arrive at a unified clincopathologic entity. Biochemical (Section 2) and immunohistochemical (Section 3) techniques are especially useful in infectious and neoplastic scenarios. When faced with complicated clinical presentations such as the blistering diseases and connective tissue diseases, other methods such as immunofluorescence (DIF) prove indispensible.

Immunobullous diseases

The most common clinical scenario in which direct immunofluorescence (DIF) testing is utilized is in the setting of the autoimmune blistering disorders. This is a diverse family of autoimmune diseases, with varying antigenic targets and clinical presentations. Differential diagnosis is aided by initial examination of a routine hematoxylin and eosin (H&E) stained slide, showing the predominant level of cleavage plane, followed by interpretation of the direct immunofluorescence pattern (Figure 10.1). These diseases are classified initially as those that exhibit a level of split beneath the basilar keratinocyte layer (subepidermal), and those in which the blister is located above the basilar keratinocyte layer (intraepidermal). Table 10.1 lists the entities and their corresponding level of cleavage.

Intraepidermal diseases

Pemphigus foliaceus

Clinical presentation

In this superficial blistering disorder, patients often develop crusted, scaly lesions without oral involvement. Their distribution favors the scalp, face, and trunk, and given the fragility of these blisters, only the residua of ruptured blisters often remain. The age range is broad, with a mean age of onset of 50–60 years (Stanley, 1998). These patients exhibit IgG autoantibodies to desmoglein 1 (160 kDa). One variant, *fogo selvagum*, occurs with high frequency in Brazil and Colombia, and desmoglein 1 antibodies may be initiated in certain haplotypes following a blackfly bite (*Simulium nigrimanum*).

Histologic (H&E) findings

If pemphigus foliaceus is present, routine histology demonstrates a superficial cleft within or adjacent to the granular layer. There is acantholysis as well, and often seen are 'clinging' partially acantholytic cells along the roof of the blister (**Figure 10.2a**). When intact, the blister cavity is typically devoid of inflammatory cells, but may exhibit adjacent eosinophilic spongiosis. With disruption, the blister may contain a neutrophilic infiltrate, raising impetigo as a diagnostic consideration. Of note, there is considerable histologic overlap between pemphigus foliaceus and staphylococcal

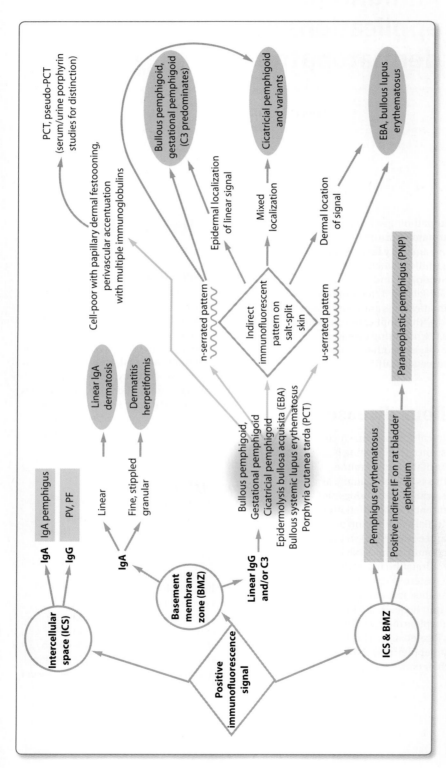

Figure 10.1 Algorithmic approach to the immunobullous diseases.

Table 10.1 Classification of the autoimmune blistering diseases

Subepidermal cleavage plane	Intraepidermal cleavage plane
Bullous pemphigoid (BP)	Pemphigus foliaceus
Epidermolysis bullosa acquisita (EBA)	Pemphigus vulgaris
Cicatricial pemphigoid	IgA pemphigus
Linear IgA bullous dermatosis (LAD)	Paraneoplastic pemphigus
Dermatitis herpetiformis (DH)	Drug induced pemphigus
Bullous lupus erythematosus	Pemphigus vegetans
Gestational pemphigoid	
Porphyria and pseudoporphyria	

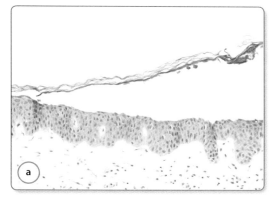

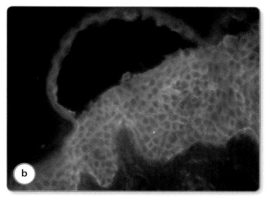

Figure 10.2 (a) Typical histologic (H&E, 100×) and (b) direct immunofluorescence (IgG) (IgG DIF, 100×) findings in pemphigus foliaceus.

scalded skin syndrome (SSS). The pathogenesis of both is similar, with a bacterial exotoxin mediating cleavage of Desmoglein 1 in the latter disease (Amagai 2000). It is particularly efficient in doing so, and unlike PF, may not leave 'clinging' acantholytic cells behind, offering a histologic clue for distinction in the absence of immunofluorescence studies.

Immunofluorescence findings

In patients with active disease, direct immunofluorescence (DIF) shows intercellular space (ICS) deposits of IgG and C3, often loosely described as a 'chicken-wire' pattern (**Figure 10.2b**). Indirect immunofluorescence (IIF) will show the same ICS pattern. Of historical interest, guinea pig epithelia offer a distinct substrate specificity for pemphigus foliaceus (Sabolinski, 1987).

Pemphigus vulgaris

Clinical presentation

A distinguishing feature of pemphigus vulgaris is the presence of oral involvement. Painful mucosal erosions will accompany flaccid blisters as well as broad areas of cutaneous erosions. These patients also exhibit lateral movement of the skin layers with rubbing (Nikolsky sign) as well as lateral spread of a blister under vertical pressure (Asboe-Hansen sign). Autoantibodies to Desmoglein 3 (130 kDa) (in mucosal dominant disease) as well as to both Desmogleins 1,3 (in mucocutaneous disease) can be demonstrated. Because these patients are at risk to losing broad areas of the barrier function of skin, they are prone to fluid loss as well as to secondary infections.

Histologic (H&E) findings

The blister cavity in pemphigus vulgaris is suprabasilar in location, with acantholytic cells often present within the cavity (**Figure 10.3a**). The naked basilar keratinocyte layer exhibits a 'tombstone' type appearance. Involvement of adnexal epithelium is a hallmark feature, and helps to distinguish between other acantholytic diseases. The superficial dermal compartment may exhibit sparse inflammatory cells, often with conspicuous eosinophils. A variant of pemphigus vulgaris, pemphigus vegetans, may also exhibit

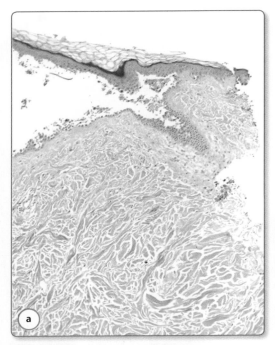

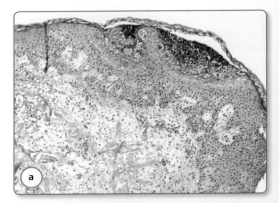

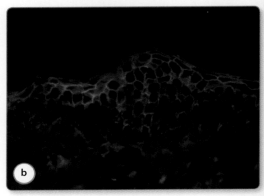

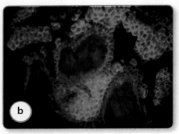

Figure 10.3 (a) Typical histologic (H&E, 100×) and (b) direct immunofluorescence (IgG) (IgG DIF, 100×) findings in pemphigus vulgaris.

Figure 10.4 (a) Typical histologic (H&E, 100×) and (b) direct immunofluorescence (IgA) (IgA DIF, 100×) findings in IgA pemphigus, SPD type.

pronounced papillomatosis of the epidermis, especially in intertriginous areas.

Immunofluorescence findings

Direct immunofluorescence (DIF) shows the classic intercellular (ICS) staining of IgG and C3 typical of the pemphigus family of immunobullous diseases (Figure 10.3b). Much like PF, PV shows the same ICS staining on indirect immunofluorescence as well, and can also be used to follow circulating antibody titers.

IgA pemphigus

Clinical presentation

There are two distinct variants of IgA pemphigus,

which usually occurs in the middle-aged to elderly population. The subcorneal neutrophilic pustular dermatosis (SPD) type and the intraepidermal neutrophilic (IEN) type both exhibit flaccid pustules or vesicles in an annular pattern, typically on the intertriginous areas as well as the trunk. In the SPD-type, IgA autoantibodies are expressed toward desmocollin 1, present within the intercellular desmosomal space (Hashimoto 1997).

Histologic (H&E) findings

As can be surmised by their names, both SPD and IEN variants of IgA pemphigus display intraepidermal aggregates of neutrophils (**Figure 10.4a**). In SPD, slight acantholysis may accompany the subcorneal pustules, and lack of adjacent spongiosis helps to distinguish this entity from mimics such as acute generalized exanthematous pustulosis (AGEP). Immunofluorescence examination is required for distinction from classic subcorneal pustular dermatosis (Sneddon-Wilkinson disease), which is DIF negative.

Immunofluorescence findings

Direct immunofluorescence classically displays intercellular (ICS) staining (**Figure 10.4b**) with IgA in the upper epidermis in the SPD type, and throughout the entire epidermis in the IEN variant (Iwatsuki, 1998). Indirect immunofluorescence may only detect circulating IgA in about 50% of cases (Mutasim 1993).

Paraneoplastic pemphigus

Clinical presentation

Described by Anhalt, paraneoplastic pemphigus (PNP) is commonly associated with neoplasms such as non-Hodgkin lymphoma and chronic lymphocytic leukemia. In adults, these two entities comprise nearly two-thirds of cases, and Castleman's disease is the most commonly associated tumor in the pediatric population. Absent from the list are adenocarcinomas (Anhalt 1990). Stomatitis with ulcerations of the oropharynx is present, accompanied by polymorphous cutaneous lesions such as blisters, EM-like lesions, or lichenoid papules.

The circulating autoantibodies in PNP are IgG directed against members of the plakin family (desmoplakin, periplakin) as well as desmogleins.

Histologic (H&E) findings

There is some variability in the corresponding histologic findings. Some lesions display suprabasilar acantholysis, others interface (EM-like) alterations, and some with combinations thereof.

Immunofluorescence findings

Direct immunofluorescence demonstrates intercellular IgG deposition with or without C3. The signal tends to be weak, and can be accompanied by homogenous deposition of both IgG and C3 at the basement membrane zone, reflecting the complicated autoantibody profile. Indirect immunofluorescence on transitional epithelium (rat bladder) is specific for PNP and shows ICS staining (Hashimoto, 2001).

Subepidermal diseases

Bullous pemphigoid

Clinical presentation

Typically a blistering disease in the elderly population, bullous pemphigoid (BP) is the most commonly encountered vesiculobullous disease. Early stage lesions may present as urticarial plaques which are intensely pruritic. The bullous stage exhibits clear fluid filled blisters, often symmetric in distribution on flexural surfaces. Oral involvement can in occur in 10–30% of patients (Di Zenzo, 2007). The antigens are well categorized, patients have circulating IgG directed against BPAg2 (180 kDa) as well as BPAg1 (230 kDa).

Histologic (H&E) findings

In the urticarial phase of BP, a blister cavity is absent, and lesions may demonstrate eosinophilic spongiosis along the BMZ or merely an eosinophilic infiltrate within the superficial perivascular compartment. The classic bullous phase will demonstrate a subepidermal blister cavity within which there are numerous eosinophils and fibrin (**Figure 10.5a**).

Immunofluorescence findings

Direct immunofluorescence (DIF) examination will demonstrate a linear pattern of deposition of IgG and/or C3 along the basement membrane zone (**Figure 10.5b**). Several other subepidermal diseases will show this pattern, and therefore, methods of distinction are required. Indirect immunofluorescence examination of patient's serum will show localization of the BMZ linear deposits to the epidermal side of salt-split human skin, as this is where BPAG1 and BPAG2 are present (**Figures 10.5c**).

Another method of distinction on direct immunofluorescence is referred to as the 'n-serrated vs. u-serrated pattern'. Although it can be sensitive to interpretation and section thickness, this pattern of serration refers to the rough 'alphabet-letter' shape of the linear DIF signal when viewed at higher magnifications. An n-serrated pattern is typical of bullous diseases with epidermal predominant antigenic targets (BP, gestational and cicatricial pemphigoid, and linear IgA disease), while a u-serrated pattern is seen in diseases with dermal targets (Type VII collagen in epidermolysis bullosa acquisita and bullous systemic lupus) (Vodegel 2004).

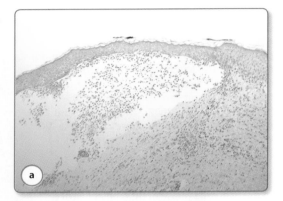

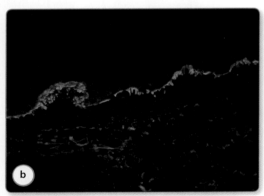

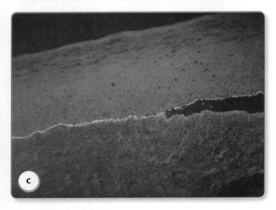

Figure 10.5 (a) Typical histologic (H&E, 100×) and (b) direct immunofluorescence (IgG) (IgG DIF, 100×) findings in bullous pemphigoid. (c) Epidermal IgG signal localization in salt-split human skin (IgG DIF, 100×).

Gestational pemphigoid

Clinical presentation

As the name implies, this variant of BP classically presents late in pregnancy, as well as within the immediate postpartum period. Blisters tend to localize on the trunk, particularly surrounding the umbilicus, and remits during the weeks following delivery. One in ten newborns can develop skin involvement due to passive transfer of antibodies. Mothers with gestational pemphigoid (GP) possess an anti-BP180 (BPAG2) IgG_1 autoantibody.

Histologic (H&E) findings

Biopsy of blisters in GP will show a subepidermal cleft with eosinophils, similar to that seen in BP.

Immunofluorescence findings

DIF in GP is unique in that a linear C3 signal predominates along the BMZ, with weak to absent IgG. Because this IgG is IgG_1, complement added indirect immunofluorescence can be performed to accentuate this weak IgG signal to exploit the strong relative avidity that IgG_1 exhibits over the IgG_4 subclass (Yancey 1991).

Cicatricial (mucous membrane) pemphigoid

Clinical presentation

True to its name, cicatricial pemphigoid (CP) often exhibits some degree of scarring. It is a heterogeneous family of diseases rather than a single entity, with varying antigenic targets (**Table 10.2**). The oral and conjunctival mucosa is involved, and the disease presents in the 60–80 year age group. Desquamative gingivitis rather than intact blisters are observed, and conjunctival

Table 10.2 Antigenic targets in mucous membrane (cicatricial) pemphigoid	
Antigenic target	**Localization in salt-split skin**
BPAG1	Hemidesmosome
BPAG2	Hemidesmosome
Laminin 332 (formerly laminin 5)	Lamina lucida/densa interface
β4 integrin	Hemidesmosome/lamina lucida

involvement can result in blindness. Concomitant cutaneous lesions may also be present in 25–30% of patients, most frequently the head and neck. One notable variant of CP that lacks mucosal involvement but can result in scarring alopecia is the Brunstig-Perry variant (Fleming 2000).

Histologic (H&E) findings

In advanced lesions of CP, scarring may predominate, but biopsy of intact early vesicles will demonstrate findings similar to that of BP.

Immunofluorescence findings

DIF studies will display a linear signal with IgG and/or C3, with a mucosal site representing a higher degree of sensitivity. Occasionally, an accompanying linear IgA signal will be present on DIF. As was mentioned previously, the heterogeneous targets of autoantibodies are reflected in indirect immunofluorescence on salt-split skin. A linear signal of IgG localizing to the epidermis is present in most patients with mucous membrane pemphigoid, while those with anti-laminin (332) CP will bind to the dermal side. An additional method of target distinction is the use of ELISA testing of patient's serum to detect specific anti-BP180, anti-laminin (332), or anti β4-integrin antibodies (Lazarova 2008).

Porphyria cutanea tarda

Clinical presentation

Patients with porphyria cutanea tarda (PCT) do not have circulating autoantibodies, but do exhibit a reduced activity of uroporphyrinogen decarboxylase (URO-D). There are both familial (autosomal dominant) and sporadic/acquired variants, the latter being the most common. In these patients, blisters occur on sun-exposed sites and are traumatically induced. Present on the back of the hands or on the face, the blisters may be accompanied by hypertrichosis or dermal sclerotic changes. The diagnosis can be confirmed by urine and plasma porphyrin studies (Frank 2012).

Histologic (H&E) findings

The blisters in PCT are subepidermal, and lack inflammatory cells. There is hyaline material surrounding the superficial vessels, which provides a structural buttress for dermal papillae,

causing them to 'festoon' or protrude into the paucicellular blister cavity. The roof of the blister can contain dense eosinophilic 'caterpillar bodies', which contain fragments of keratinocytes, intermediate keratin filaments, and basement membrane material (**Figure 10.6a**).

Immunofluorescence findings

Despite the lack of a demonstrable circulating autoantibody, the DIF pattern in PCT shows a perivascular 'donut' like accentuation, with increased signal density along the BMZ with multiple immunoreactants (IgG and C3 most commonly) (**Figure 10.6b**). Indirect

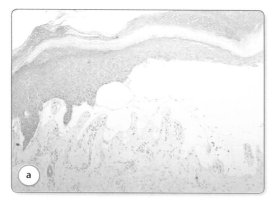

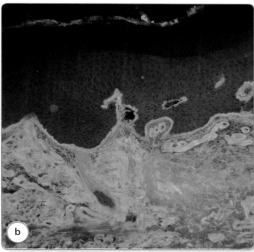

Figure 10.6 (a) Histologic findings in porphyria cutanea tarda (H&E, 100×) and (b) perivascular signal accentuation on DIF (IgG DIF, 100×).

immunofluorescence on patient serum is negative, and typically not performed.

Linear IgA dermatosis

Clinical presentation
Two variants of linear IgA dermatosis (LAD) exist, the childhood variant, and the adult onset. In the childhood variant, flexural areas and the lower trunk exhibit areas of annular erythema and blisters, referred to as a 'crown of jewels'. In adults, the eruption can involve the trunk and limbs in a similar annular pattern of blisters. Certain drugs (**Table 10.3**) have been associated with the development of LAD. Within the patient's serum, there is a circulating IgA autoantibody directed against a cleaved ectodomain of BPAG2, known as LABD97 (97 kDa).

Histologic (H&E) findings
LAD is a subepidermal blistering disease that characteristically is neutrophil rich. Early lesions may show areas of predominant neutrophils within dermal papillae, mimicking dermatitis herpetiformis (**Figure 10.7a**). Immunofluorescence allows distinction.

Immunofluorescence findings
DIF in patients with LAD shows a linear IgA signal along the basement membrane zone (**Figure 10.7b**). IIF is positive for IgA in 60–70% of patients, unlike dermatitis herpetiformis.

Dermatitis herpetiformis (DH)

Clinical presentation
Another IgA mediated disease, DH is a consequence of gluten sensitivity. It is associated

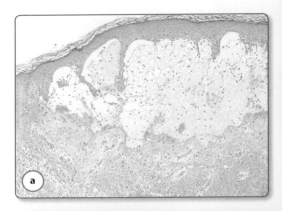

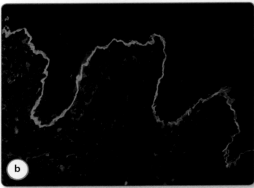

Figure 10.7 (a) Typical histologic (H&E, 100×) and (b) direct immunofluorescence (IgA) (IgA DIF, 100×) findings in linear IgA dermatosis.

with the HLA-DQ2 haplotype, and anti IgA endomysial antibodies are produced. These are IgA1 antibodies directed against epidermal transglutaminase (TG3), and localize in the dermal papillae (Sardy 2002). Patients develop pruritic papules and vesicles on the elbows, buttocks, and knees classically.

Histologic (H&E) findings
Biopsy of an intact vesicle will demonstrate a subepidermal blister with discrete aggregates of neutrophils within dermal papillae (**Figure 10.8a**).

Immunofluorescence findings
DIF will demonstrate granular deposits of IgA within dermal papillae in a majority of cases, while a continuous fine granular band may also be seen in a minority. Areas of

Table 10.3 Drugs associated with linear IgA dermatosis
Vancomycin
Penicillin
Cephalosporins
NSAIDs
ACE inhibitors
Phenytoin
Sulfonamide antibiotics

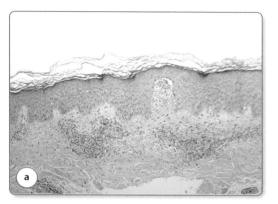

Figure 10.8 (a) Typical histologic (H&E, 100×) and (b) direct immunofluorescence (IgA) (IgA DIF, 100×) findings in dermatitis herpetiformis.

papillary dermal accentuation of this signal are invariably also present (**Figure 10.8b**). Indirect immunofluorescence does not demonstrate circulating antibodies that deposit in skin, unlike LAD.

Epidermolysis bullosa acquisita (EBA)

Clinical presentation

Not to be confused with the mechanobullous disease, epidermolysis bullosa acquisita is mediated by circulating autoantibodies to the non-collagenous (NC1) domain of type VII collagen. Patients present with skin fragility, blisters, and scarring on trauma-prone extensor skin surfaces. Equally affected are males and females, usually afflicted in the fourth and fifth decades. There is an association with

other autoimmune diseases, including Crohn's disease and systemic lupus erythematosus (Woodley 2005).

Histologic (H&E) findings

Biopsies of EBA demonstrate a paucicellular subepidermal blister similar to that seen in PCT, but lacking caterpillar bodies and papillary dermal festooning.

Immunofluorescence findings

DIF displays a thick linear band of IgG and or C3 along the basement membrane zone. As mentioned earlier, the pattern is u-serrated rather than n-serrated when viewed on higher power. Indirect immunofluorescence is also positive, and examination of salt-split skin will show a characteristic linear band that localizes to the dermal side of the cleft, where the targeted type VII collagen resides.

Bullous lupus erythematosus

Clinical presentation

True BSLE shares with EBA a circulating autoantibody toward type VII collagen. There are other blistering eruptions that occur in the setting of lupus that originate not from autoantibody production, but from underlying confluent interface change or even vasculitis. Patients with true BSLE will fulfill American College of Rheumatology criteria for SLE, demonstrate sub epidermal blisters with neutrophils, and exhibit a positive DIF with circulating anti-type VII collagen antibodies. It is rare (fewer than 0.5 cases per million population), however, African American females are more commonly affected, and present in the second through fourth decades of life (Gammon 1993).

Histologic (H&E) findings

Histologically, BSLE differs from EBA in that it is a neutrophil rich subepidermal blistering process.

Immunofluorescence findings

DIF in true BSLE is positive in a pattern identical to that of EBA, a strong linear band of IgG and/or C3 along the dermoepidermal junction. IIF examination of salt split skin will also show localization of immunoreactants to the dermal side of the cleft. ELISA testing for detection of anti-type VII collagen (NC1) domain antibodies is also available.

Connective tissue diseases

The term connective tissue disease is a broad reference to a group of diseases in which autoimmunity primarily affects collagen and the interstitium, but may also involve epithelial structures. Entities considered in the discussion of immunofluorescence techniques will include acute, subacute, and chronic lupus erythematosus, as well as dermatomyositis. Immunofluorescence is an important diagnostic aid in these diseases, but it should be emphasized that a thorough integration of all physical, serologic, and histologic findings is often required for definitive diagnosis. There are broad ranges of published positive/negative DIF rates which are highly dependent on biopsy site and disease time course (Mutasim 2001). A negative DIF finding does not in and of itself exclude a connective tissue disease.

Discoid lupus erythematosus

Clinical presentation

Patients with discoid lupus erythematosus (DLE) are typically females in the fourth decade of life. On the scalp, face, and ears, they exhibit well-defined macules or papules with adherent scale, which often extends into patulous follicles, resulting in follicular hyperkeratosis (plugging). Scarring and dyspigmentation manifest with chronicity, but progression to systemic disease (SLE) is rare. Serologic testing for circulating antibodies is negative.

Histologic (H&E) findings

Routine histology of DLE typically shows vacuolar alteration along the basilar layer with dyskeratosis and a thickened basement membrane. Follicular plugging, hyperkeratosis, and a concomitant perivascular as well as periadnexal lymphocytic infiltrate is seen; eosinophils are conspicuously absent. Interstitial mucin deposition is also present (**Figure 10.9a**).

Immunofluorescence findings

Direct immunofluorescence examination of lesional tissue demonstrates numerous cytoid bodies, most frequently with IgG and IgM. In addition, there is a granular band of immunoreactants along the DEJ, comprised of one or more immunoglobulins (IgG, IgM,

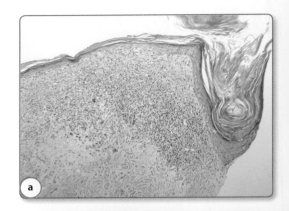

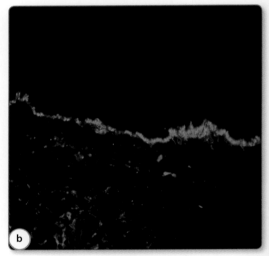

Figure 10.9 (a) Histologic (H&E, 100×) and (b) immunofluorescence (IgM) (IgM DIF, 100×) findings in discoid lupus erythematosus.

IgA) in addition to complement (C3) and fibrin deposition (**Figure 10.9b**).

Systemic lupus erythematosus

Clinical presentation

This manifestation of LE is most often associated with acute cutaneous LE and characterized by transient malar erythema following sun exposure with an occasional accompanying papular component. These lesions heal without scarring, and patients will fulfill American College of Rheumatology Criteria for SLE (**Table 10.4**) (Petri, 2005).

Table 10.4 American College of Rheumatology criteria for systemic lupus erythematosus

Clinical feature	Description
Malar rash	Fixed, flat, or raised erythema
Discoid rash	Erythema with keratotic scale, follicular plugging, scarring
Photosensitivity	UV exposure causes rash
Oral ulcers	Includes nasopharyngeal lesions
Arthritis	Two or more joints, non-erosive
Serositis	Pericarditis or pleuritis
Renal disorder	>0.5 g/day proteinuria, casts
Neurologic disorder	Seizures, psychosis
Hematologic disorder	Cytopenias
Immunologic disorder	Anti-dsDNA antibodies, anti-Sm, antiphospholipid antibodies
Antinuclear antibody	Abnormal titer, not drug related

Histologic (H&E) findings

In acute cutaneous LE, the histologic findings tend to be less pronounced than in DLE. There is more subtle basilar vacuolar change, and a milder perivascular lymphocytic infiltrate. Mucin deposition is also present.

Immunofluorescence findings

Direct immunofluorescence examination of lesional tissue will show features similar to that seen in DLE, with fewer cytoid bodies. There is granular, band-like deposition of immunoreactants along the DEJ. In addition, patients with SLE may also exhibit vascular deposition of immunoglobulins IgG and IgM in the setting of vascular injury that can be associated with systemic disease (Mutasim 2001).

Subacute cutaneous lupus erythematosus

Clinical presentation

This variant of LE is also more frequent in women and tends to be photosensitive. Patients present with an annular, scaly eruption on the head/neck, trunk, but lack severe systemic disease. These patients have an associated Ro/SSA and or La/SSB autoantibody. Other clinical presentations include a papulosquamous variant, in which patients develop more psoriasiform plaques (Sontheimer 1979).

Histologic (H&E) findings

Lesions of subacute cutaneous lupus erythematosus (SCLE) will demonstrate interface alteration with epidermal atrophy, and a perivascular lymphocytic infiltrate accompanied by dermal mucin.

Immunofluorescence findings

As can be seen in any interface dermatosis, DIF examination of SCLE will also demonstrate cytoid bodies with multiple immunoreactants. Granular deposition of IgG and IgM +/- C3 is present. A pattern peculiar to SCLE is stippled granular deposition of IgM and/or IgG within basilar epithelium (**Figure 10.10**). This is thought to arise from anti-Ro autoantibodies depositing within the skin (Mutasim 2001).

Dermatomyositis (DM)

Clinical presentation

As can be surmised by its name, DM combines cutaneous features with additional skeletal muscle manifestations. In the absence of cutaneous findings, this would be termed polymyositis. Classic skin findings include heliotrope rash, periorbital edema, and Gottron papules on the proximal interphalangeal joints. Erythema, scale, dyspigmentation, and atrophy (poikiloderma) may also be present. Elevated muscle enzymes (CK, aldolase, LDH) and circulating autoantibodies (anti-aminoacyl-tRNA synthetase and anti-Jo-1) and electromyographic findings aid in definitive diagnosis.

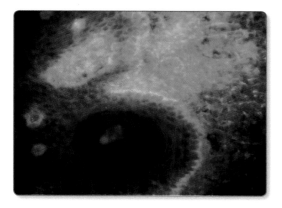

Figure 10.10 Cytoplasmic stippling (IgG) within basilar keratinocytes in subacute lupus erythematosus (SCLE) (IgG DIF, 100×).

Histologic (H&E) findings

DM histologically is best described as poikiloderma, with epidermal atrophy, interface change, telangiectasia, and pigment incontinence. Mucin deposition may be quite pronounced, and a biopsy of DM is difficult to distinguish from SCLE.

Immunofluorescence findings

Direct immunofluorescence in DM is usually weak to negative, and may consist of cytoid bodies and weak granular deposition of IgG/IgM/C3 along the BMZ. Immunofluorescence testing with anti-C5b-9 antibodies however, will demonstrate intramural deposition within vessels, supporting the hypothesis that microvascular injury plays a role in pathogenesis of DM (Magro 1997).

Other diseases

Vasculitis

Clinical presentation

Infiltration and destruction of blood vessels has a broad range of causes. Cutaneous vasculitis is separated into primary and secondary etiologies, but presents with palpable purpura, ulcers, or necrosis in severe cases. Henoch–Schöenlein purpura (HSP), connective tissue disease, infections, drug reactions, paraneoplastic processes, and autoimmune processes (Wegener's granulomatosis, Churg–Strauss syndrome) are all considerations, along with idiopathic manifestations. Injury to the vessel wall may be direct (bacteria/viruses), or indirect through the deposition of antibodies and activation of complement. An important point of distinction is the immunoglobulin class present in the setting of vascular injury, IgA versus non-IgA. Detection of IgA within vessel walls can be seen in Henoch–Schöenlein purpura, a systemic disease with involvement of renal function, abdominal pain, and arthritis. Treatment and prognosis differ in the IgA versus non-IgA mediated vasculitides, making immunofluorescence distinction important (Chen 2008; Alawani 2014).

Histologic (H&E) findings

Key to the diagnosis of vasculitis is the identification of fibrinoid destruction of vessel walls by inflammatory cells. Often present are extravasated RBCs, as well as an accompanying inflammatory background of lymphocytes, neutrophils, neutrophilic debris (leukocytoclasia), and/or eosinophils. Although there is significant histologic overlap, the presence or absence of eosinophils or granulomas should be noted, as they can raise or lower the possibility of HSP, Wegener's granulomatosis, or Churg–Strauss syndrome. Secondary surface changes of ulceration and fibrinoinflammatory exudate may also be observed, particularly in older stage lesions, biopsy of which should be avoided if at all possible.

Immunofluorescence findings

DIF examination of a fresh lesion of vasculitis will demonstrate deposition of immunoreactants within the vessel wall, often very crisp and punctate. Fibrinogen signal accentuation of these vessels is also observed. Interpretation of DIF should pay careful attention to the presence or absence of intramural IgA (**Figure 10.11**). Indirect immunofluorescence examination is non-contributory, but examination of serum for anti-endothelial antibodies is offered in some laboratories (Belizna 2006).

Oral lichen planus

Clinical presentation

Patients with classic cutaneous lichen planus (LP) rarely require ancillary studies for diagnosis, however, when patients present with isolated oral involvement, direct immunofluorescence techniques can provide a diagnostic aid. The most common presentation of oral LP is that of reticular, whitish, linear lines on the buccal mucosa. Other presentations include an ulcerative variant, and isolated gingival erosions can be seen in 10% of cases. Associated vulvovaginal LP can be seen in these patients (Goldstein 2005), emphasizing the importance of a thorough examination.

Histologic (H&E) findings

Histologically, classic LP will show features similar to those seen in its cutaneous counterpart: irregular acanthosis, dyskeratosis, and an obscuring band-like lymphocytic infiltrate (**Figure 10.12a**). This H&E pattern overlaps with several other diseases, including contact mucositis, connective tissue diseases, and chronic

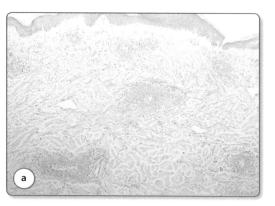

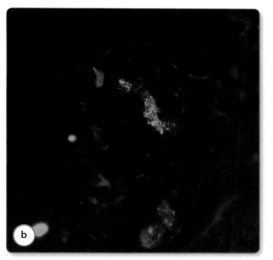

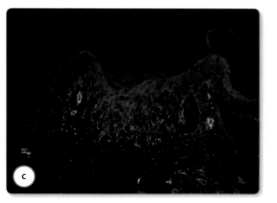

ulcerative stomatitis. In the erosive variant of LP, clinicians must take care to sample intact adjacent erythematous mucosa, as the central erosion will demonstrate only secondary findings (ulceration and fibrinoinflammatory exudate).

Immunofluorescence findings

In intact mucosa, a lesion of oral lichen planus will demonstrate bright globular cytoid bodies, positive for a broad array of immunoreactants (IgM, IgG, IgA and C3). Cytoid bodies are not specific for LP, and can be seen in any disease manifesting as an interface or lichenoid dermatitis. Therefore, more helpful in intact mucosa is the presence of fibrinogen on immunofluorescence (**Figure 10.12b**), whose

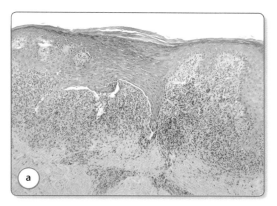

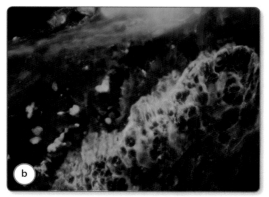

Figure 10.11 (a) Immune-complex mediated small vessel leukocytoclastic vasculitis (H&E, 100×) (b) IgM mediated (IgM DIF, 200×). (c) IgA mediated, showing punctate intramural deposition within small caliber vessels (IgA DIF, 100×).

Figure 10.12 (a) Typical histology (H&E, 100×) and (b) fibrillary fibrinogen deposition (Fibrinogen DIF, 200×) in lichen planus.

signal often extends into the submucosa in a feathery, finger-like pattern. This submucosal extension is more pronounced in buccal mucosa, and quite attenuated in gingival mucosal biopsies, where the submucosa is more dense and fibrotic than the permissive buccal region.

Chronic ulcerative stomatitis

Clinical presentation

Like erosive oral lichen planus, chronic ulcerative stomatitis (CUS) primarily affects middle aged women and presents as painful ulcerations and erosions that can come and go. Often, these patients have undergone treatment with corticosteroids, but the erosions prove recalcitrant to this approach. There have been described circulating autoantibodies to $\Delta NP63\alpha$, a protein component of stratified epithelia (Solomon, 2008). Therapy with hydroxychloroquine is beneficial in many cases, leading some to assume this may be a connective tissue disease variant.

Histologic (H&E) findings

The histologic manifestations of CUS are identical to erosive LP; namely, acanthosis with an obscuring band-like lymphocytic infiltrate.

Immunofluorescence findings

The only way to distinguish CUS from LP is via direct immunofluorescence examination of erythematous but non-ulcerated mucosa. DIF will demonstrate the presence of an in vivo anti-nuclear antibody signal (ANA), and will lack the characteristic fibrillar fibrinogen signal typically seen in LP (**Figure 10.13a**).

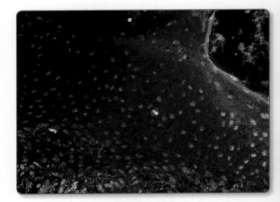

Figure 10.13 Positive in vivo ANA (IgG DIF, 100×) in chronic ulcerative stomatitis (CUS).

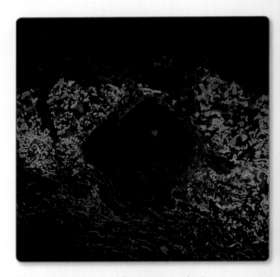

Figure 10.14 Incidental fluorescence of ochronosis deposits (FITC, 100×).

Mechanobullous diseases

As mentioned in Chapter 9, immunomapping using direct immunofluorescence techniques on a fresh blister (see **Figure 9.7**) can elucidate cleavage planes in the mechanobullous diseases. Complex cocktails of antibodies to BMZ antigenic targets can obviate the need for electron microscopy (EM) in certain instances. However, with the advent of sequencing and other molecular techniques, these nascent technologies may in turn supplant DIF in identifying defective structural proteins.

Miscellany

Occasionally, immunofluorescence examination will reveal the presence of unexpected fluorescent substances. For example, the irregular elongated deposits of ochronosis will exhibit a positive immunofluorescent signal (**Figure 10.14**). In addition, subtle amyloid deposits can be stained with thioflavin T (or thioflavin S), a more sensitive method to detect their presence under a fluorescent microscope.

Summary

The complexity of diseases encountered in dermatopathology practice often warrants the use of many ancillary studies, as demonstrated throughout this text. These diseases are complex, and their salient findings are summarized in Table 10.5. For the practicing dermatopathologist, a working knowledge of the complex macromolecular architecture of skin serves them well, and enlisting the aid of immunofluorescence examination will enable crucial diagnostic distinction.

Table 10.5 Summary of immunofluorescence findings and antigenic targets in selected immunobullous and connective tissue diseases		
Disease	**Findings**	**Target antigen(s)/notes**
Pemphigus vulgaris	Intercellular deposition of IgG and/or C3	Desmoglein 3, desmoglein 1 and 3 in mucocutaneous disease
Pemphigus foliaceus	Intercellular deposition of IgG and/or C3	Desmoglein 1
IgA pemphigus	Intercellular deposition of IgA	Desmocollin 1
Paraneoplastic pemphigus	Intercellular as well as homogenous BMZ deposition of IgG, C3. Cytoid bodies may also be present Antibodies also directed to simple or transitional epithelium (rat bladder)	Desmoplakin I/II, BPAG1(230kDa), desmogleins
Bullous pemphigoid	Linear basement membrane staining with IgG and/or C3. Salt split samples will localize to the epidermal side	BPAG1(230kDa), BPAG2(180kDa)
Cicatricial pemphigoid (MMP)	Linear basement membrane staining with IgG and/or C3. Salt split samples show variable localization	BPAG2, Laminin 332, integrins
Gestational pemphigoid	Linear basement membrane staining with C3, IgG is generally less pronounced	BPAG1(230kDa), BPAG2(180kDa)
Epidermolysis bullosa acquisita	Linear IgG and/or C3 along the basement membrane zone. Salt split samples will localize to the dermal side	Type VII collagen
Dermatitis herpetiformis	Granular IgA within dermal papillae	Anti- transglutaminase 3
Lichen planus	Clumps of cytoid bodies and fibrinogen in the basement membrane zone	N/A
Chronic ulcerative stomatitis	In vivo ANA signal	Autoantibodies to ΔNP63α
Discoid lupus erythematosus (DLE)	Granular deposition of IgG, IgM, and/or IgA along the basement membrane zone in conjunction with cytoid bodies	Lesions less than 6 weeks may show false negative immunofluorescence
Systemic lupus erythematosus	Same as for DLE	Greater sensitivity in active disease
Subacute lupus erythematosus	Similar to DLE, may also find stippled cytoplasmic deposition within basilar epithelial cells	The cytoplasmic stippling may be due to endogenous anti-Ro antibodies
Bullous lupus erythematosus	Linear IgG and/or C3 along the basement membrane zone	Type VII collagen, similar to EBA
Vasculitis	Perivascular IgA: Henoch-Schöenlein purpura Perivascular IgM/IgG/C3: other forms of vasculitis	Circulating immune complex deposition, anti-endothelial antibodies
Linear IgA dermatitis	Linear IgA deposition at the basement membrane zone	LAD-1 (97kDa): a cleaved ectodomain of BPAG2
Porphyria/pseudoporphyria cutanea tarda	Linear IgG, IgM, and C3 around vessels and dermal-epidermal junction	Elevated urine porphyrins in porphyria

References

Alawani M et al. Clinical significance of Immunoglobulin Deposition in Leukocytoclastic vasculitis: A 5-year retrospective study of 88 patients at Cleveland Clinic. Am J Dermatopathol 2014; 36:723–729.

Amagai M et al. Toxin in bullous impetigo and staphylococcal scalded skin syndrome targets desmoglein 1. Nature Medicine 2000; 6:1275–1277.

Anhalt GJ et al. Paraneoplastic pemphigus. An autoimmune mucocutaneous disease associated with neoplasia. N Engl J Med 1990; 323:1729–1735.

Belizna A et al. Antiendothelial cell antibodies in vasculitis and connective tissue disease. Ann Rhem Dis 2006; 65:1545–1550.

Chen KR et al. Clinical approach to cutaneous vasculitis. Am J Clin Dermatol 2008; 9:71–92.

Di Zenzo. Bullous pemphigoid: physiopathology, clinical features, and management. Adv Dermatol 2007; 23:237–88.

Fleming TE et al. Cicatricial pemphigoid. J Am Acad Dermatol 2000; 43:571–591.

Frank J et al. Porphyria. In: Bolognia J, Dermatology. Philadelphia: Elsevier/Saunders 2012:717–727.

Gammon WR. Epidermolysis bullosa acquisita and bullous systemic lupus erythematosus. Dermatol Clin 1993; 11:535–547.

Goldstein AT et al. Vulvar lichen planus. Clin Obstet Gynecol 2005; 48:818–823.

Hashimoto T. Human desmocollin 1 (DSC1) is an autoantigen for the subcorneal pustular dermatosis type of IgA pemphigus. J Invest Dermatol 1997; 109:127–131.

Hashimoto T et al. Immunopathology of pananeoplastic pemphigus. Clin Dermatol 2001; 19:675–682.

Iwatsuki K. IgA pemphigus. In: Vassileva S, Kanitakis J. Diagnostic immunohistochemistry of skin. London: Chapman and Hall Medical, 1998:95–104.

Lazarova Z et al. IgG anti-laminin 332 autoantibodies are present in a subjet of patients with mucous membrane, but not bullous, pemphigoid. J Am Acad Dermatol 2008; 58:951–958.

Magro CC. The immunofluorescent profile of dermatomyositis: a comparative study with lupus erythematosus. J Cutan Pathol 1997:543–552.

Mutasim DF et al. Established methods in the investigation of bullous diseases. Dermatol Clin 1993; 11:399–418.

Mutasim DA. Immunofluorescence in dermatology. J Am Acad Dermatol 2001; 45:803–822.

Pemphigus SJ. In: Freedberg IE, Dermatology in General Medicine. New York: McGraw-Hill, 1998: 654–666

Petri M. Review of classification criteria for systemic lupus erythematosus. Rheum Dis Clin North Am 2005; 31:245–254.

Sabolinski MB. Substrate specificity of anti-epithelial antibodies of pemphigus vulgaris and pemphigus foliaceus sera in immunofluorescence tests on monkey and guinea pig esophagus sections. J Invest Dermatol 1987; 88:545–549.

Sardy M et al. Epidermal transglutaminase (TGase 3) is the autoantigen of dermatitis herpetiformis. J Exp Med 2002; 195:747–757.

Solomon L. Chronic ulcerative stomatitis. Oral Dis 2008; 14:383–389.

Sontheimer RT. Subacute cutaneous lupus erythematosus: a cutaneous marker for a distinct lupus erythematosus subset. Arch Dermatol 1979; 115:1409–1415.

Vodegel RM et al. U-serrated immunodeposition differentiates type VII collagen targeting bullous diseases from other subepidermal bullous autoimmune diseases. Br J Dermatol 2004; 151:112–118.

Woodley DT et al. Evidence that anti-type VII collagen antibodies are pathogenic and responsible for the clinical, histological, and immunological features of epidermolysis bullosa acquisita. J Invest Dermatol 2005; 124:958–964.

Yancey KB et al. Herpes gestationis. In: Jordan RE, Immunologic diseases of the skin. Norwalk: Appleton & Lange, 1991:315–320

Section 6

Electron microscopy

11

Electron microscopy: background

Matthew Lewin

The creation of the first electron microscope is attributed to the German electrical engineer Max Knoll and physicist Ernst Ruska in 1931. Their microscope was capable of 400× magnification. Ernst Ruska was later awarded the Nobel Prize in 1986 for his work in electron optics. As opposed to light microscopy which uses light photons, electron microscopy (EM) uses a beam of electrons which is passed through a thin slice of the tissue sample, enabling better resolution and 4000× the magnification of conventional light microscopy.

Since the discovery of the electron by J.J. Thompson and the invention of the first transmission electron microscope in 1931 there have been many advances that have improved the quality and accessibility to ultrastructural studies (**Table 11.1**). Electron microscopy has been widely utilized in the fields of biological and medical research as well as medical diagnosis.

Types and principles of electron microscopes

There are two types of electron microscopes. The transmission electron microscope uses a beam of electrons passing through a thin tissue sample to produce a two dimensional black and white image (**Figure 11.1**). The scanning electron microscope detects secondary electrons emitted from the surface of objects to produce three-dimensional topographical information. The transmission electron microscope (TEM) is the technology more commonly used in the study of dermatologic tissue specimens. The usefulness of TEM in the study of biological tissue is that it enables high power examination of cell structures and cellular organelles not visible by routine light microscopy. The use of the TEM can aid in establishing cellular differentiation and in identifying viral particles.

Specimen handling

If it is known at the time of the biopsy that electron microscopy studies are desired, procurement of tissue for EM should be executed at the time of the biopsy. As an example, with a 3.0 mm punch biopsy (not advised to use smaller tissue samples) the specimen can be bisected with one half placed in formalin for routine paraffin embedding and processed for light microscopy. The other half should be divided into small 1.0 mm square samples. Each of these 1.0 mm samples should contain epidermis and dermis (a dissecting microscope may be beneficial in dividing the tissue) and placed in EM fixative such as glutaraldehyde or Trumps fixative and submitted to the electron microscopy laboratory for ultrastructural studies.

It is often the case that fresh tissue is not available once it is determined that electron microscopy is needed to aid in the diagnosis. In those instances, reprocessing paraffin embedded tissue for electron microscopy can be performed and the paraffin embedded tissue can be embedded in plastic for EM studies. The quality of the tissue is diminished but in most cases the tissue is of good enough quality to aid in the diagnosis.

Electron microscopy in dermatology

TEM aids in ultrastructural evaluation of skin disorders including the study of tumors, pigmentation disorders, viral infections, and blistering diseases. With the advent of other ancillary techniques including immunohistochemistry and immunofluorescence, electron microscopy is infrequently used. There are, however, rare winstances in which ultrastructural evaluation can aid in establishing the correct diagnosis in dermatologic cases.

Table 11.1 Milestones in the history of electron microscopy	
1897	Discovery of the electron by J. J. Thompson
1924	P. De Broglie: particle/wave dualism
1927	Hans Busch: electron beams can be focused in an inhomogeneous magnetic field
1931	Ernst Ruska and Max Knoll built the first TEM
1938	First scanning transmission electron microscope (M. von Ardenne)
1939	First commercial TEM by Siemens (Ruska, von Borries)
~1940	Basic theoretical work on electron optics and electron lenses (W. Glaser, O. Scherzer)
1943	Electron energy-loss spectroscopy EELS (J. Hillier)
1948	First TEM at ETH Zurich (report)
1951	X-ray spectroscopy (R. Castaing)
1956	First lattice image (J. Menter)
1957	Multi-slice method (J. Cowley, A. Moodie)
1964	First commercial SEM by Cambridge Instruments
~1970	First HRTEM microscopes with a resolution better than 4 Å
1986	Nobel prize for E. Ruska (together with G. Binning and H. Rohrer, who developed the Scanning Tunneling Microscope)
~2000	Development of aberration-corrected TEM (H. Rose, M. Haider, K. Urban)

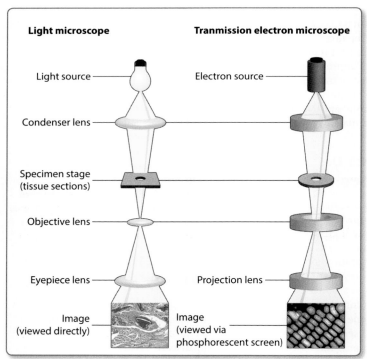

Figure 11.1 Light microscope versus transmission electron microscope.

Further reading

Stirling WS, Cury A, Eyden B, Eds. Diagnostic Electron Microscopy. London: John Wiley & Sons Ltd, 2013.

Zelickson AS. The Clinical Use of Electron Microscopy in Dermatology. Minneapolis: Bolger Publications, Inc, 1985.

Gregory A. Hosler

Electron microscopy (EM) has been extremely useful over the past century, mainly in the 1960s and 1970s, to help characterize numerous dermatologic diseases (Zelickson, 1985). Walter F. Lever (1909-1992) and Gundula Schaumburg brought EM to the forefront of dermatopathology in the 5th of many editions of Lever's *Histopathology of the Skin* (Lever & Schaumburg-Lever, 1990). In the mid-1970s, EM was coupled with immunolabeling (immunoelectron microscopy) to increase specificity and resolution of the technique, specifically for the detection of in vivo-bound immunoglobulins (Schaumburg-Lever, 1995). Today, in most cases, EM has been replaced by more cost-effective methods and/or more modern methods for diagnostic purposes. For example, cultures, immunohistochemistry, and genetic tests are now preferred over EM when characterizing tumors, inflammatory conditions, infections, and genodermatoses. In addition to the challenges in justifying the cost of EM, payers may not reimburse EM services and there is a waning supply of EM expertise, especially with non-kidney specimens. While inclusion of EM in this body of work is mainly for historical purposes, there are a few practical applications for EM in dermatopathology that still remain.

Applications

Tumor pathology

EM has played an important role for ultrastructurally characterizing tumors (Eyden, 2013). Most every tumor type, at one point, has been examined by EM in an attempt to determine lineage and ultimately shape classification schemes (**Table 12.1**). Features of the cell membrane, cell junctions, cytoplasmic shape, quantity and type of organelles and filaments, nuclear elements, and stroma all contribute to the determination of tumor lineage. Immunohistochemistry and genetic markers can now serve this function in most settings, but a few uses of EM in tumor pathology still remain. Because EM is used only as a last resort, testing often needs to be performed off paraffin sections, which can impact clarity and interpretation.

Melanoma

Occasionally, poorly differentiated tumors yield ambiguous results by immunohistochemistry. For example, a poorly differentiated or spindle cell neoplasm, based on epidermal involvement or other features, may be concerning for melanoma but immunohistochemistry is not conclusive (**Figure 12.1**). The tumor cells may have lost some combination of MART-1, S-100, SOX-10, and HMB-45 expression making distinction from a malignant peripheral nerve sheath tumor or other poorly differentiated tumor challenging, or perhaps immunohistochemistry is not possible for technical reasons. In this scenario, EM may be used to search for melanosomes, offering the only clue to tumor lineage. Type II (unmelanized) and type III (partially melanized) melanosomes are the most reliable ultrastructural melanocytic markers, although type II melanosomes have been reported in some neural, neuroendocrine and smooth muscle tumors (confirmed by immunohistochemistry). Type IV melanosomes are fully melanized and very electron dense, difficult to distinguish from lysosomes.

Langerhans cell histiocytosis

Until recently, EM was the only definitive test for Langerhans cells when characterizing histiocytic infiltrates. Both Langerhans cells and indeterminate cells are positive by S-100 and CD1a immunohistochemistry, but only

Table 12.1 Examples of EM findings in tumor pathology

Tumor category	Tumor	Finding
Adnexal tumors	Benign mixed tumor	Ducts with ductal epithelium and a myoepithelial layer, the latter likely producing stroma
	Cylindroma	Hyaline material is basal lamina with anchoring fibrils
	Hidradenoma papilliferum	Decapitation secretion and abundant secretory granules
	Hidroacanthoma simplex	Few desmosomes, decreased tonofilaments, abundant glycogen
	Hidrocystoma	Bilayer with microvilli along luminal border, typical of eccrine duct
	Myoepithelioma	Desmosomes, tonofibrils, lamina, myofilaments
	Papillary eccrine adenoma	Contains basal and luminal cells, the latter with intracytoplasmic cavities and no secretory granules
	Pilomatricoma	Ghost cells are keratin swirls surrounding nuclear remnants
	Poroma	Numerous desmosomes, eccrine duct formation with luminal microvilli
	Sebaceous carcinoma	Cytoplasmic lipid vacuoles, tonofilaments inserting into desmosomes
	Spiradenoma	Clear polygonal cell with abundant mitochondria most common cell, hyaline material is basal lamina with anchoring fibrils
	Steatocystoma	Keratinization without keratohyaline granules, typical of sebaceous duct
	Syringofibroadenoma	Features of developing acrosyringium, abundant glycogen
	Trichoepithelioma	May have perinuclear glycogen, not seen in BCC
Neuroendocrine and melanocytic tumors	Carcinoid	Cytoplasmic electron dense core granules
	Ewings sarcoma/PNET	Glycogen, neuroendocrine granules, filaments, cell processes
	Merkel cell carcinoma	Electron dense cytoplasmic neurosecretory granules, paranuclear whorls of intermediate filaments
	Cellular blue nevus	Melanosomes in both pigmented and larger more pale cells
	Dysplastic nevi	Incomplete and uneven melanization of spherical melanosomes
	Melanoma (poorly-differentiated)	Melanosomes
Hematopoietic and histiocytic tumors	Mycosis fungoides and Sézary syndrome	Cells with convoluted cerebriform nuclei and clumped chromatin
	Plasmacytoma	Immature cells with decreased rough ER
	Cutaneous atypical histiocytosis	Cytoplasmic giant multivesicular bodies, pleomorphic granules
	Indeterminate cell histiocytosis	Absent Birbeck granules
	Langerhans cell histiocytosis	Birbeck granules present
	Congenital self-healing histiocytosis	Birbeck granules in 5-25% of cells, plus concentrically laminated electron dense core bodies
	Histiocytic sarcoma	Numerous organelles, no Birbeck granules
	Interdigitating dendritic cell sarcoma	Interdigitating processes, without desmosomes or Birbeck granules
	Follicular dendritic cell sarcoma	Interdigitating processes and desmosomes, no Birbeck granules

Table 12.1 *(continued opposite)*

	Table 12.1 *(continued)* Examples of EM findings in tumor pathology	
Tumor category	**Tumor**	**Finding**
	Aggressive angiomyxoma	Prominent intermediate filaments
	Angiolipoma	Lipid vacuoles in mature adipocytes, endothelial cells without Weibel-Palade bodies
	Angiomyofibroblastoma	Lamina, attached plaques, plasmalemmal caveolae
	Angiosarcoma	Lumina without microvilli, bordered by pinocytotic vesicles
	Epithelioid sarcoma	Abundant filaments, tonofibrils, myofilaments, no desmosomes or lamina
	Hibernoma	Numerous lipid droplets and mitochondria
	Kaposi sarcoma	Tubuloreticular inclusions, siderosomes
	Liposarcoma	Lipoblasts with cytoplasmic lipid vacuoles admixed with lipid-free cells
	Spindle cell lipoma	Spindle cells resemble fibroblasts, with few lipid vacuoles
	Granular cell tumor	Granules are phagolysosomes, cell processes coated in lamina
	Neurofibroma	Mix of Schwann cells, fibroblasts, perineurial cells separated by collagen bundles and matrix
	Neurothekeoma	Features of Schwann cell, smooth muscle, fibroblast, and myofibroblast differentiation
	PEComa	Melanosomes, attachment plaques, lamina, myofilaments
	Perineurioma	Spindle cells with few organelles, pinocytic vesicles along plasmalemma
	Schwannoma	Schwann cells have entangled cytoplasmic processes but only few cell junctions
	Malignant peripheral nerve sheath tumor (MPNST)	Features of Schwann cell and perineurial differentiation
Soft tissue tumors	Glomus tumor	Resembles smooth muscle, with basal lamina encasing each cell, intermediate filaments, pinocytotic vesicles
	Epithelioid hemangioendothelioma	Immature cell junctions with intermediate filaments and Weibel-Palade bodies, intracellular lumens
	Angiofibroma	Fibroblast or fibrohistiocytic origin, endothelium with microvilli on luminal surface, stroma with banded structures, no myofibroblasts
	Giant cell tumor of tendon sheath	Features of synovial, fibrohistiocytic, and osteoblastic differentiation in stroma, giant cells with osteoclastic features
	Juvenile hyaline fibromatosis	Fibroblasts with numerous vesicles containing fibrillogranular material, same material in matrix
	Epithelioid sarcoma	Filapodia-like surface extensions, intermediate filaments, features of epithelial and myofibroblastic differentiation
	Atypical fibroxanthoma (AFX)	Fibroblastic or myofibroblastic differentiation with abundant rough ER, nuclear indentations, small cytoplasmic vesicle and cytoplasmic filaments
	Sclerotic fibroma	Widened tightly-packed collagen bundles, spindle cells around vessels have myoid features
	Fibrous hamartoma of infancy	Myofibroblastic and fibroblastic differentiation, primitive mesenchymal cells in immature areas
	Digital fibromatosis of infancy	Myofibroblastic differentiation, inclusions are masses of actin and degradation products
	Infantile myofibromatosis	Myofibroblastic differentiation with primitive vascular formation and irregular clefts between cells
	Myopericytoma	Myopericytes are elongated with irregularly thickened and duplicated basement membranes, 'peg-and-socket' junctions with endothelium, numerous pinocytotic vesicles, electron dense bodies, poorly developed rough ER and Golgi

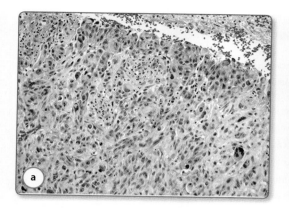

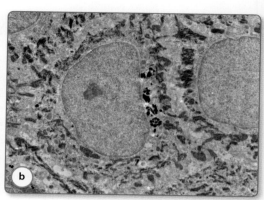

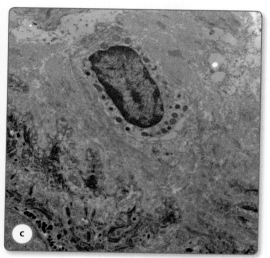

Figure 12.1 EM in the diagnosis of poorly-differentiated melanoma. On rare occasions, EM may be useful to diagnose melanoma when immunohistochemistry is inconclusive or not available. (a) This poorly-differentiated epithelioid neoplasm was negative for S-100, SOX-10, MART-1, HMB-45, and tyrosinase immunohistochemistry (not shown) (H&E, 200×). (b) Electron microscopy of the epidermis shows a keratinocyte with electron dense mature type IV melanosomes (center cell, 7100×). (c) Within the poorly-differentiated tumor cells with early (type I and II) round and ovoid melanosomes were present (center cell, 7100×).

Langerhans cells have Birbeck granules (**Figure 12.2**). Birbeck granules are cytoplasmic organelles with tennis racket or rod shapes. The rod is striated and there is often an attached electron lucent bubble, giving the appearance of a tennis racket The Birbeck granule was named after the British electron microscopist Michael Birbeck (1925-2005). The presence of these granules may help distinguish Langerhans cell histiocytosis from indeterminate cell histiocytosis or may help diagnose a pleomorphic malignancy as having Langerhans cell origin (Langerhans cell sarcoma). CD207, or langerin, is localized to Birbeck granules and its corresponding immunohistochemical test has obviated the need to perform EM, in most cases.

Mechanobullous disease

For decades, EM has been an integral part of the diagnostic algorithm for mechanobullous diseases, along with routine histology and clinical presentation (**Figure 12.3**). EM is still used today but with decreased frequency, as many institutions are moving to immunomapping (immunohistochemistry or immunofluorescence to map the split and defect) or straight to gene sequencing for diagnosis (see Chapters 10 & 16). EM's primary role is determining the level of the split (**Table 12.2**).

Metabolic diseases

The metabolic disorders affect multiple organ systems, often including the skin, which provides

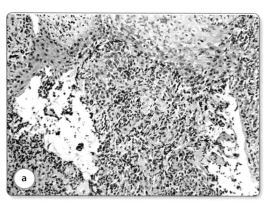

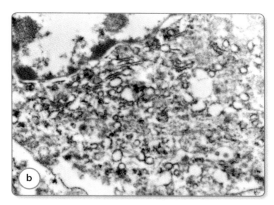

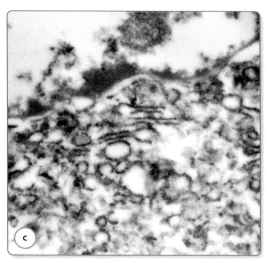

Figure 12.2 EM in the distinction of Langerhans cell and indeterminate cell infiltrates. On rare occasions, ultrastructural analysis may be required to distinguish Langerhans cell infiltrates/tumors from non-Langerhans cell infiltrates/tumors. (a) This ulcerating poorly-differentiated epithelioid neoplasm was positive for S-100 and CD1a immunohistochemistry but Langerin expression was equivocal (not shown) (H&E, 200×). (b, c) Tubular and tennis racket-shaped Birbeck granules were identified by EM, confirming Langerhans cell origin (18,000×; 36,000× respectively).

easy access for tissue diagnosis. Most of these are lysosomal storage diseases, which are typically metabolic enzyme defects ultimately leading to the accumulation of various substances within cytoplasmic organelles. Some metabolic disorders are acquired. Regarding lysosomal storage disease, there are numerous types. EM is not as useful for the specific diagnosis, but can be very helpful for excluding non-lysosomal storage diseases in the clinical differential diagnosis and can be helpful by identifying the category of lysosomal storage disease by characterizing the accumulating substance (glycolipids, mucopolysaccharides, glycoproteins, etc.) and directing further testing, such as genetic testing (**Table 12.3**) (Alroy, et al., 2013). For example, lysosomes with electron-lucent or fine fibrillar material likely contain oligosaccharides or free sialic acids, such as is observed in the mucopolysaccharidoses. If the lysosomes have lamellated membrane structures (zebra bodies, for example), the material is more likely glycolipids, which accumulate in the gangliosidoses and mucolipidoses (**Figure 12.4**).

CADASIL

Cerebral autosomal dominant arteriopathy with subcortical infarcts and leukoencephalopathy (CADASIL) is a neurologic disorder caused by mutations in *NOTCH3* (Joutel et al., 1996). Patients with CADASIL have migraines, recurrent strokes and progressive dementia. CADASIL is not a dermatologic disease but is included here because EM remains the gold standard

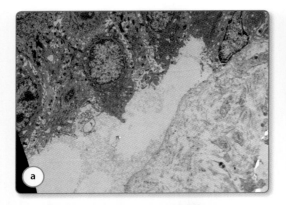

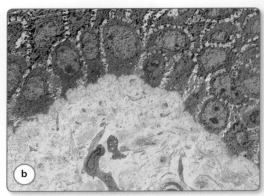

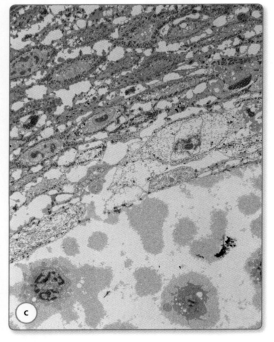

Figure 12.3 EM in mechanobullous disease. EM remains important in the ultrastructural characterization of anatomic splits in mechanobullous disease. (a, b) As an example, this newborn baby girl with mucocutaneous blistering underwent skin biopsy and EM analysis. H&E showed a paucicellular subepidermal bullous dermatosis (not shown). EM revealed retention of the lamina densa while the epidermis had fine granularity attached to its basal aspect (consistent with lamina rara remnants), suggesting a lamina lucida split (1200×; 800× respectively). A diagnosis of junctional epidermolysis bullosa was rendered. (c) In contrast, a different child presented with acral blisters and was biopsied to rule out mechanobullous disease. H&E showed mild spongiosis and prominent dermal edema with a subepidermal split (not shown). By EM, the basement membrane was intact and there was prominent dermal and intra-keratinocytic edema with retained desmosomes, excluding mechanobullous disease and consistent with a diagnosis of dyshidrosis (700×).

to detect pathologic findings and is performed on a skin biopsy. A full-thickness punch or excisional biopsy from the upper arm (non-sun-damaged) is recommended. Light microscopic examination may be normal or unremarkable, but there are distinctive EM findings. Extracellular, granular, osmiophilic material is found within the basement membranes of vascular smooth muscle cells, often causing an indentation of the membranes of pericytes and/or smooth muscle cells (**Figure 12.5**). The deposits may be ovoid or have a mushroom-like or jelly fish-like

morphology. These are best found by screening small arterioles, followed by larger vessel examination. Future diagnosis of CADASIL may shift to *NOTCH3* direct sequencing.

Other

Many other dermatologic diseases have been characterized by EM, but use of EM in the diagnostic setting is restricted to unique settings, and often as a last resort (**Figure 12.6**). Examples of EM features in select dermatologic disease are listed in **Tables 12.4–12.11**.

Table 12.2 Mechanobullous diseases

Disorder	Other names	Level of split	Other EM findings	Inheritance pattern	Gene defect(s)	Protein(s)
Epidermolysis bullosa (EB)	EB lethal acantholytic	Suprabasal		AR	DSP	Desmoplakin
	McGrath Ectodermal dysplasia-skin fragility			AR	PKP1	Plakophilin 1
Epidermolysis bullosa simplex (EBS)	Dowling-Meara	Basal	Clumping of tonofilaments	AD	KRT5	Keratin 5
					KRT14	Keratin 14
	Weber-Cockayne localized			AD	KRT5	Keratin 5
					KRT14	Keratin 14
					ITGB4	β4-integrin
	Koebner generalized			AD	KRT5	Keratin 5
					KRT14	Keratin 14
	EBS with mottled pigmentation			AD	KRT5	Keratin 5
	EBS-AR			AR	KRT14	Keratin 14
	EBS with muscular dystrophy			AR	PLEC1	Plectin 1
	EBS with pyloric atresia			AR	PLEC1	Plectin 1
	Ogna			AD	PLEC1	Plectin 1
	EBS with migratory circinate erythema			AD	KRT5	Keratin 5
Junctional epidermolysis bullosa (JEB)	JEB-Herlitz	Lamina lucida	Sub-basal dense plates absent	AR	LAMA3	Laminin-5 (α3)
					LAMB3	Laminin-5 (β3)
					LAMC2	Laminin-5 (γ2)
	JEB-non-Herlitz inversa, progressive, severe non-lethal, disentis, generalized benign, localized			AR	COL17A1 (BPAG2)	Collagen XVII (α1)
					LAMA3	Laminin-5 (α3)
					LAMB3	Laminin-5 (β3)
					LAMC2	Laminin-5 (γ2)
					ITGB4	β4-integrin
	JEB with pyloric atresia Carmi			AR	ITGA6	α6-integrin
					ITGB4	β4-integrin
Epidermolysis bullosa dystrophica, autosomal dominant (DDEB)	Pasini, Cockayne-Touraine	Sublamina densa		AD	COL7A1	Collagen VII (α1-chain)
	DDEB-pretibial			AD		
	DDEB-pruruginosa			AD/AR/sporadic		
	DDEB-toenails only			AD		
	DDEB-transient bullous dermolysis of the newborn		Perinuclear stellate inclusions	AD/AR		
	Bart			AD		

(continues overleaf)

Table 12.2 (continued) Mechanobullous diseases

Disorder	Other names	Level of split	Other EM findings	Inheritance pattern	Gene defect(s)	Protein(s)
Recessive dystrophic epidermolysis bullosa (RDEB)	Hallopeau-Siemans	Sublamina densa		AR	COL7A1	Collagen VII (α1-chain)
	Non-Hallopeau-Siemens			AR		
	RDEB-inversa			AR		
	RDEB-centripetalis			AR		
Kindler syndrome	Kindler	Variable		AR	FERMT1 (KIND1)	Kindlin-1
Laryngo-onycho-cutaneous syndrome	LOCS Shabbir	Lamina lucida		AR	LAMA3	Laminin-5 (α3)
Skin fragility-wooly hair syndrome	SFWHS	Suprabasal		AR	DSP	Desmoplakin
Nephropathy with pretibial epidermolysis bullosa and deafness		Sublamina densa		AR	CD151	Platelet-endothelial cell tetraspanin antigen 3
Macular-type hereditary bullous dystrophy	Mendes da Costa	Variable		XR	?	?

AR, autosomal recessive; AD, autosomal dominant; XR, X-linked recessive

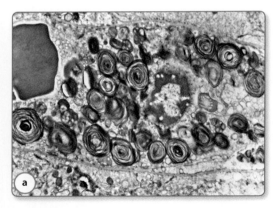
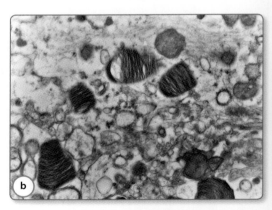

Figure 12.4 EM in the diagnosis of lysosomal storage disease. (a) This endothelial cell is filled with ~2 micron concentric membranous bodies in a patient with Niemann-Pick disease. An erythrocyte is present in the top left of the image. (b) Zebra bodies can be observed in lysosomal storage disease, such as Tay Sachs. © SynapseWeb (Kristen M. Harris and Josef Spacek, Atlas of Ultrastructural Neurocytology).

Conclusion

Electron microscopy continues to have a small but diminishing role in dermatopathology. Immunohistochemistry and molecular studies have replaced EM for most applications, but there remain select settings where ultrastructural analysis cannot be substituted. While EM may ultimately disappear from dermatopathologists' armamentarium, its historical contribution to the characterization of dermatologic disease cannot be disputed.

Table 12.3 Examples of EM findings in metabolic diseases		
Disorder	Target cell or other microanatomic compartment	Finding
Cystinosis	Fibroblasts in papillary dermis	Hexagonal cystine crystal deposits
Disseminated lipogranulomatosis	Fibroblasts, endothelium, Schwann cells	Curvilinear (Farber) bodies, zebra bodies, and banana bodies (Schwann cells)
Fabry disease	Endothelium, pericytes, fibroblasts, macrophages, myoepithelial cells	Lamellar intracytoplasmic or membrane-bound lipid bodies around vessels
Fucosidosis	Endothelium macrophages, fibroblasts, melanocytes, eccrine glands, Schwann cells	Membrane-bound granular vacuoles, lamellated bodies (Schwann cells, myoepithelial cells)
GM2-gangliosidoses	Endothelium, Schwann cells, pericytes, eccrine secretory cells, axons (Tay-Sachs disease)	Membrane bound inclusions, zebra bodies
GM1-gangliosidoses	Endothelium, Schwann cells, fibroblasts, eccrine secretory cells	Empty vacuoles
Glycogenosis	Many cell types	Glycogen granules
I-cell disease	Endothelium, fibroblasts, and many others	Electron-dense ringed vacuoles
Krabbe disease	Schwann cells	Crystalloid and tubular inclusions
Lafora disease	Eccrine/apocrine ducts	Round-to-oval juxtanuclear electron dense inclusions containing filamentous material
Mannosidosis	Many cell types	Membrane-bound granular vacuoles
Metachromatic leukodystrophy	Schwann cells	Membrane-bound herring-bone inclusions
Mucopolysaccharidoses (Hunter, Hurler, etc.)	Fibroblasts, endothelium, Schwann cells, macrophages, eccrine glands	Multiple membrane-bound cytoplasmic vacuoles with amorphous and granular material, occasional lamellar inclusions (Schwann cells)
Neuronal ceroid lipofuscinoses	Endothelium, eccrine glands, smooth muscle, macrophages	Membrane-bound curvilinear or fingerprint inclusions
Niemann-Pick disease	Fibroblasts	Membrane-bound myelin-like inclusions
Oculocutaneous tyrosinosis	Keratinocytes	Lipid-like inclusions in upper epidermis, increase in tonofibrils
Porphyria	Variable	Reduplication of basal laminae and encasement of vessels, also at DEJ (PCT and variegate porphyria), caterpillar bodies (PCT) are degenerating keratinocytes and basement membrane material, bullae have a dermal split
Sialidosis	Fibroblasts	Cytoplasmic vacuoles, lamellar inclusions (galactosialidosis)

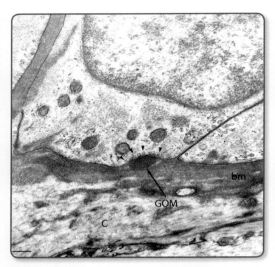

Figure 12.5 EM in the diagnosis of CADASIL. A diagnosis of CADASIL can be made by identifying granular osmiophilic material (GOM) around vascular smooth muscle cells (courtesy of Morroni M, Marzioni D, Ragno M, et al. Role of electron microscopy in the diagnosis of Cadasil syndrome: a study of 32 patients. PLoS ONE 2013; 8(6): e65482).

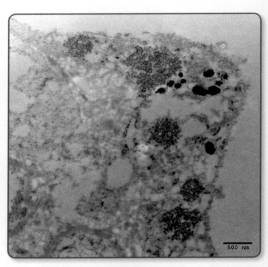

Figure 12.6 EM in the diagnosis of infection. EM can be used in discovery or as a last resort in diagnosing infectious disease. This is an example of polyomavirus virion assembly detected in the skin of a patient with an unusual undiagnosed eruption (direct magnification 22000X) (Nguyen et al. 2016).

Table 12.4 Examples of EM findings in the ichthyoses	
Disorder	**Finding (in keratinocytes or stratum corneum)**
Bullous ichthyosis (EHK)	Clumping of tonofilaments near cell membrane, prominent perinuclear endoplasmic reticulum without tonofilaments, numerous keratohyaline granules in upper layers
CHILD syndrome	Abnormal cytoplasmic lamellar inclusions in prickle layer
Erythrokeratodermia variabilis	Reduced keratinosomes in stratum granulosum, clumped tonofilaments in dyskeratotic cells
Harlequin ichthyosis	Thickened stratum corneum with lipid and vacuoles, dense core granules and loss of lamellar granules
Ichthyosis vulgaris	Defective keratohyaline synthesis with small degenerative granules
Netherton syndrome	Increased mitochondria, electron dense oval lipoid bodies in stratum corneum, premature degradation of corneodesmosomes
Refsum disease	Non-membrane-bound vacuoles in basal and suprabasilar keratinocytes
Sjögren-Larsson syndrome	Abnormal cytoplasmic lamellar inclusions of cells in granular and horny layer

Table 12.5 Examples of EM findings in infections

Infection	Finding
Cryptococcosis	Electron dense wall surrounded by clear space (and capsule)
Erythrasma	Dissolution of keratin fibers at sites of organisms
Granuloma inguinale	Organisms within phagolysosomes
Hansen disease (leprosy)	Organisms are within macrophages, eccrine glands, Schwann cells and endothelium
Herpesvirus	Enveloped icosahedral capsid with protruding tubular capsomeres
Histoplasmosis	Large eccentric nucleus and cell wall but no capsule, organisms in phagolysosomes
Malakoplakia	Michaelis-Guttmann bodies are intracytoplasmic electron-dense (and calcified) inclusions, presumed giant lysosomes, often with a concentrically layered or targetoid appearance
Monkeypox	Large, oval viral particle with laminated capsule, electron dense core with cross-hatched appearance
Molluscum contagiosum	'Brick' shaped with rounded ends, surface threading more clear than with orthopoxviruses
Papovaviruses (HPV)	Icosahedral capsid with prominent capsomeres
Parapoxviruses (ORF, Milker's nodule)	Large, 'sausage'-shaped with surface spiral threading, electron dense core with cross-hatched appearance
Pitted keratolysis	Polymorphous bacteria with a 'hairy' surface forming tunnel-like spaces between keratin fibers
Polyomaviruses	40 nm regular capsid virion particles collect in nucleus and cytoplasm
Poxviruses (cowpox, smallpox)	'Brick' shaped with thread-like structures over surface
Rhinoscleroma	Mikulicz cells are macrophages with phagolysosomes containing bacteria
Syphilis	Located in intercellular space in vicinity of vessels, and within macrophages and endothelium

Table 12.6 Examples of EM findings in hair disorders

Disorder	Target cell or other microanatomic compartment	Finding
Acquired progressive kinking	Hair shaft	Longitudinal canalicular grooves
Alopecia areata	Various	Apoptosis in outer root sheath of catagen follicles anagen hair bulbs and matrix keratinocytes, exclamation mark hairs have asymmetric cortical disintegration below frayed tip
Anagen defluvium	Huxley and Henle layers	Intercellular edema in Huxley layer, abnormal keratinization of Henle layer
Bubble hair	Hair shaft	Large cavity in shaft
Hair casts	Root sheaths	Incomplete inner layer and thicker less compact outer layer
Monilethrix	Cortex	Deviated axis of microfibrils, homogeneous nonfibrillar material
Pili annulati	Cortex, follicles	Small holes in cortex, disorder of cuticular scales, reduplicated lamina densa of follicles
Pili canaliculati et triaguli	Hair shaft and inner root sheath	Longitudinal canal in shaft, inner root sheath tonofilament-desmosomal detachment
Trichorrhexis invaginata	Cortex	Cleavages in hair and electron dense deposits in cortex
Trichothiodystrophy	Hair shaft	Cuticle scales damaged or absent, abnormal ridging of hair surface

Table 12.7 Examples of EM findings in melanin/melanocyte disorders

Category	Disorder	Finding
Hypopigmentation	Chédiak-Higashi syndrome	Giant melanosomes, large keratinocytic pigment granules
	Giscelli syndrome	Reduced type IV melanosomes, hair shafts with clumped melanin
	Hypomelanosis of Ito	Reduced melanosomes with immature forms, keratinocytes have decreased melanin granules
	Idiopathic guttate hypomelanosis	Reduced melanosomes and shortened dendritic processes, degenerative changes
	Nevus depigmentosus	Melanosomes appear normal but aggregate, decreased melanin granules in keratinocytes
	Oculocutaneous albinism	Lack of stage III/IV melanosomes (type 1A), shortened dendritic processes
	Progressive macular hypomelanosis	Aggregates of types I-III melanosomes, reduced type IV melanosomes
	Sulfonamide depigmentation	Absence of melanocytes
	Tuberous sclerosis	Reduced number and size of melanosomes, some aggregation of melanosomes
	Vitiligo	Absence of melanocytes, in transition areas, intracellular edema and vacuoles of melanocytes/keratinocytes
Hyperpigmentation	Becker nevus	Increased number and size of pigment granules in basal and prickle layers
	Café-au-lait spots	Macromelanosomes, increased subepidermal and intra-epidermal nerve fibers
	Dowling-Degos disease	Increased melanosomes
	Familial gigantic melanocytosis	Numerous stage IV melanosomes
	Laugier-Hunziker syndrome	Macromelanosomes

Table 12.8 Examples of EM findings in acquired blistering disorders

Disorder	Finding
Bullous lupus erythematosus	Deposits deep to anchoring fibrils in upper dermis
Bullous pemphigoid	Split at lamina lucida, extensive damage in cases with abundant eosinophils
Anti-p200 pemphigoid	Split at lamina lucida-lamina densa interface
Cicatricial pemphigoid	Split below basal lamina
Deep lamina lucida pemphigoid	Lower lamina lucida
Mucous membrane pemphigoid	Split in lower lamina lucida
Dermatitis herpetiformis	Split within or below lamina lucida, immunoglobulin aggregates in dermal papillae
Epidermolysis bullosa acquisita	Split within or below lamina lucida, electron dense deposits beneath lamina densa at anchoring fibrils
Friction blister	Intracellular edema with cell rupture and collections in intercellular space
IgA bullous dermatosis	Split within lamina lucida or sublamina densa
IgA pemphigus	Deposits on cell surface, not limited to desmosomes
Pemphigus (vulgaris and foliaceus)	Dissolution of desmosomes, desmosomal plaques, location depends on antigen
Paraneoplastic pemphigus	Cytoplasmic plaques
Peeling skin syndrome	Keratin filaments are not fully aggregated in area of split, keratohyaline granules poorly formed, cleavage of corneocytes
Staph scalded skin syndrome	Disruption of desmosomes, widening of intercellular space

Table 12.9 Examples of EM findings in the histiocytoses

Disorder	Finding
Benign cephalic histiocytosis	Coated vesicles, comma-shaped inclusions
Congenital self-healing histiocytosis	Birbeck granules in 5-25% of cells, plus concentrically laminated electron dense core bodies
Generalized eruptive histiocytoma	Cytoplasmic electron dense bodies, some with myelin laminations, some comma-shaped bodies
Indeterminate cell histiocytosis	Absent Birbeck granules
Juvenile xanthogranuloma	Collection of lipids, cholesterol clefts
Langerhans cell histiocytosis	Birbeck granules present
Multicentric reticulohistiocytosis	Numerous cytoplasmic rounded electron dense bodies, intracytoplasmic elastin and collagen
Progressive mucinous histiocytosis	Cytoplasmic zebra and myeloid bodies (Wong, Killingsworth, Crosland, & Kossard, 1999)
Progressive nodular histiocytosis	Cytoplasmic laminated inclusions, some comma-shaped inclusions, some inclusions with electron-lucent centers
Xanthomas (multiple types)	Numerous cytoplasmic lipid inclusions
Xanthoma disseminatum	Cytoplasmic lipid, microvilli on plasma membranes

Table 12.10 Examples of EM findings in connective tissue disease disorders

Category	Disorder	Finding
Increased elastic tissue	Colloid milium	Amorphous and granular material with wavy filaments associated with elastic fibers (adult form), whorling fibrillary masses of keratin tonofilaments (juvenile)
	Elastofibroma	Abnormal elastic fibers collecting around original fibers, adjacent large fibroblasts
	Elastoma	Increased branched elastic fibers, with sequential maturation, and without fragmentation
	Elastosis perforans serpiginosa	Increased large convoluting and branching elastic fibers
	Elastosis perforans serpiginosa (penacillamine-induced)	Thorn-like protrusions on surface of elastic fibers
	Pseudoxanthoma elasticum	Calcification of elastic fibers and collagen fibers, elastogenesis, twisted collagen fibers
	Solar elastosis	Increased tangled and degenerating elastic fibers
Decreased elastic tissue	Acrokeratoelastoidosis	Disaggregation of elastic fibers, microfibril fragmentation
	Anetoderma	Reduced and fragmented elastic fibers, elastophagocytosis
	Cutis laxa	Fragmented elastic fibers surrounded by macrophages and fibroblasts, accumulation of granular material
	Menkes syndrome	Decrease in central amorphous component of elastic fibers in reticular dermis
	Mid-dermal elastolysis	Degenerated elastic fibers and elastophagocytosis in mid dermis
Other connective tissue disorders	Corticosteroid atrophy	Variably sized and disorganized collagen fibers, microfibril globules
	Ehlers-Danlos syndrome	Variable disordered fibril aggregation and orientation (depending on subtype)
	Focal dermal hypoplasia	Fine filamentous tropocollagen within and between collagen fibers, diminished rough ER and Golgi in fibroblasts, immature fat cells, decreased elastic fibers
	Lichen sclerosus	Degeneration and regeneration of superficial dermal collagen
	Marfan syndrome	Increase in fine, fragmented elastin fibers
	Prolidase deficiency	Irregular collagen, fragmented elastic fibers
	Restrictive dermopathy	Degenerating fibroblasts, small and irregular collagen fibers with granulofilamentous deposits
	Scleroderma	Disarray and variable thickness of collagen at advancing border, endothelium contains vacuoles
	Scurvy	Defective collagen formation, alterations of endothelial cell junctions

Table 12.11 Examples of EM findings in miscellaneous dermatologic disease

Disorder	Target cell or other microanatomic compartment	Finding
Acrodermatitis enteropathica	Keratinocytes	Cytoplasmic vacuoles and lipid droplets in upper epidermis, decreased desmosomes
Amiodarone pigmentation	Macrophages	Variable electron dense deposits
Amyloidosis	Superficial dermis and epidermis	Randomly-arranged, straight, non-branching filaments, may be within keratinocytes as tonofilaments in keratin-derived amyloidosis
Argyria	Eccrine glands, macrophages	Electron dense cytoplasmic granules
Atrophie blanche	Vessels	Luminal fibrin
CADASIL	Vessels	Granular, electron dense osmiophilic material in basement membrane of vascular smooth muscle cells
Chrysiasis	Macrophages	Electron dense particles in phagolysosomes
Circumscribed acral hypokeratosis	Keratinocytes and stratum corneum	Intracytoplasmic splitting of corneocytes, with intact cell-cell attachments
Confluent and reticulated papillomatosis	Keratinocytes and stratum corneum	Increase in Odland bodies in the granular layer
Cryoglobulinemia	Vessels	Mixture of tubular microcrystals, filaments, and cylindrical and annular bodies, depending on type of cryo
Darier disease	Keratinocytes	Corp ronds have perinuclear halo surrounded by tonofilaments and keratohyaline granules, corp grains are premature tonofilament aggregates, basal keratinocyte processes extend into dermis
Follicular mucinosis	Follicles	Detached keratinocytes with intercellular granular and flocculent material
Glucagonoma	Keratinocytes	Widening of intercellular space and decreased desmosomes, vacuolar degeneration, dyskeratosis
Granuloma annulare	Dermis	Collagenolytic areas show fibrin and loss of periodic banding and fragmentation, degenerative elastic fibers
Hailey-Hailey disease	Keratinocytes	Separating and invaginating desmosomes
Hydrargyriasis (mercury)	Dermis	Large electron dense extracellular deposits
Hyperkeratosis lenticularis perstans	Stratum corneum	Persistence of desmosomal components, loss of keratohyaline granules
Incontinentia pigmenti	Keratinocytes and melanophages	Melanin phagocytosis by macrophages, dyskeratotic cells in epidermis with tonofilament clumping
Lichen planus	Basal keratinocyte	Surface cytoplasmic budding, organelle degeneration, aggregates of tonofilaments in dyskeratotic cells
Lipoid proteinosis	Dermal connective tissue	Fine collagen fibers embedded in an amorphous granular matrix, reduplication of basal lamina at the DEJ and around vessels
Malignant atrophic papulosis (Degos disease)	Vessels	Endothelial swelling with tubular aggregates and degenerative changes
Mastocytosis	Mast cells	Prominent surface projections, giant cytoplasmic granules, numerous endocytic and autophagic vacuoles
Minocycline pigmentation	Macrophages	Variable electron dense deposits
Multiple minute digitate keratoses	Keratinocytes and stratum corneum	Odland bodies present, reduced keratohyaline content
Ochronosis	Dermis	Electron dense extracellular deposits
Palmoplantar keratoderma	Keratinocytes	Variable findings, filaggrin-keratin association abnormalities, nuclear hypertrophy (punctate), lipid-like vacuoles and abnormally shaped keratohyaline granules (Papillon-Lefèvre) , membrane-coating vesicles (Vohwinkel)

(continues opposite)

Table 12.11 *(continued)* Examples of EM findings in miscellaneous dermatologic disease

Disorder	Target cell or other microanatomic compartment	Finding
Phenothiazine pigmentation	Macrophages	Variable electron dense deposits
Pityriasis rosea	Keratinocytes	Aggregates of tonofilaments in dyskeratotic cells, occasional case with viral particles
Pityriasis rubra pilaris	Keratinocytes	Numerous lipid-like vacuoles in parakeratotic areas, basal lamina contains gaps
Porokeratosis	Keratinocytes	Cytoplasmic budding at active edge, variable degenerative changes
Pretibial myxedema	Dermal connective tissue	Fragmented elastic fibers, glycosaminoglycans and glycoproteins on fibroblasts and intercellular space
Psoriasis	Keratinocytes, stratum corneum	Keratinocytes have abundant organelles, reduced keratohyaline granules
Relapsing polychondritis	Chondrocytes	Abundant electron dense granules and vesicles in matrix around chondrocytes
Reticular erythematous mucinosis	Dermal connective tissue	Fragmented elastic fibers, tubular aggregates in endothelium
Scleredema	Dermal connective tissue	Thickened collagen fibers with widening of inter-fiber space, fibroblasts with abundant rough ER
Scleromyxedema	Dermal connective tissue	Fibroblasts with abundant rough ER, proteoglycans in intercellular space
Subcutaneous fat necrosis of newborn	Adipocytes	Radially arranged or parallel needle-shaped crystals and granules within intact and necrotic fat cells
Tangier disease	Macrophages, Schwann cells	Electron lucent spherical and crystalline deposits in foam cells, lipid in Schwann cells
Waldenström macrogammaglobulinemia	Vessels	Hyaline is electron-dense granular material, no fibrils
Wells syndrome	Dermis	Eosinophil granules coat collagen fibers

References

Alroy J, Pfannl R, Ucci AA. Electron microscopy as a useful tool in the diagnosis of lysosomal storage diseases. In: Stirling JW, Curry A, Eyden B (Eds.), Diagnostic Electron Microscopy. London: John Wiley & Sons, Ltd, 2013, pp. 237–268.

Eyden B. The diagnostic electron microscopy of tumours. In: Stirling JW, Curry A, Eyden B (Eds.), Diagnostic Electron Microscopy. London: John Wiley & Sons, Ltd, 2013; 153–180

Joutel A, Corpechot C, Ducros A, et al. Notch3 mutations in CADASIL, a hereditary adult-onset condition causing stroke and dementia. Nature 1996; 383:707–710.

Lever WF, Schaumburg-Lever G, Eds. Histopathology of the Skin, 5th ed. Philadelphia: J. B. Lippincott Company, 1990.

Morroni M, Marzioni D, Ragno M, et al. Role of electron microscopy in the diagnosis of Cadasil syndrome: a study of 32 patients. PLoS ONE 2013;8:6.

Nguyen KD, Lee EE, Yue Y, et al. Novel strains of HPyV6 and HPyV7 are associated with a pruritic and dyskeratotic dermatosis (2016, in press).

Schaumburg-Lever G. New applications of electron microscopy techniques in dermatopathology. Journal of Cutaneous Pathology 1995; 22:483–487.

Wong D, Killingsworth M, Crosland G, Kossard S. Hereditary progressive mucinous histiocytosis. British Journal of Dermatology 1999; 141:1101–1105.

Zelickson AS. (Ed.). The Clinical Use of Electron Microscopy in Dermatology, 4th ed. Minneapolis: Bolger Publications, Inc., 1985.

Section 7

Molecular testing

13 In situ hybridization (non-FISH)

Pamela Aubert

The purpose of in situ hybridization (ISH) is to localize specific gene sequences while preserving cell and tissue integrity. Chromogenic in situ hybridization (CISH), bright-field in situ hybridization (BRISH) and fluorescence in situ hybridization (FISH) are essentially all the same method with different detection systems. CISH is most commonly used to detect genetic sequences unique to infectious agents whereas FISH is used to detect human germline and somatic genetic alterations. BRISH is a fairly new detection system used to evaluate for light chain restriction in tissue B-cell neoplasms. The major advantage of ISH is the preservation of tissue histology permitting anatomically meaningful interpretations in a semi-quantitative manner. One of the disadvantages for all ISH technologies is that only probe-directed sequences can be identified, requiring prior knowledge of the target and its sequence for detection. However, what ISH sacrifices in comprehensiveness it gains in specificity. In dermatology, CISH is used to detect the presence of human papilloma virus (HPV) in condylomata acuminata and Epstein-Barr virus (EBV) in cutaneous lymphoproliferative disorders. BRISH has been recently introduced as a more sensitive detection system for HPV as well as light chain restriction in cutaneous B-cell lymphomas. Both CISH and BRISH applications in dermatology are discussed in the subsequent paragraphs. FISH is discussed separately in Chapter 14 due to its expanding role in the challenging diagnosis of melanocytic neoplasms and soft tissue pathology.

Principles of ISH

ISH is the process by which a specific labeled nucleic acid probe anneals to a complementary sequence in cells of either fresh frozen tissues (stored at –70°C) or formalin-fixed tissues. One can have DNA–DNA, DNA–RNA, RNA–DNA, and RNA–RNA ISH, depending on various types of probes and targets concerned (Jin & Lloyd, 1997). Complementary RNA probes, or riboprobes, are prepared by in vitro transcription using the cDNA sequences as a template. cRNA probes are very sensitive and can be used for detection of low copy numbers during gene expression. Experimental conditions for annealing and separating the two bound strands must be optimized for each target reaction. Once bound, the hybridized probe is visualized using a detection system. In the case of CISH, the probe is labeled with an enzyme such as biotin to which a substrate such as avidin or streptavidin conjugated to alkaline phosphatase (AP) or horseradish peroxidase (HPO) is added to create a color product in a process similar to IHC. Digoxigenin-labeled probes with higher sensitivity and less background staining were recently introduced and are rapidly becoming more widely used. A positive control is always used to assess the preservation and integrity of target mRNA/DNA. Negative controls are used to test for background staining. Results of CISH can be scored using a bright field microscope. Bright-field ISH (BRISH) technology (RNAscope, Advanced Cell Diagnostics, Hayward, CA) is very similar to CISH except it uses an additional sequence-specific amplification step (of DNA or RNA targets) after a probe-hybridization step and prior to the detection step. In this way BRISH increases the sensitivity of RNA ISH signals by detecting low levels of mRNA previously undetectable by standard CISH. The final step is similar to CISH, using chromogens and bright field microscopy for visualization. Additionally, BRISH can be performed as a dual-color detection method with two targets on one slide.

This is particularly useful for comparing levels of κ and λ mRNA for assessment of light chain restriction in B-cell proliferations. BRISH uses target probes for IGLL5 and the bacterial gene dapB, on a separate slide, as a negative control and to assess background staining.

Applications

Human papilloma virus

Human papilloma virus (HPV) is a double stranded DNA virus with over 100 types that infect human skin and mucosa. In dermatology, persistent HPV infection with particular strains is associated with a number of clinical presentations (**Table 13.1**). HPV strains are divided into low-risk or high-risk types based on their propensity to cause cervical dysplasia and dysplasia in other organ systems. High risk HPV integration into human cells is tumorigenic. The E7 gene product of HPV binds to retinoblastoma protein, causing its functional inactivation leading to progression of the cell cycle (Dyson et al. 1989). In dermatology, low-risk HPV types are associated with benign cutaneous lesions such as condylomata acuminata (HPV 6, 11) whereas high-risk HPV types are implicated in carcinomas such as in squamous cell carcinoma in situ, Bowen's disease (HPV 16, 18). Exceptions to this rule include verrucous carcinoma and its variants including oral florid papillomatosis, Buschke-Lowenstein tumor and epithelioma cuniculatum,

which are low-grade malignancies associated with low-risk HPV types 6 and 11.

HPV cannot be cultured and serologic tests do not distinguish between previous exposure and active disease. Therefore, the only method to detect the virus is to analyze lesional tissue. CISH with RNA probes has been the most effective method to date to detect HPV in cutaneous samples. Immunohistochemistry against p16 can also be used for high risk HPV types. p16 is a cyclin-dependent kinase required for cell cycle regulation that is increased through a negative feedback loop after functional inactivation of retinoblastoma protein by E7 (Dyson et al. 1989). Commercially available HPV ISH assays are available; however, none have been FDA approved. These include GenPoint HPV Probes (Dako, Glostrup, Denmark), ZytoFast HPV Probes (Zyto Vision, Bremerhaven, Germany), PathoGene HPV probes (Enzo Life Sciences, Plymouth Meeting, PA), Pan Human Papillomavirus Probe (Life Technologies, Thermo Fisher Scientific, Waltham, MA), and INFORM HPV (Ventana, Tuscon, AZ). These assays are cocktails of probes specific to low-risk, high-risk or a combination of low-risk and high-risk viral types, so called pan-HPV assays. While the most common high- and low- risk types are included, some of the less common types are omitted, resulting in potential false-negative reactions and decreasing the assay's utility in conditions caused by rare HPV types such as Heck's disease

Table 13.1 Clinical manifestations associated with HPV infection	
Clinical manifestation	Most common HPV types
Verruca vulgaris	1, 2, 4
Butcher's wart	7
Verruca plana	3, 10
Verruca palmoplantaris	1, 4
Condyloma acuminatum	6, 11
Giant condyloma of Buschke and Lowenstein	6, 11
Squamous papilloma (oral)	6, 11
Focal epithelial hyperplasia (Heck's disease)	13, 32
Epidermodysplasia verruciformis	5, 8
Bowen's disease, Bowenoid papulosis	16, 18, 31, 33, 51
Squamous cell carcinoma	5, 8, 16, 18, 31, 33, 51

(HPV 13, 32). Nonetheless, low-risk cocktails have been useful for differentiating condylomata acuminata from seborrheic keratoses and skin tags (**Figure 13.1**). HPV assays have suffered from low sensitivity when assessing older senescent condylomas with low viral copy numbers. However, more recent advances in RNA ISH technology, namely the BRISH technique discussed in more detail in the section on light chain detection, have improved sensitivity and specificity in the 90% range (Schache et al., 2013). High risk HPV ISH can be useful when the histologic differential diagnosis includes both reactive changes and high grade HPV driven lesions. This particular attribute of high risk HPV ISH is exploited for the diagnosis of cervical

neoplasia, vulvar neoplasia, anal neoplasia, and oropharyngeal squamous cell carcinomas (Ukpo et al. 2011). Furthermore, the detection of the HPV in oropharyngeal SCC has prognostic implications (Fakhry et al. 2008).

As mentioned, commercially available ISH assays for HPV detection use cocktails of probes to HPV subtypes. The desire to detect HPV, from a diagnostic perspective, usually can be satisfied by using low-risk, high-risk and/or pan HPV cocktails or probes. Rarely, there are situations when detection of a specific HPV subtype is warranted, such as epidemiological tracking of an infection or detecting an unusual HPV subtype and/or disorder, such as Heck's disease. For these purposes, specific lab-developed tests (more likely by PCR-based assays or next-generation sequencing, see Chapter 16) must be used and may not be currently available outside of the research setting.

Epstein–Barr virus

Epstein–Barr Virus (EBV) is a double stranded DNA member of the gamma herpesvirus family of viruses. It is a B-cell lymphotropic virus and its incorporation into the nucleus of B cells can lead to B-cell immortalization. Even in healthy persons, small numbers of EBV-infected B cells are detectable but latent, with possible reactivation at a later time. EBV-infected lymphocytes are more susceptible to other genetic mutations including those of proto-oncogenes. With immunosuppression, there is a decreased ability of the cytotoxic T lymphocyte to respond to the viral antigen, leading to unsuppressed growth of the virus and of transformed lymphocytes. EBV infections are associated with a broad range of lymphoproliferative disorders: Hodgkin lymphoma, Burkitt lymphoma, other specific non-Hodgkin lymphomas, post-organ transplantation lymphoproliferative disorders, nasopharyngeal carcinoma and gastric carcinoma. During latent EBV infection of lymphocytes, the virus expresses a small number of EBV nuclear antigens (EBNAs) and latent membrane proteins (LMPs). Immunohistochemical stains are available against EBNA1, EBNA2, LMP1 and LMP2 and are a reasonable cost-effective method of EBV detection. *EBER1* and *EBER2* genes are EBV genes that are also expressed early during latent EBV infection of lymphocytes and code

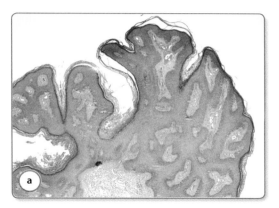

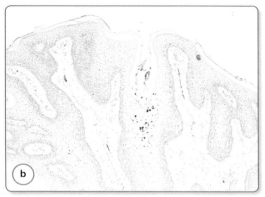

Figure 13.1 HPV ISH in a condyloma acuminatum. (a) This condyloma acuminatum is papillomatous, without definitive viral cytopathic effect (H&E, 20×). (b) HPV in situ hybridization highlights nuclear positivity of spinous layer keratinocytes within the dells of the thickened papillomatous epidermis (HPV ISH, 40×).

for small mRNAs (EBERs) that are expressed in high amounts throughout the course of latent infection. ISH with nonisotopic-labeled oligonucleotides, or riboprobes, have been developed to detect EBERs (Chang et al. 1992). Detection of EBV within hematopoietic and epithelial proliferations by EBER ISH techniques is a more sensitive method as compared to EBNA or LMP immunohistochemistry. Select neoplastic disorders are discussed in more detail below as they can present in the skin either as a primary cutaneous disease or secondarily as metastatic spread (**Table 13.2**).

Hydroa vacciniforme-like lymphoma

Hydroa vacciniforme-like lymphoma (HVLL) is a cutaneous T-cell lymphoma afflicting children and adolescents from Asia, Mexico, and Central and South America. In addition to the vesicular sun-induced facial eruption typical of hydroa vacciniforme, HVLL presents with marked facial edema, ulceration, and facial disfigurement in both photo-exposed and photo-protected areas. Systemic symptoms can occur late in its course and portend a poor prognosis. The infiltrate is composed of small to medium sized lymphocytes expressing a CD8+ cytotoxic profile (TIA-1+, perforin+ or granzyme B+) and less commonly CD56+ indicating an NK/T cell phenotype. There is prominent angiocentricity and angiodestruction throughout the dermis with overlying ulceration. EBV chronic infection likely plays a pathogenic role, and as such, EBER ISH

positivity is required for diagnosis (Quintanilla-Martinez et al. 2013a). There is marked morphologic and histologic overlap between hydroa vacciniforme and HVLL, however all cases with positive TCR rearrangements (see Chapter 15) in this differential diagnosis should be classified as HVLL (Quintanilla-Martinez et al. 2013b).

Hodgkin lymphoma

Hodgkin lymphoma (HL) is a lymphoma of B-cell origin with a bimodal distribution, peaking in both young adults and the elderly. It is characterized by painless lymphadenopathy with frequent mediastinal involvement and constitutional B symptoms. HL is classified into nodular lymphocyte predominant HL and classical HL, the latter making up >95% of cases of HL in the USA and all cases with cutaneous involvement. Classical HL is further subdivided into 4 categories:

1. Nodular sclerosis
2. Mixed cellularity
3. Lymphocyte rich
4. Lymphocyte depleted

Cutaneous involvement is uncommon and occurs most often on the trunk in advanced stages as direct extension from mediastinal disease or lymphatic retrograde spread. Primary cutaneous HL is exceedingly rare and has been debated as a real entity. Some reported cases in the literature may have been T-cell rich CD30-positive large B-cell lymphoma and others have been reclassified as EBV mucocutaneous ulcers. In the setting of the human immunodeficiency virus (HIV), primary cutaneous HL can have an aggressive course, depending on the underlying immune status of the host. The role of EBV in the evolution of HL is well established, identified in 40–50% of cases of classical HL, most commonly in the mixed cellularity subtype and in immunosuppressed patients (Glaser et al. 1997). Classical HL cutaneous lesions are similar histologically to their nodal counterparts with a dense nodular infiltrate composed mostly of reactive inflammatory cells and few scattered neoplastic Hodgkin Reed-Sternberg (HRS) cells. The diagnosis rests on identifying the HRS, which are Pax5+, CD30+ and CD15+, but CD45- and CD20+/-. EBV associated cases will be positive for EBV ISH in malignant HRS cells.

Table 13.2 EBV+ lymphoproliferative disorders with cutaneous manifestations
Hydroa vacciniforme-like lymphoma (HVLL)
Hodgkin lymphoma (HL)
Lymphomatoid granulomatosis (LG)
EBV-positive diffuse large B cell lymphoma (DLBCL) of the elderly
Nasal and (related) extranodal NK/T-cell lymphoma
Post-transplant lymphoproliferative disease (PTLD)
Methotrexate/cyclosporin A (CsA) associated lymphoproliferative disease
HIV-related lymphomas
Endemic Burkitt lymphoma
Angioimmunoblastic T-cell lymphoma

Lymphomatoid granulomatosis

Lymphomatoid granulomatosis (LG) results from a dysregulated CD4 T-cell response to EBV-infected B cells. There is frequent malignant transformation into a large B-cell lymphoma in middle-aged adults. LG invariably affects the lungs and up to 50% of patients will develop skin lesions including subcutaneous nodules, plaques, ulcers or erythroderma. Histopathologically, there are small and large angiocentric lymphocytes causing marked angiodestruction. Histiocytes are present but well-formed granulomas, despite its name, are not observed. In the background there is a small population of large atypical EBV+ B cells thought to represent the neoplastic population. EBV positivity is best demonstrated by ISH over latent membrane protein-1 (LMP1) immunohistochemistry. EBV positivity is found more frequently in pulmonary lesions than cutaneous ones (Angel et al. 1994; Beaty et al. 2001). While the clinical course of LG can wax and wane, its overall prognosis is poor.

Diffuse large B cell lymphoma

EBV-positive diffuse large B cell lymphoma (DLBCL) of the elderly is an EBV+ lymphoma arising in patients at a median age of 71 years with no history of previous lymphoma or immunosuppression. The majority of patients present with extranodal disease affecting the skin and soft tissue, bone and bone marrow, oropharyngeal cavities, lungs and gastrointestinal system. The infiltrate is monomorphic, filled with large neoplastic cells, or polymorphic, containing admixed reactive inflammatory cells. Neoplastic B cells express CD19 and CD20 in addition to MUM1/IRF4, BCL2 and EBER ISH. EBV-positive DLBCL of the elderly runs an aggressive course, particularly as compared to its EBV-negative counterpart, making the identification of EBV positivity important for prognostication (Oyama et al. 2003).

Nasal (and related) extranodal NK/T-cell lymphoma

Extranodal NK/T-cell lymphoma is an aggressive neoplasm afflicting patients from East Asia and Central and South America. It is rare in Europeans and North Americans. Natural killer (NK) cells and cytotoxic T cells are closely related as cytotoxic T cells can express CD56 and NK cells can display a cytotoxic T-cell phenotype (CD2, CD7, CD8). For this reason, a distinction in NK/T cell lymphoma is not made, although most neoplastic cells appear to be derived from the NK cell. Most commonly, the tumor arises in the nasal cavity and upper aerodigestive tract and is termed nasal type. Extra-nasal types occur in the skin and soft tissue, gastrointestinal tract and testes. Cutaneous lesions frequently occur and they can be solitary or multifocal in presentation. Associated constitutional symptoms are usually present. Skin biopsies show a dense dermal angiocentric infiltrate with necrosis extending into the subcutaneous compartment (**Figure 13.2**). Epidermotropism is rare. Tumor cells are variable in size and large reactive cells may be present, causing diagnostic confusion. The tumor is invariably positive for EBER ISH and a negative test should put the diagnosis into question. The link between EBV and NK/T cell lymphoma is so strong that PCR analysis of plasma EBV DNA parallels the clinical course and can be used for prognostication at presentation (Au et al. 2004).

Immunosuppression-associated EBV lymphoproliferative disorders

Immunosuppression-associated EBV lymphoproliferative disorders fall into 3 categories: 1) post-transplant lymphoproliferative disease (PTLD), 2) other iatrogenic immunodeficiency associated lymphoproliferative disorders and 3) HIV-related lymphomas. PTLD occurs in hematopoietic (bone marrow, stem cell) and solid organ transplant patients secondary to the post-transplant immunosuppression regimen. The majority of cases are B cell in origin and over 90% are associated with EBV. PTLD is divided into early plasmacytic hyperplasia, polyclonal PTLD and monoclonal PTLD, all of which have demonstrable EBV by ISH. Cutaneous disease is rare and typically restricted to the skin portending a better prognosis (Beynet et al. 2004). Other iatrogenic immunodeficiency associated lymphoproliferative disorders occur most commonly in patients with autoimmune disease undergoing therapy, specifically rheumatoid arthritis (RA) patients treated with methotrexate. PTLD in psoriasis and dermatomyositis patients has also been reported. These lymphoproliferative disorders most closely mimic DLBCL, HL and PTLD. Cases with cutaneous involvement tend to

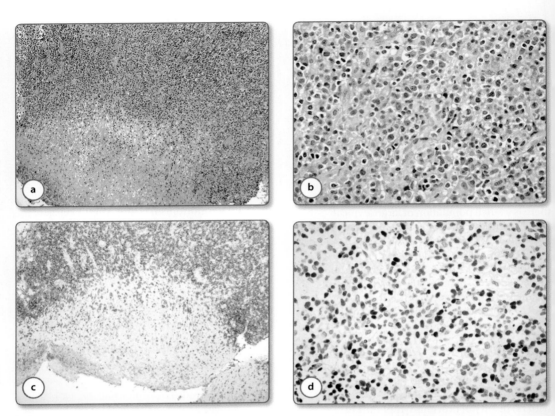

Figure 13.2 NK/T-cell lymphoma with EBER+ ISH. (a) This example of NK/T-cell lymphoma contains a dense pan-dermal infiltrate, with angiodestruction (H&E, 100×). (b) Pleomorphism within the infiltrate is evident at higher magnification (H&E, 400×). The tumor cells are positive for (c) CD56 (CD56, 100×) and (d) EBER ISH (EBER ISH, 400×).

be CD30-positive DLBCL. It is difficult to ascertain how much immunosuppression plays a role in the development of lymphoma since RA patients have a 2 to 20-fold increase risk of developing lymphoma at baseline and are often treated concomitantly with multiple immunomodulating drugs (Thomas et al. 2000). Similarly, the frequency of EBV infection in these lymphoproliferative disorders of autoimmune patients is variable, being more common in HL types (80%) than other B-cell lymphoma types (Swerdlow S.H. 2008). Spontaneous regression may occur after drug withdrawal, particularly in EBV+ cases (Salloum et al. 1996). Patients with HIV can developed a number of EBV–related lymphomas including central nervous system lymphoma (nearly 100% EBV+), primary effusion lymphoma (concomitant EBV+ and HHV8+), Burkitt lymphoma, DLBCL, and

Hodgkin lymphoma. Some of these, as previously discussed, can involve the skin (**Figure 13.3**). For a thorough review on EBV-related lymphomas in the HIV-positive patient, the reader is directed to Pinzone et al (Pinzone et al. 2015). In addition to HIV-associated Burkitt lymphoma (BK), BK can be sporadic or endemic; the latter type is most commonly associated with EBV. Cutaneous involvement is rare and is characterized by an atypical lymphocytic infiltrate containing numerous tingible body macrophages with apoptotic lymphocytes giving it a 'starry sky' appearance. BK is the fastest growing tumor in humans but has a high cure rate (90%) with chemotherapy.

Angioimmunoblastic T-cell lymphoma

Angioimmunoblastic T-cell lymphoma (AITL), also known as

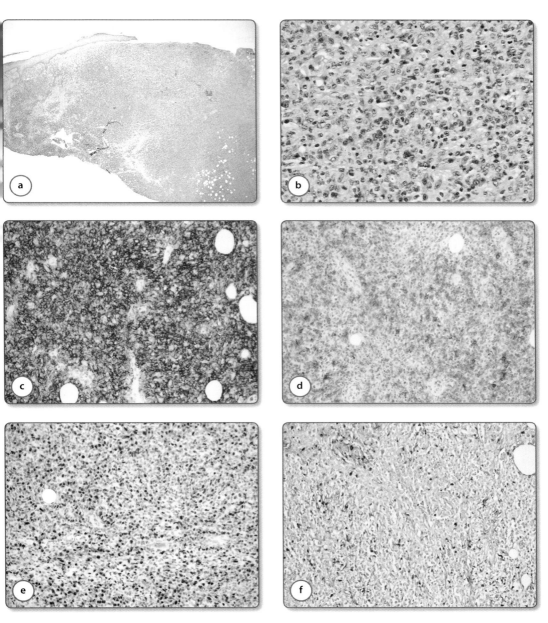

Figure 13.3 Cutaneous diffuse large B-cell lymphoma. (a, b) DLBCL in an HIV patient, with sheets of centroblasts and immunoblasts and numerous mitoses (H&E, 20×; H&E, 200× respectively). Tumor cells are positive for (c) CD20 (CD20, 100×), (d) CD30 (CD30, 100×) and (e) MUM1/IRF4 (MUM1/IRF4, 100×). (f) EBV ISH highlights nuclear positivity in large tumor cells (EBER ISH, 100×).

angioimmunoblastic lymphadenopathy with dysproteinemia, is a neoplastic disorder characterized by lymphadenopathy, hepatosplenomegaly, hemolytic anemia, and hypergammaglobulinemia. Males and females are affected equally, most commonly in the 5th and 6th decade. Cutaneous lesions may occur in 50% of patients. Skin involvement most frequently manifests as a pruritic maculopapular eruption on the trunk, but nodules, plaques and ulcerations can also be present. Histologically the cutaneous infiltrate is composed of dense superficial or superficial and deep perivascular T lymphocytes with a CD4+ T-helper cell profile. Leukocytoclastic vasculitis and granulomatous inflammation may be seen. While AITL is a subtype of peripheral T-cell lymphoma, EBV+ B cells are identified by EBER ISH in >90% of lymph node biopsies and some cutaneous biopsies (Weiss et al. 1992). Additionally EBV is demonstrated early in the course of disease. Given the frequency and timing of EBV, the virus has been hypothesized to have an integral role in pathogenesis. Current hypotheses suggest EBV+ B cells stimulate follicular helper T cells which further stimulate infected B cells creating an immunostimulatory loop and subsequent unregulated expansion of neoplastic T-helper cells (Dunleavy et al. 2007). Monoclonal T-cell receptor rearrangements are invariably detected. While patients may have an initial response to therapy, the overall prognosis is poor.

Light chain restriction in B-cell lymphoproliferative disorders

Most B-cell lymphomas involving the skin are cutaneous in origin (primary cutaneous) and include follicle center cell lymphoma, marginal zone lymphoma, and diffuse large B-cell lymphoma. Systemic/nodal non-Hodgkin lymphomas can occasionally secondarily involve the skin and include chronic lymphocytic leukemia/small lymphocytic lymphoma (CLL/SLL) and mantle cell lymphoma (MCL), among others. One of the most important questions when faced with a dense cutaneous infiltrate of predominantly B lymphocytes is whether it is cutaneous lymphoid hyperplasia (CLH) versus a primary or secondary B-cell lymphoma. Molecular clonality testing by PCR can be instrumental in answering the question

of benignity versus malignancy, but has its limitations, including its variable sensitivity and inability to determine the anatomic relationship of clones (see Chapter 15). Immunohistochemistry can act as a surrogate for clonality, looking for light chain expression restricted to kappa or lambda, but is only useful with tumors that express these light chains in high quantities, such as lymphomas with plasmacytic differentiation (some marginal zone lymphomas) and plasmacytomas. CISH is more sensitive than IHC because it detects κ/λ mRNA levels instead of surface proteins, but still lacks sufficient sensitivity to detect most cutaneous B-cell neoplasms. Furthermore, high background for both IHC and CISH impacts the sensitivity of these assays and limits their interpretation. The recently adapted BRISH technique, through the use of its amplification system, enables sensitive detection of low levels of mRNA (**Figure 13.4**) (Tubbs et al. 2013). Measured against standard flow cytometric data, BRISH had a 99% concordance rate of light chain restriction in hematopoietic B-cell neoplasms from lymphoid tissue (Tubbs et al. 2013). A similar study was conducted for cutaneous lymphomas including follicle center cell lymphomas, marginal zone lymphomas, large B-cell lymphomas and cutaneous lymphoid hyperplasias. All specimens were in FFPE and were measured against PCR clonality results. The concordance rate was 96% with PCR and all CLH specimens were negative by BRISH (Minca et al. 2015).

Conclusion

In situ hybridization is a powerful, DNA/RNA probe-based technology, which can be used as a diagnostic and prognostic tool for infection and tumors by targeting microbial-specific and tumor-specific DNA and RNA, while maintaining the anatomic relationships of cells with positive signals. In dermatopathology, ISH offers supplemental information to the dermatopathologist at critical junctures in specific scenarios. As examples, it can confirm the diagnosis of condylomata acuminata and it can offer prognostic information such as in DLBCL of the elderly. For certain entities,

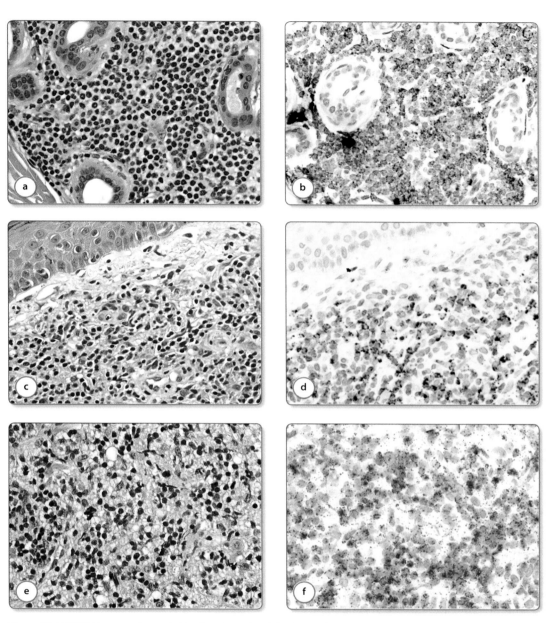

Figure 13.4 BRISH. Hematoxylin-eosin histology (a, c, e) and dual BRISH for kappa/lambda light chain mRNA (b, d, f; kappa signals black chromogen, lambda signals red chromogen) were performed on samples of benign lymphoid hyperplasia (a, b: 100×), kappa-restricted marginal zone lymphoma (c, d: 100×), and lambda-restricted follicle center lymphoma (e, f: 100×). Courtesy of Minca EC & Ma XJ, 2015.

demonstration of EBV positivity is a requirement for diagnosis. The new techniques for ISH have led to increased sensitivity with decreased background staining making interpretation more straightforward and reliable. Given the similarities of ISH to immunohistochemistry,

every dermatopathologist should feel comfortable with the technique and interpretation of the stain and, as such, have no difficulty including it in their armamentarium. Specific roles for fluorescence in situ hybridization (FISH) are discussed in the next chapter.

References

Angel CA, Slater DN, Royds JA, Nelson SN, Bleehen SS. Epstein–Barr virus in cutaneous lymphomatoid granulomatosis. Histopathology 1994; 25:545–548.

Au WY, Pang A, Choy C, Chim CS, Kwong YL. Quantification of circulating Epstein-Barr virus (EBV) DNA in the diagnosis and monitoring of natural killer cell and EBV-positive lymphomas in immunocompetent patients. Blood 2004; 104:243–249.

Beaty MW, Toro J, Sorbara L, et al. Cutaneous lymphomatoid granulomatosis: correlation of clinical and biologic features. Am J Surg Pathol 2001; 25:1111–1120.

Beynet DP, Wee SA, Horwitz SS, et al. Clinical and pathological features of posttransplantation lymphoproliferative disorders presenting with skin involvement in 4 patients. Arch Dermatol 2004; 140:1140–1146.

Chang KL, Chen YY, Shibata D, Weiss LM. Description of an in situ hybridization methodology for detection of Epstein–Barr virus RNA in paraffin-embedded tissues, with a survey of normal and neoplastic tissues. Diagn Mol Pathol 1992; 1:246–255.

Dunleavy K, Wilson WH, Jaffe ES. Angioimmunoblastic T cell lymphoma: pathobiological insights and clinical implications. Curr Opin Hematol 2007; 14:348–353.

Dyson N, Howley PM, Munger K, Harlow E. The human papilloma virus-16 E7 oncoprotein is able to bind to the retinoblastoma gene product. Science 1989; 243:934–937.

Fakhry C, Westra WH, Li S, et al. Improved survival of patients with human papillomavirus-positive head and neck squamous cell carcinoma in a prospective clinical trial. J Natl Cancer Inst 2008; 100:261–269.

Glaser SL, Lin RJ, Stewart SL, et al. Epstein-Barr virus-associated Hodgkin's disease: epidemiologic characteristics in international data. Int J Cancer 1997; 70:375–382.

Jin L, Lloyd RV. In situ hybridization: methods and applications. J Clin Lab Anal 1997; 11:2–9.

Minca EC, Wang H, Wang Z, et al. Detection of immunoglobulin light-chain restriction in cutaneous B-cell lymphomas by ultrasensitive bright-field mRNA in situ hybridization. J Cutan Pathol 2015; 42:82–89.

Oyama T, Ichimura K, Suzuki R, et al. Senile EBV+ B-cell lymphoproliferative disorders: a clinicopathologic study of 22 patients. Am J Surg Pathol 2003; 27:16–26.

Pinzone MR, Berretta M, Cacopardo B, Nunnari G. Epstein–Barr virus- and Kaposi sarcoma-associated herpesvirus-related malignancies in the setting of human immunodeficiency virus infection. Semin Oncol 2015; 42:258–271.

Quintanilla-Martinez L, Jansen PM, Kinney MC, et al. Non-mycosis fungoides cutaneous T-cell lymphomas: report of the 2011 Society for Hematopathology/European Association for Haematopathology workshop. Am J Clin Pathol 2013a; 139:491–514.

Quintanilla-Martinez L, Ridaura C, Nagl F, et al. Hydroa vacciniforme-like lymphoma: a chronic EBV+ lymphoproliferative disorder with risk to develop a systemic lymphoma. Blood 2013b; 122:3101–3110.

Salloum E, Cooper DL, Howe G, et al. Spontaneous regression of lymphoproliferative disorders in patients treated with methotrexate for rheumatoid arthritis and other rheumatic diseases. J Clin Oncol 1996; 14:1943–1949.

Schache AG, Liloglou T, Risk JM, et al. Validation of a novel diagnostic standard in HPV-positive oropharyngeal squamous cell carcinoma. Br J Cancer, 2013; 108:1332–1339.

Swerdlow SH, Harris N, Jaffe ES, et al. WHO Classification of Tumours of Haematopoietic and Lymphoid Tissues, 4th ed. Lyon, France: International Agency for Research on Cancer (IARC), 2008.

Thomas E, Brewster DH, Black RJ, Macfarlane GJ. Risk of malignancy among patients with rheumatic conditions. Int J Cancer 2000; 88:497–502.

Tubbs RR, Wang H, Wang Z, et al. Ultrasensitive RNA in situ hybridization for detection of restricted clonal expression of low-abundance immunoglobulin light chain mRNA in B-cell lymphoproliferative disorders. Am J Clin Pathol 2013; 40:736–746.

Ukpo OC, Flanagan JJ, Ma XJ, et al. High-risk human papillomavirus E6/E7 mRNA detection by a novel in situ hybridization assay strongly correlates with p16 expression and patient outcomes in oropharyngeal squamous cell carcinoma. Am J Surg Pathol 2011; 35:1343–1350.

Weiss LM, Jaffe ES, Liu XF, Chen YY, Shibata D, Medeiros L J. Detection and localization of Epstein–Barr viral genomes in angioimmunoblastic lymphadenopathy and angioimmunoblastic lymphadenopathy-like lymphoma. Blood 1992; 79:1789–1795.

14 Fluorescence in situ hybridization

Pamela Aubert

History

Fluorescence in situ hybridization (FISH) was developed by researchers in the 1980s to detect the location of specific gene sequences in chromosomes as well as changes in gene copy number and chromosomal structural alterations. The earliest in situ hybridization assays did not use fluorescence but rather radioisotope labeled probes, a labor intensive and hazardous technique with poor resolution. With these limitations in mind, fluorescently labeled nucleic acid probes were developed, improving the speed, resolution and safety of the detection system. In 1980 the first application of FISH used a radiolabeled ribonucleic acid (RNA) probe to bind in situ specific deoxyribonucleic acid (DNA) sequences. At this time FISH was primarily a research tool. A decade later, in the 1990s, improved labeling and hybridization techniques of single stranded DNA probes allowed direct detection of DNA sequences and an increase in the number of detectable targets (Levsky & Singer, 2003). These changes opened up the applications of FISH to the field of molecular diagnostics, with detection of microdeletion syndromes, translocations in hematologic malignancies, and later chromosomal abnormalities in solid tumors. However, it was only recently that FISH entered the field of dermatopathology as a commercially available test with diagnostic value. For a broad and comprehensive overview of the role of molecular tests in dermatopathology see Hosler and Murphy *Molecular Diagnostics for Dermatology* (Hosler, 2014).

Principles of fluorescence in situ hybridization (FISH)

FISH can be performed on bone marrow, peripheral blood smears, frozen tissue or formalin-fixed paraffin-embedded (FFPE) sections. One of the advantages of FISH is the possibility to study non-dividing cells for chromosomal aberrations in tissue sections and cytological specimens, giving it a practical edge over cytogenetics. The direct detection of nucleic acids in tissue sections on slides allows for the preservation of tissue histology. This is particularly useful with skin biopsies of atypical melanocytic lesions with a nevus component or background inflammation. The atypical area can be isolated for analysis for a more accurate assessment of potential biologic activity of the lesion as a whole. FISH utilizes specific fluorescently labeled single-stranded DNA nucleic acid probes that are complementary to portions of the genes of interest. The labeled probe and the target DNA are denatured to yield ssDNA. They are then combined, allowing the annealing of complementary DNA sequences between the target tissue DNA and the probe. This process is called hybridization and is performed under specific optimized conditions to ensure a sensitive and specific reaction. If the target sequence of interest is present, the labeled probe will hybridize to it. Unbound probes are washed away prior to the detection step. The probes are then visualized using a fluorescence microscope. Multiple probes can be used in combination in a single analysis. In dermatopathology FISH is most frequently used to detect chromosomal gains and losses in the work-up of melanocytic lesions. A normal cell is diploid and should contain only two copies of each genetic target. Gains and losses are detected by the presence of more or fewer than the normal two copies. FISH can also be used to detect inversions and translocations using fusion probes or break-apart probes, more complex techniques used to detect characteristic recurrent translocations present in certain soft tissue tumors.

Applications

Melanoma

In the field of dermatopathology FISH is used primarily for diagnosis of ambiguous melanocytic lesions. Clinical evaluation and biopsy with standard histochemical analysis remains the gold standard for the identification of melanoma. However, it is well known that the diganosis of melanoma is plagued by diagnositic ambiguity and interobserver variability. While immunohistochemistry can classify a lesion into the melanocytic category, the distinction between benign and malignant with such stains as HMB-45 and Ki-67 is limited. Molecular testing is a recent addition to the diagnostic armamentarium which has the potential to increase diganostic accuracy for melanoma. The development of molecular assays followed the discovery that benign nevi and melanoma differ in the presence or absence of chromosomal alterations. These differences were exploited to devise a FISH-based assay to help the pathologist distinguish between atypical nevi and melanoma. The FISH melanoma assay was developed Dr Pedram Gerami, Dr Boris Bastian, and their colleagues at Northwestern University (Chicago, IL), University of California San Francisco (San Francisco, CA) and Abbott Molecular (Abbott Park, IL). In their 2009 study they used existing comparative genomic hybridization (CGH) data of 13 identified oncogene amplifications and tumor suppressor gene deletions to develop and test multiple probe sets of four (fluorophore wavelength restrictions limit the number of usable probes to four) (Gerami et al., 2009). Each probe set was validated against a set of unequivocal melanomas and benign nevi. The best perfoming set was then applied to a second and third cohort of unequivocal melanomas and benign nevi to establish cutoff values for the positive and negative results and performance characteristics. Lastly the probe set was applied to a set of histologically ambiguous melanocytic lesions with long-term follow-up data to determine whether the assay could predict patient outcomes. All 6 of 6 patients with metastases were FISH positive while only 6/21 of the patients without recurrence had a positive result. Overall the sensitivity and specificity were 87% and 95% respectively. However, these test attributes varied with histologic subtype of melanoma being analyzed. Sensitivity for acral melanomas reached 100%, but decreased to 81% for superficial spreading, 70% for spitzoid melanomas and down to 50% for desmoplastic melanomas (Gammon et al. 2012; Gerami et al. 2011; Gerami et al. 2010). This first generation FISH assay also had false-positive rates particularly in Spitz nevi. Many of these false positives were due to tetraploidy which is found in up to 10% of Spitz nevi (Isaac et al. 2010). Tetraploidy occurs when the entire genome is duplicated causing four copies of every gene and chromosome instead of the normal two copies. This can be due to errors during normal mitosis and does not necessarily represent malignancy. However, the presence of tetraploidy can cause difficulty in interpretation of the FISH assay leading to false-positive results.

A second generation FISH assay has been developed to address some of these shortcomings (Gerami et al. 2012). The new panel added 9p21 (*CDKN2A*) and 8q24 (*MYC*) to two members of the original panel, 6p25 (*RREB1*) and 11q13 (*CCND1*) (**Table 14.1**). New cutoff values were determined and new scoring rules were adopted to account for Spitz nevus-associated tetraploidy. In the current assay melanomas are associated with any of the following: homozygous loss of 9p21 or gains of 8q24, 6p25 or 11q13 (**Figure 14.1**). Studies in spitzoid melanomas have shown a relatively high frequency of p16 loss, a protein encoded by the *CDKN2A* gene located at the 9p21 locus. Therefore, the homozygous loss of 9p21 was added to the melanoma assay to improve the diagnostic accuracy for spitzoid melanomas (**Figure 14.1c, d**). Importantly, the deletion must be homozygous to be considered positive as heterozygous deletion of 9p21 occurs in benign nevi and nevi with architectural disorder. These refinements improved the performance characteristics to a sensitivity of 94% and specificity of 98%, giving the assay better overall discriminatory power and a better ability to exclude tertraploidy, which increased the diagnostic accuracy for spitzoid melanomas. The specific parameters of the second generation assay with respect to the different melanoma histologic subtypes are still being evaluated. Notably, despite these changes FISH still has limited applicability in purely intraepidermal melanomas and markedly inflamed melanomas

Table 14.1 Published second generation FISH probe set for the diagnosis of melanoma (Gerami et al. 2012).

Region	Gene	Function	Criteria	Cutoffs (%)	Histologic subtype*
9p21	CDKN2A	Locus for p16/p14 tumor suppressors	Homozygous deletion	>29	Spitzoid melanoma
6p25	RREB1	Zinc finger protein	>2 signals	>29	Blue nevus-like melanoma Nevoid melanoma
11q13	CCND1	Cyclin D1 (bcl-1), cell cycle regulator	>2 signals	>29	Significant in any subtype
8q24	MYC	Transcription factor	>2 signals	>29	Amelanotic melanoma

* These are reported associations between histologic subtypes and genetic abnormalities, but they are not 100% sensitive or 100% specific

due to difficulty in identification of neoplastic cells from surrounding benign cells.

Given the very recent changes to the assay most of the published studies using FISH for melanocytic lesions were performed using the first generation assay. Nevertheless, it has proved to be a useful tool in a variety of diagnostic settings including differentiating between atypical nevi and melanoma (Gerami et al. 2009), conjunctival nevi and melanoma (Busam et al., 2010), and blue nevi and metastatic melanoma (Gammon et al. 2011; Pouryazdanparast et al. 2009). It has also been used in the lymph node to distinguish subcapsular and intranodal nevi from lymph node metastasis (Dalton et al. 2010). A few diagnostic scenarios are discussed below to highlight the assay's clinical utility.

One of the most difficult diagnostic dilemmas in dermatopathology is the distinction between a benign blue nevus and a blue nevus-like metastatic melanoma. Histomorphologically these two entities can be identical. Cases of metastatic melanoma can have a symmetric bland appearance whereas cases of benign blue nevi can contain atypical pleomorphic melanocytes with a variable mitotic index. While the clinical history and presentation can be helpful, without the history of a prior advanced stage melanoma, arriving at a definitive diagnosis can be challenging. Nonetheless, the importance of distinguishing the two cannot be overstated as it is the difference between stage IIIB disease qualifying for systemic adjuvant treatment and simple reassurance. The first generation FISH assay has been applied in this clinical context

and has proved to be a useful diagnositic aid in the diffentiation between epithelioid and cellular blue nevi and blue nevus-like metastatic melanomas. In a recent study nine out ten blue nevus-like melanomas were FISH positive whereas all 10/10 epithelioid blue nevi were negative (Pouryazdanparast et al. 2009). In another similar study all five cases of blue nevus-like melanomas were FISH positive and all 12 cellular blue nevi were negative (Gammon et al. 2011). Interestingly in both these studies the positive FISH assay was driven by chromosomal copy gains in 6p25, the locus for the *RREB* gene lending further credence to the validity of the assay (**Figure 14.1e, f**).

Another challenging distinction is that between nevoid melanoma and mitotically active nevi. The lack of a significant epidermal component and pagetoid spread combined with the symmetric silhouette and banal growth pattern of nevoid melanomas mimic that of a benign compound or intradermal nevus. While nevoid melanomas are usually characterized by their lack of maturation, they can have some degree of maturation and may lack significant nuclear pleomorphism and mitotic activity. As such, no single criterion can be used to distinguish malignancy from benignity. The first generation melanoma FISH assay was used in a study of ten nevoid melanomas compared to ten compound and intradermal banal nevi (Gerami et al. 2009). Histologically the nevoid melanomas had worrisome clinical and histologic features including cellular confluence, deep mitoses and a history of metastasis. On the other hand, aside

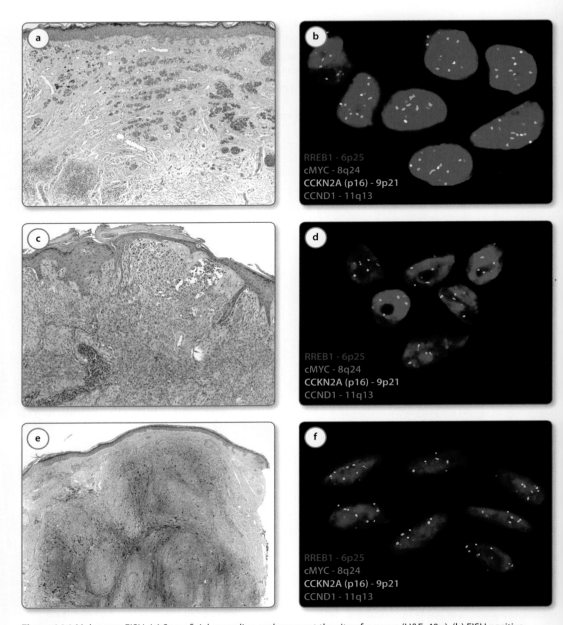

Figure 14.1 Melanoma FISH. (a) Superficial spreading melanoma at the site of a nevus (H&E, 40×). (b) FISH positive with increased numbers of RREB1, MYC, and CCND1 above cutoff limits for positivity. Notably, the nevus cells in the bottom left hand corner were FISH negative (not shown in FISH panel). (c, d) Spitzoid melanoma confirmed by FISH with homozygous loss of 9p21, CDKN2A (H&E, 20x; H&E, 40×, respectively). (e) Blue-nevus like melanoma in a patient with known melanoma (H&E, 20×) and (f) confirmed by loss of RREB1 by FISH.

from the increased mitotic rate, the benign nevi matured and lacked cytologic atypia. FISH was positive in 10/10 nevoid melanomas and negative in 10 of 10 mitotically active nevi. All ten genetic aberrations were in the *RREB1* gene at the 6p25 locus.

Kinase fusions in spitzoid neoplasms

Spitzoid neoplasms are some of the most challenging lesions to differentiate from melanoma. As previously mentioned, the second-generation FISH assay has a relatively good sensitivity and specificity now that the homozygous loss of 9p21 has been added to the panel. Recently, a study by Weisner et al. demonstrated the frequency of kinase fusions in the biologic spectrum of spitzoid lesions (Wiesner et al. 2014). Up to 50% of Spitz nevi, atypical Spitz tumors and spitzoid melanomas harbored kinase fusions of *ROS1, NTRK1, ALK, BRAF* or *RET* in a mutually exclusive pattern. While the identification of these fusion products does not help with the differentiation of benign versus malignant biologic potential, their presence was shown to stimulate oncogenic signaling pathways. As we learn more about the role of these fusion proteins in tumorigenesis, the identification of kinase fusions by FISH may become important for selection of kinase inhibitor therapy.

Soft tissue tumors

The fluorescence in situ hybridization technique can also be used as a tool for the diagnosis of soft tissue tumors, albeit the particular detectable molecular events differ from those of melanoma. Even though soft tissue tumors are infrequently encountered in routine dermatopathology they cause a disproportionate amount of anxiety for many dermatopathologists. While patient age and location can make a diagnosis more or less likely, the clinical presentation alone is rarely diagnostic. Histologically soft tissue tumors can have variable histomorphology depending on the proportion of the different components of the tumor present. Immunohistochemistry can help categorize a tumor into a certain lineage but more specific markers are largely lacking. Interestingly as opposed to other solid tumors, many sarcomas harbor distinct recurrent molecular defects, which can be exploited for diagnostic and even

prognostic intents (**Tables 14.2 and 14.3**). By far the most common genetic events are reciprocal translocations in which there are no gains or losses in genetic material. These balanced translocations can result in either transcriptional deregulation of an oncogenic fusion gene or aberrant signaling of pathways responsible for cell cycle and growth. Other less frequent molecular events include amplification of oncogenes, activating mutations of oncogenes or inactivating mutations of tumor suppressor genes, and the formation of ring chromosomes. The presence of ring chromosomes in osteosarcoma, atypical lipomatous tumors and dedifferentiated liposarcomas leads to additional genetic material and amplification of tumorigenic genes *CDK4, MDM2* and *CPM* (Arrigoni & Doglioni 2004; Yang & Zhang 2013). While some of the molecular defects in soft tissue tumors are unique and defining, others are shared by various unrelated tumors. As such, molecular findings should not be used in isolation but rather combined with histomorphologic, immunohistochemical and clinical data to culminate in a final diagnosis.

FISH is a powerful tool for identification of translocations, ring chromosomes and amplifications, which together comprise the largest group of molecular defects in soft tissue tumors. Most of the translocations are balanced without net gains or losses and therefore not detectable by CGH. The numerous breakpoints within a particular translocated gene make RT-PCR testing tedious and a less attractive approach over FISH. However, uncommon activating and silencing genetic mutations will require other techniques for identification such as RT-PCR, IHC and next generation sequencing and are discussed in their respective chapters. For the purposes of identifying translocations there are two main types of FISH: break-apart FISH and dual-fusion FISH. In break-apart FISH, two probes with different fluorochromes (red and green) are directed to the same locus to flank a known chromosomal breakpoint and gene of interest. When no translocation is present, the two signals, red and green, overlap appearing as a yellow signal. When a translocation is present they are separated and the cell has two separate and distinct red and green signals (**Figure 14.2a**). In break-apart FISH, only one translocation partner is probed. This technique is acceptable if

Table 14.2 Select superficial soft tissue tumors with molecular defects

Tumor	Chromosomal abnormality	Gene fusion product	FISH sensitivity *†
Angiomatoid fibrous histiocytoma	t(2;22)(q33;q12) t(12;22)(13;q12) t(12;16)(q13;q11)	EWSR1-CREB1 EWSR1-ATF1 FUS-ATF1	72% 21% 7%
Angiosarcoma (radiation-induced and lymphedema-induced)	8q24	MYC amp	80-100%
Atypical lipomatous neoplasm/ well-differentiated liposarcoma	12q13-15	Amp of MDM2, HGMIC, TSPAN31, CDK4 Amp of GLI, DDIT3	>95% Rare
Clear cell sarcoma	t(12;22)(13;q12) t(2;22)(q33;q12)	EWSR1-ATF1 EWSR1-CREB1	90% 10%
Dermatofibrosarcoma protuberans (DFSP) and giant cell fibroblastoma	t(17;22)(q21;q13)	COL1A1-PDGFB	>90%
Epithelioid hemangioendothelioma	t(1;3)(p36;q25) t(X;11)(p11;q22)	WWTR1-CAMTA1 YAP1-TFE3	>95% Rare
Ewings sarcoma / primitive neuroectodermal tumor (PNET)	t(11;22)(q24;q12) t(21;22)(q22;q12) t(7;22)(q21;q12) t(2;22)(q35;q12) t(17;22)(q21;q12) t(16;21)(q11;q22) t(2;22)(q35;q11)	EWSR1-FLI1 EWSR1-ERG EWSR1-ETV1 EWSR1-FEV EWSR1-ETV4 FUS-ERG FUS-FEV	90% 5% <1% <1% <1% <1% <1%
Ewing-like sarcoma	t(20;22)(q13;q12) t(4;19)(q35;q13) t(10;19)(q26;q13) inv(X)(p11.4p11.22)	EWSR1-NFATC2 CIC-DUX4 CIC-DUX4 BCOROCCNB3	Low Low Low Low
Low-grade fibromyxoid sarcoma	t(7;16)(q33;p11) t(11;16)(p11;p11)	FUS-CREB3L2 FUS-CREB3L1	>95% <5%
Myoepithelioma	t(6;22)(p21;q12) t(1;22)(q23;q12) t(19;22)(q13;q12)	EWSR1-POU5F1 EWSR1-PBX1 EWSR1-ZNF444	15% 15% Rare
Myxoid/round cell liposarcoma	t(12;22)(q13; p11) t(12;22)(q13;q12)	DDIT3-FUS DDIT3-EWSR1	95% 5%
Nodular fasciitis	t(17;22)(p13;q12)	MYH9-USP6	90%

*Sensitivities were determined by testing a sample of tumors for the molecular defect of interest by FISH and calculating the percentage of positive cases [test +/ total cases].
†References in main text

there is only one main translocation for a given tumor (DFSP, for example) or if the identity of the fusion partner is inconsequential. However, if the translocation partner is important for diagnosis, the dual fusion FISH technique is required. Dual-fusion FISH probes identify both genes involved in a translocation. In contradistinction to the break apart probe, the presence of a juxtaposition of red and green signals (two different genes) appearing as a yellow signal identifies a translocation compared with two separate red and two separate green signals typical of a normal diploid cell (**Figure 14.2b**). Dual-fusion FISH is useful when a commonly translocated gene (*EWSR1*) has multiple potential fusion partners and the identity of the partner is required to favor one diagnosis over another (*EWSR1-NR4A3* in extraskeletal myxoid chondrosarcoma vs *EWSR1-WT1* in desmoplastic small round cell tumor). Most laboratories utilize the break-apart FISH

Table 14.3 Additional soft tissue tumors with molecular defects

Tumor	Chromosomal abnormality	Gene fusion product	FISH sensitivity*
Alveolar rhabdomycosarcoma	t(2;13)(q35;q14) t(1;13)(p36;q14) t(X;2)(q13;q36)	PAX3-FOXO1 PAX7-FOXO1 PAX3-FOXO4	75% 10% (RT-PCR) Low (RT-PCR)
Alveolar soft part sarcoma	t(X;17)(p11;q25)	ASPSCR1-TFE3	N/A
Chondroid lipoma	t(11;16)(q13;p13)	C11orf95-MKL2	N/A
Congenital infantile fibrosarcoma	t(12;15)(p13;q25)	ETV6-NTRK3	75%
Desmoplastic small round cell tumor	t(11;22)(p13;q12)	EWSR1-WT1	>95%
Endometrial stromal sarcoma	t(7;17)(p15;q11) t(6;7)(p21;p15) t(6;10)(p21;p11) t(10;17)(q23;p13)	JAZF1-SUZ12 JAZF1-PHF1 EPC1-PHF1 YWHAE-FAM22	50% 10% Low Low
Extraskeletal myxoid chrondrosarcoma	t(9;22)(q22;q12) t(9;17)(q22;q12) t(9;15)(q22;q21) t(3;9)(q12;q22)	EWSR1-NR4A3 TAF15-NR4A3 TCF12-NR4A3 TFG-NR4A3	80% Low Low Low
Fibroma of tendon sheath	t(2;11)(q31-32;q12)	Unknown	N/A
Inflammatory myofibroblastic tumor	t(1;2)(q21;p23) t(2;19)(p23;p13) t(2;17)(p23;q23) t(2;2)(p23;q12) t(2;11)(p23;p15) inv(2)(p23;p35) t(2;4)(p23;q21)	TPM3-ALK ALK- TPM4 ALK -CLTC ALK -RANBP2 ALK- CARS ALK-ATIC ALK-SEC31A	N/A
Malignant gastrointestinal neuroectodermal tumor	t(12;22)(q13;q12) t(2;22)(q33;q12)	EWSR1-ATF1 EWSR1-CREB1	45% 25%
Mesenchymal chondrosarcoma	t(8;8)(q13;q21)	HEY-NCOA2	80%
Myxoinflammatory fibroblastic sarcoma/ hemosiderotic fibrolipomatous tumor	t(1;10)(p22;q24) 3p11-12 (ring)	TGFBR3-MGEA5 Amp of VGLL3, CHMP2B	80%
Ossifying fibromyxoid tumor	t(6;12)(p21;q24.) t(X;22)(p11;q13) t(1;6)(p35;p21) t(6;10)(p21;p11)	EP400-PHF1 ZC3H7B-BCOR MEAF6-PHF1 EPC1-PHF1	40% Low Low Low
Osteosarcoma	12q14-15 (ring)	Amp of CDK4, MDM2, CPM, others	60%
Pericytoma	t(7;12)(7p22;q13)	ACTB-GLI1	N/A
Pulmonary myxoid sarcoma	t(2;22)(q34;q12)	EWSR1-CREB1	70%
Sclerosing fibroepithelioid fibrosarcoma	t(7;16)(q33;p11) t(11;16)(p13;p11)	FUS-CREB3L2 FUS-CREB3L1	N/A N/A
Solitary fibrous tumor	12q13 inversion	NAB2-STAT6	90% (RT-PCR)
Subungual exocytosis	t(X;6)(q22;q13-q14)	COL12A1-COL4A5	N/A
Synovial sarcoma	t(X;18)(p11;q11)	SS18-SSX1 SS18-SSX2 SS18-SSX4	60% 35% (RT-PCR) Rare
Giant cell tumor of tendon sheath	t(1;2)(p13;q35-36) other t with 1p13	CSF1-COL6A3 CSF1	N/A N/A

N/A little or no data available

*Sensitivities were determined by testing a sample of tumors for the molecular defect of interest either by FISH or RT-PCR and calculating the percentage of positive cases [test +/ total cases].

(adapted from Hosler 2014 & Goldblum 2014)

technique as is obviates some of the technical difficulties present in dual-fusion FISH and is adequate for the majority of diagnostic dilemmas. If a translocation is identified with break-apart FISH and the identity of the fusion partner is required, break apart FISH can reflex to dual-probe FISH. Identification of amplifications is straightforward and requires a single probe to the target gene. The number of signals of the target gene per cell is compared to a centromere probe, to control for aneuploidy/polyploidy. The presence of more than two signals (normal is one signal for each allele) is considered a positive result. Typically the signal amplification is much greater than 2 signals and interpretation is obvious (**Figure 14.2c**).

A discussion of all soft tissue tumors and their respective molecular defects is beyond the scope of this book and the practice of most dermatologists and dermatopathologists. For detailed descriptions of the multitude of soft tissue tumors the reader is directed to review texts on soft tissue pathology (Goldblum 2014). The following selected soft tissue tumors are discussed in further detail as they can present superficially in the subcutis or dermis and may therefore be first diagnosed by dermatologists and dermatopathologists. While standard diagnostic methods, including histomorphologic and immunophenotypic characteristics, are first line approaches in these cases, molecular findings can aid in confirming a suspected diagnosis of a rare tumor or cases with unusual histologic/immunophenotypic features.

Angiomatoid fibrous histiocytoma (AFH)

Previously termed *angiomatoid malignant fibrous histiocytoma*, this tumor was renamed to reflect its favorable prognosis. The tumor typically presents in children and young adults as a several centimeter asymptomatic nodule arising from the dermis or subcutis on an extremity. There can rarely be accompanying systemic symptoms such as fever, anemia and weight loss due to tumor cytokine overproduction. However, this tumor rarely metastasizes and most patients have an excellent clinical course. Histologically, the tumor is characterized by a triad of irregular solid masses of histiocyte-like

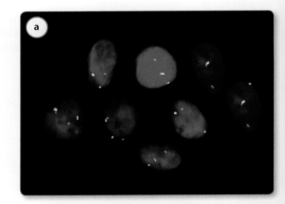

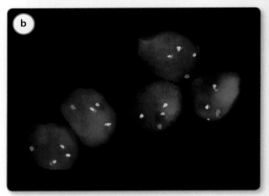

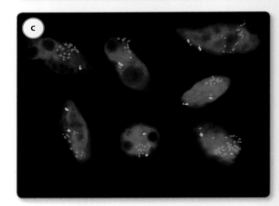

Figure 14.2 FISH techniques. (a) In break-apart FISH, a yellow signal represents the overlap of one red and green signal directed to the same locus (wild type), and separate red and green signals represent a positive translocation. (b) In dual-fusion FISH, separate red and green signals signify normal (wild type) and yellow signals signify the presence of a translocation. Amplifications are detected by probing the gene of interest and comparing the number of signals per cell with a centromere probe. (c) An example of MDM2 high amplification (MDM2 red, centromere 12 green).

cells and cystic areas of hemorrhage at the center and chronic inflammation at the periphery (**Figure 14.3a, b**). While in the majority of cases the histiocyte-like cells are bland without cytologic atypia, occasionally these cells can be atypical with hyperchromatic nuclei; a feature that does not correspond to aggressive behavior. The histiocyte-like cells frequently contain hemosiderin or lipid. Multifocal hemorrhage is uniformly present leading to cystic change and the appearance of pseudovascular spaces. The lesion can sometimes resemble a lymph node due to the surrounding fibrous pseudocapsule and prominent lymphoid cuff. Immunohistochemistry is relatively unhelpful as only half the cases stain with a lineage specific marker such as CD68 (KP-1 clone) or desmin.

CD99 is positive in 50% of cases. However, the tumor does possess several translocations, the identification of which can aid in making the diagnosis. The most common fusion transcript is *EWSR1-CREB1* present in over 70% of cases. The second most common is *EWSR1-ATF* and *FUS-ATF* is the least common fusion gene found in less than 10% of cases (Antonescu et al. 2007; Waters et al. 2000). Importantly, up to one quarter of cases do not have a demonstrable translocation. The commonly available FISH *EWSR1* break-apart probe is the most common probe used to identify AFH with a sensitivity of 76% (**Figure 14.3c, d**) (Tanas et al. 2010). While *FUS* rearrangements would be missed with the *EWSR1* break apart probe, these translocations appear to be rare events.

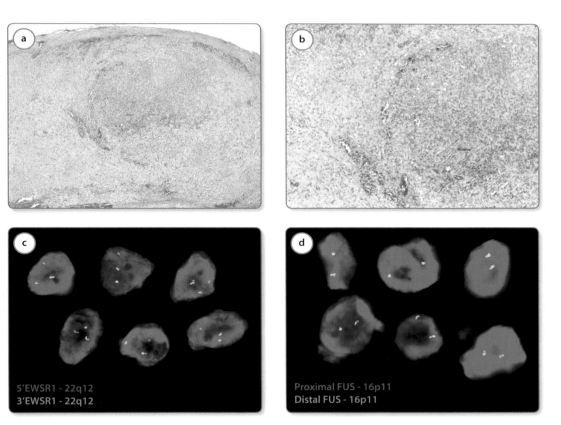

Figure 14.3 Angiomatoid fibrous histiocytoma. (a) This tumor has a triad of solid masses of histiocyte-like cells, cystic areas of hemorrhage at the center, and chronic inflammation at the periphery (H&E, 20×). (b) Hemorrhage is uniformly present leading to cystic change and the appearance of pseudovascular spaces (H&E, 40×). (c) Positive EWSR1 break–apart FISH. (d) Negative FUS break–apart FISH.

Radiation-induced angiosarcoma

While the overall incidence of developing angiosarcoma after radiation is low, 0.05–0.14% of all patients, up to one quarter of angiosarcomas diagnosed occur following radiation (Fodor et al. 2006; Marchal et al. 1999). Traditionally this tumor was seen exclusively in patients with previous radiation treatment for visceral cancers with a mean latency of 10 years following exposure. However, with the increasing commonality of breast-sparing surgery combined with radiation for the treatment of breast cancer, the incidence of radiation-induced angiosarcoma on breast skin is rising. This type of angiosarcoma has a much shorter latency than radiation-induced angiosarcoma of other sites, with tumors developing within 3-5 years of radiation exposure (Fodor et al. 2006; Marchal et al. 1999). The reason for this shortened latency is not known. There is a spectrum of vascular lesions that can develop in irradiated skin, from atypical vascular lesions (AVLs) with some atypia but a relatively benign clinical course to malignant angiosarcomas with marked cellular atypia and a poor prognosis (**Figure 14.4a**). Histomorphologically radiation-induced angiosarcoma is identical to standard cutaneous angiosarcoma (**Figure 14.4b**). The actual diagnostic dilemma lies in the distinction of radiation-induced angiosarcoma from AVLs. Both lesions will mark with immunohistochemical stains for vascular lineage (CD34 and ERG) and both will have elevated proliferative indices by Ki-67 (MIB-1) immunohistochemistry. An important distinction is the presence of *MYC* amplifications (>8 signals per diploid cell) in 50-100% of radiation-induced angiosarcomas whereas all AVLs studied to date lack this amplification (Guo et al. 2011). Additionally, angiosarcomas without a history of radiation also lack the *MYC* amplification (Manner et al. 2010). FISH is useful for the detection of *MYC* amplification (**Figure 14.4c**). Preliminary data suggests good correlation between the presence of FISH *MYC* amplification and nuclear positivity of c-myc immunohistochemical staining (Fernandez et al. 2012). It is important to keep in mind that *MYC* amplifications can be seen in many cancers and

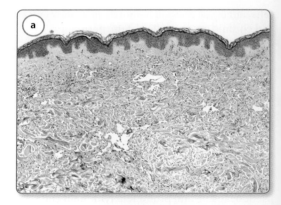

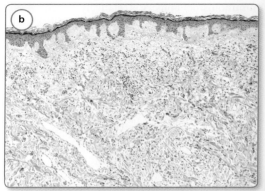

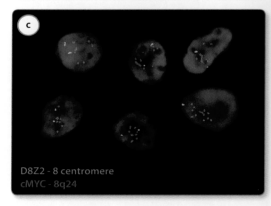

D8Z2 - 8 centromere
cMYC - 8q24

Figure 14.4 FISH use in vascular tumors. (a) Atypical vascular lesion (AVL) of the breast (H&E, 20×) and (b) radiation-induced angiosarcoma of the breast (H&E, 20×) can look very similar by histomorphology. (c) A diagnosis of post-radiation angiosarcoma was confirmed by MYC amplification (FISH).

is not unique to radiation-induced angiosarcoma. However, most of these other entities do not enter the differential diagnosis of an atypical vascular lesion. *MYC* amplification in angiosarcoma arising in the context of chronic lymphedema has recently been described (Harker et al. 2016 in press).

Clear cell sarcoma

Clear cell sarcoma (CCS) is an aggressive tumor arising from the deep soft tissues and commonly involving the tendons and aponeuroses. Its previous designation as *malignant melanoma of soft parts* reveals the tumor's close relationship to melanoma. However clear cell sarcoma and melanoma are clinically and genetically distinct tumors, a distinction confirmed by the identification of a characteristic translocation in CCS not found in melanoma. CCS occurs in young adults between the ages of 20–40 commonly affecting the foot and ankle region. The head, neck and trunk regions are unusual sites. Lesions are typically painless and slow growing, reaching several centimeters prior to diagnosis. Patients have a protracted course with multiple recurrences followed by metastasis and death. However, tumors confined to the superficial skin appear to have better clinical outcomes. Histologically, CCS is composed of nests and fascicles of spindled or fusiform cells separated by thin fibrocollagenous septa. Lesional cells have vesicular nuclei and cleared out cytoplasm. Multinucleated cells with up to 10–15 peripheral nuclei are a characteristic finding while pleomorphism and mitoses are uncommon. Melanin pigment is present in half the cases and melanocytic differentiation is consistently present when immunohistochemical analysis is performed. S100 is uniformly positive and HMB-45, MART-1 (melan-A), tyrosinase and MiTF are usually positive. As a result, the most common entity in the histologic differential diagnosis is clear cell melanoma which can be histomorphologically and immunohistochemically identical. As such, molecular testing can be an invaluable diagnostic aid. The most common molecular event in CCS is a t(12,22)(q13;q12) translocation leading to the fusion of *EWSR1-ATF1*, present in 70-80% of cases (Zucman et al. 1993). A minority of cases (<5%) have a t(2,22) translocation resulting in the *EWSR1-CREB1* fusion gene (Antonescu et al. 2006). The latter translocation is more common in CCS tumors of the gastrointestinal tract. All fusion variants can be detected using a *EWSR1* break-apart FISH assay. Even though many other soft tissue tumors have *EWSR1* rearrangements, all melanomas are negative for *EWSR1* translocations, making it a useful test for the distinction between CCS and clear cell melanoma (Patel et al. 2005). Additionally, many melanomas have *BRAF* or *NRAS* mutations, both of which are rarely seen in CCS.

Dermatofibrosarcoma protuberans and giant cell fibroblastoma

Dermatofibrosarcoma protuberans (DFSP) is an intermediate grade fibrohistiocytic tumor with frequent local recurrence but rare metastasis. It affects the trunk and proximal extremities of young to middle age adults. Giant cell fibroblastoma is a clinical and histologic variant of DFSP occurring in children. Histologically, DFSP tumor cells are bland elongated fibroblast-like cells diffusely involving the dermis in a storiform pattern (**Figure 14.5a, b**). The tumor infiltrates the subcutis in a distinctive honeycomb pattern around individual adipocytes. The giant cell fibroblastoma variant seen in children has giant cells and pseudovascular spaces. Both DFSP and giant cell fibroblastoma are characterized by diffuse uniform staining with CD34. Additionally, virtually all DFSPs and giant cell fibroblastomas share the same molecular rearrangements of either a linear unbalanced or ring translocation t(17;22)(q21;q13) (**Figure 14.5c–e**) (Patel et al. 2008; Simon et al. 1997). The presence of a ring versus a linear translocation may be related to age as they are more commonly seen in adult cases (Sirvent et al. 2003). This leads to a fusion of collagen type I α-1 *(COL1A1)* gene on chromosome 17 and platelet-derived growth factor β *(PDGFB)* gene on chromosome 22. This translocation places *PDGFB* under the control of the *COL1A1* promoter leading to overproduction of the PDGF-β protein. The growth factor then binds to its cell surface receptor ultimately stimulating cell proliferation (Shimizu et al., 1999). The fusion product can be easily detected by FISH *PDGFB* break-apart or by dual-probe technique (Salgado et al., 2011). Focally, DFSP

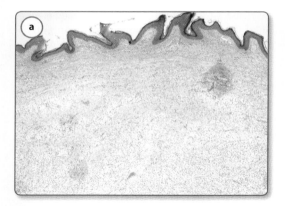

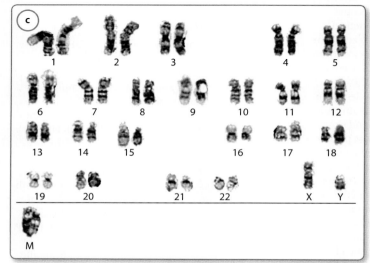

Figure 14.5 (a, b) Dermatofibrosarcoma protuberans infiltrating the dermis and subcutis with cytologically bland elongated fibroblast-like cells (H&E, 20x; H&E, 100x, respectively). (c) Karyotype from tumor cells reveals an abnormal profile with a superfluous ring chromosomes. The ring chromosomes contain material from (d) Chr 17 and (e) Chr 22.

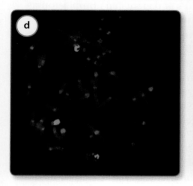

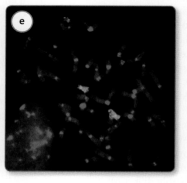

can have fibrosarcomatous change with areas of atypical spindle cells in a herringbone pattern with increased mitotic activity. Whether the presence of these areas signifies more aggressive behavior has not been established (Mentzel et al. 1998). The area of fibrosarcomatous change typically abuts an area of low grade classical DFSP. However, some can recur or metastasize as pure fibrosarcoma. These fibrosarcomatous areas have diminished CD34 staining making FISH testing for the *COL1A1-PDGFB* translocation particularly useful in this situation (Ha et al., 2013). The PDGF-β receptor is a tyrosine kinase receptor and as such tyrosine kinase inhibitors such as imatinib can inhibit its downstream signaling. While wide local excision or Mohs remains the standard of care for DFSP, targeted tyrosine kinase receptor inhibitors such as imatinib have been successful as a therapeutic alternative for large, inoperable or rare metastatic tumors (Rutkowski et al. 2010). Nevertheless, up to 50% of patients are initially resistant or progress while on imatinib therapy (Stacchiotti et al. 2011).

Epithelioid hemangioendothelioma

The term hemangioendothelioma denotes a group of vascular tumors with intermediate malignancy lying somewhere on the spectrum between hemangioma and angiosarcoma. Epithelioid hemangioendothelioma (EHE) is the most aggressive of this group of tumors. It occurs at any age, albeit rarely in children. The tumor arises within the superficial or deep soft tissues anywhere on the body but with a predilection for the extremities. At least half of cases appear to arise from a vessel. The tumor is composed of cords and chains of epithelioid cells with intracytoplasmic vascular lumens. The stroma can vary from myxoid to hyalinized. On standard histology, the vascular nature of the tumor may not be obvious and, as such, other entities such as epithelioid sarcoma enter the differential diagnosis. Immunohistochemistry can be helpful but requires a broad panel as 25% of EHEs can stain with cytokeratins despite its vascular origin while other tumors such as epithelioid sarcoma can stain with vascular markers such as CD34. However, there is a unique translocation t(1;3)(p36;q25) resulting in a fusion *WWTR1-CAMTA1* gene that has been reported in almost all EHEs tested and reported to date (Errani et al. 2011; Tanas et al. 2011). The *WWTR1-CAMTA1* fusion gene has not been reported in any other soft tissue tumor making it a disease defining translocation. Calmodulin-binding transcription activator 1 *(CAMTA1)* is a transcription factor that becomes activated under the *WWTR1* promoter. This fusion product leads to cell proliferation and

tumorigenesis although the exact mechanistic details are still unknown. Studies have attempted to use an anti-CAMTA1 immunohistochemistry antibody to exploit the overexpression of the CAMTA1 protein with varied results (Shibuya et al. 2015; Yusifli & Kosemehmetoglu 2014). A small subset of *WWTR1-CAMTA1* negative EHEs has been found to harbor a *YAP1-TFE3* translocation detectable by break–apart *TFE3* or, less commonly, a *YAP1* probe (Antonescu et al. 2013). This subset of tumors has a solid growth pattern with minimal intervening stroma and prominent mature lumen formation. All cases had strong nuclear immunoexpression of TFE3, a useful screening tool for *TFE3* rearrangements.

Ewing sarcoma

The Ewing family of tumors (EFT) encompasses three entities previously thought to be distinct: extraskeletal Ewing sarcoma, primitive neuroectodermal tumor and Askin tumor. Identification of a common translocation involving the *EWSR1* on 22q12 in all three tumors supports the concept of a shared histogenesis (de Alava & Pardo 2001). Extraskeletal Ewing sarcoma originates from the deep soft tissues most commonly in the upper thigh and buttock although EFTs have been documented at every anatomic site. Rarely the tumor is primary to the dermis or subcutis where it can be encountered by dermatopathologists. Ewing sarcoma is a small round blue cell tumor with solidly packed uniform round cells with distinct nuclear membranes, finely dispersed chromatin and ill-defined cytoplasm. Occasionally there can be accumulation of intracellular glycogen giving the cells a cleared out appearance. Immunohistochemically a few stains are highly sensitive for EFTs including CD99 and FLI-1. However, many of the entities in the small round blue cell differential diagnosis such as Merkel cell carcinoma, alveolar rhabdomyosarcoma and lymphoma also stain focally with these markers (Folpe et al. 2000; Ozdemirli et al. 2001). Diagnosis can be greatly facilitated by the identification of defining translocations of the *EWSR1* gene on 22q12 with one of several members of the ETS family of transcription factors (Delattre et al. 1992) (**Table 14.2**). The t(11;22)(q24;q12) translocation resulting in the *EWSR1-FLI1* fusion gene is observed in over 90% of cases (Turc-Carel et al. 1988). In 5% of cases, a t(11;22) (q24;q12) translocation occurs between *EWSR1* and *ERG* (Sorensen et al. 1994). The *EWSR1* gene can fuse with any gene member of the ETS (E-twenty-six) family (*ETV1, FEV, ETV4*, etc.) but this is much less common than the previously mentioned translocations (Shing et al. 2003). There is a category of soft tissue tumors termed Ewing-like sarcoma, histologically resembling extraskeletal Ewing sarcoma or EFTs but without the characteristic *EWSR1* translocation. Most commonly these tumors harbor a translocation substituting *FUS* for *EWSR1* to form *FUS-ERG* and *FUS-FEV* fusion genes. *FUS* translocated tumors are biologically identical to EFTs and are currently treated similarly. There are a few other tumors classified under Ewing-like sarcoma, most of which are found in the bone or abdominal cavity. One tumor termed an undifferentiated small round cell sarcoma with *CIC-DUX4* translocation occurs in the deep soft tissue of the extremities in young adults. It is composed of nodules of small round blue cells with vesicular nuclei and prominent nucleoli (**Figure 14.6a**). Mitoses are frequent and the tumor contains broad zones of necrosis. While it stains poorly with immunohistochemical lineage stains the tumor is identifiable by characteristic translocations, t(4,19)(q35;q13) or t(10;19) (q26.3;q13), both leading to a *CIC-DUX4* fusion gene (Kawamura-Saito et al., 2006). These tumors are best detected with a FISH break-apart *CIC* probe (**Figure 14.6b**).

Liposarcoma

Liposarcoma is the most common type of soft tissue tumor. If there is subcutaneous or dermal involvement it is more commonly due to extension from a deep soft tissue origin rather than arising out of the dermis or subcutaneous compartment. As such, they will be only briefly discussed below. Liposarcomas can be classified into four main categories:

1. Atypical lipomatous neoplasm/ well-differentiated liposarcoma (ALN/WDL) and de-differentiated liposarcoma (DL)
2. Myxoid/round cell liposarcoma (MRCL)
3. Pleomorphic liposarcoma
4. Liposarcomas of mixed or unclassifiable type

ALN/WDL is the most common type of liposarcoma and characterized histologically by mature fat and variable atypical spindled stromal cells with hyperchromatic nuclei and lipoblasts (**Figure 14.6c**). At times, the atypical stromal cells are rare and only mature fat is seen on initial biopsy. For this reason the diagnosis is often made on recurrences. Long marker chromosomes and ring chromosomes containing amplified sequences of 12q are identifiable by FISH in almost all ALN/WDL (**Figure 14.6d**) (Italiano et al. 2008; Sirvent et al. 2007). These cytogenetic alterations lead to the amplification of genes *MDM2* and *CDK4*, among others, leading to cell proliferation through inhibition of apoptosis (Leach et al. 1993). De-differentiated liposarcomas are a subset of ALN/WDL tumors with the same molecular defect but displaying histologic progression. They contain areas of typical well-differentiated liposarcoma abutting areas of poor differentiation resembling fibrosarcoma or undifferentiated pleomorphic sarcoma. These areas import more aggressive biologic behavior as compared to ALN/WDL. While ALN/WDLs can be encountered in the subcutaneous and deep soft tissue compartment, DLs are more commonly located in the retroperitoneum. MRCL also exist on a spectrum of differentiation. Well-differentiated myxoid liposarcoma is a multinodular mass; each nodule containing small fusiform or round cells with small nuclei and low mitotic activity surrounded by a richly myxoid stroma. There is a delicate capillary network, a feature allowing distinction from a benign myxoma. With histologic progression, the tumor accumulates areas of primitive round cells with high nuclear to cytoplasmic ratios either as clearly delineated nodules or more commonly as gradual areas of increased cellularity. Nearly all MRCL contain the balanced translocation t(12,22)(q13; p11) leading to the *DDIT3-FUS* fusion transcript (Crozat et al. 1993). A small percentage of cases contain a variant translocation, t(12;22)(q13;q12), in which *DDIT3* fuses with *EWSR1* (Panagopoulos et al. 1996). This molecular aberration leads to the tumor's ability to evade cell cycle checkpoints leading to unregulated growth (Kuroda et al., 1997). While pleomorphic liposarcoma is the least common type, up to 25% develop in skin or subcutis (Hornick et al., 2004). Histologically

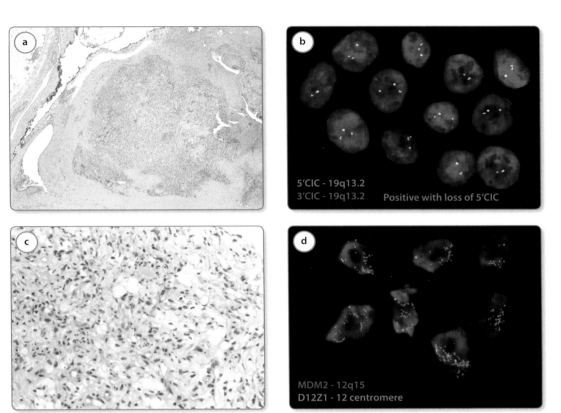

Figure 14.6 Undifferentiated small round cell sarcoma and atypical lipomatous neoplasm/well-differentiated liposarcoma. (a) Undifferentiated small round cell sarcoma has distinct nodules of small round blue cells and zones of necrosis (H&E, 40×). (b) It is positive for the FISH break–apart CIC probe. (c) Atypical lipomatous neoplasm/well-differentiated liposarcoma has mature fat and variable atypical spindled stromal cells with hyperchromatic nuclei and lipoblasts (H&E, 200×). (d) In this tumor, amplification of 12q and the MDM2 gene is identified by FISH.

they most commonly resemble undifferentiated pleomorphic sarcomas (malignant fibrous histiocytomas) with intervening giant lipoblasts with hyperchromatic atypical nuclei. A rare variant can have a more epithelioid morphology mimicking a carcinoma or melanoma. Pleomorphic liposarcoma is an aggressive tumor with complex genetic rearrangement but without a known characteristic translocation or amplification.

Low grade fibromyxoid sarcoma

Evans in 1987 initially described low grade fibromyxoid sarcoma (LGFS) arising in the deep soft tissues of two young women (Evans, 1987). Due to shared histology and molecular defects,

hyalinizing spindle cell tumor with giant rosettes is now considered a histologic variant of LGFS (Reid et al. 2003). LGFS occurs in young adults on the trunk and extremities, most commonly the thigh. Most tumors arise in the skeletal muscle or subcutis, but occasionally can be more superficially located and involve the dermis. Histologically, LGFS is a deceptive tumor with bland cytology but an ability to metastasize. It is composed of spindle cells set in a myxoid and fibrous stroma in varying proportions in different areas within the same tumor (**Figure 14.7a, b**). There can be abrupt or gradual transitions from myxoid to fibrous areas. The tumor has low to moderate cellularity and low mitotic activity. Cases previously diagnosed as hyalinizing spindle cell tumor with giant rosettes feature a variable number of giant rosettes with peripheral ovoid cells and central brightly eosinophilic collagen on a background of typical LGFS. Immunohistochemically, LGFS can have focal positivity for smooth muscle markers, EMA, claudin-1 and CD99. A recent study found strong and diffuse expression of MUC4 in all LGFS and absence of expression in tumors commonly in the differential diagnosis, such as myxofibrosarcoma, neurofibroma, myxomas, desmoid fibromatoses and perineurioma (Doyle et al. 2011). LGFS has a characteristic translocation between the *FUS* gene on chromosome 7 and the *CREB3L2* on chromosome 16 resulting in the *FUS-CREB3L2* fusion gene. A very high proportion of cases (~70–90%) have this *FUS-CREB3L2* translocation which is detectable by FISH *FUS* break-apart probe or RT-PCR (**Figure 14.7c**) (Mertens et al. 2005; Rose et al. 2011). None of the common fibrous or myxoid entities in the differential test positive for the translocation supporting the high sensitivity and specificity of the FISH assay for the detection of LGFS.

Myoepithelioma

Myoepithelioma, also known as mixed tumor of soft tissue, arises in patients of all ages, most commonly in the deep soft tissues of the extremities and the head and neck region. Occasionally the tumor can extend to involve the dermis. Myoepitheliomas are considered related to mixed tumors with the latter designation reserved for tumors with true ductular formation. Myoepithelial carcinoma can be used when malignant histologic foci are present within the lesion signifying an increased risk of metastasis. Myoepthelial carcinoma is seen more commonly in the pediatric population in which it can have an aggressive clinical course (Gleason & Fletcher 2007). The histomorphologic appearance of myoepithelioma varies from reticulated cords of cells to nests, sheets or mixed architectural patterns. At the periphery there can be infiltrating small nests and single cells with a surrounding desmoplastic stromal response. The tumor stroma can also vary from myxochondroid to hyalinized. Lesional cells are both epithelioid and spindled with little to no nuclear atypia and

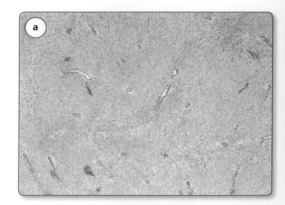

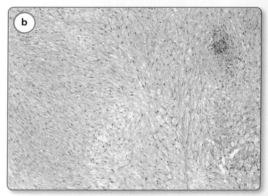

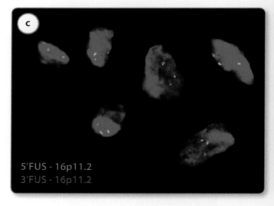

5'FUS - 16p11.2
3'FUS - 16p11.2

Figure 14.7 Low-grade fibromyxoid sarcoma. (a) This tumor has moderate cellularity with a fibrous and myxoid stroma of varying density and a network of curvilinear blood vessels (H&E, 20×). (b) The tumor is composed of bland spindle-shaped cells with small hyperchromatic nuclei (H&E, 40×). (c) The FISH FUS break-apart probe is positive.

rare mitoses. The tumor consistently expresses epithelial markers (cytokeratins and/or EMA) with more frequent positivity with broad spectrum cytokeratins (i.e. AE1/AE3) and low-molecular weight cytokeratins (i.e. Cam 5.2) over high molecular weight cytokeratins (CK 5/6). Molecular studies may be helpful in instances with varied morphology and an inconsistent immunohistochemistry profile. Similar to other soft tissue tumors, myoepitheliomas have translocations involving *EWSR1* and much less commonly *FUS* (Cristina R. Antonescu et al., 2010). The fusion partners are different from other *EWSR1* soft tissue tumors and most frequently include *POU5F1* resulting in the *EWSR1-POU5F1* fusion gene from a t(6;22)(p21;q12) translocation. The related mixed tumors have a different molecular signature with *PLAG1* rather than *EWSR1* rearrangements (Bahrami et al. 2012). Distinguishing myoepithelioma from extraskeletal myxoid chondrosarcoma based on standard histomorphology can be difficult and often necessitates additional immunohistochemical or molecular testing. Since *EWSR1* rearrangements are also found in extraskeletal myxoid chondrosarcoma, testing for the partner gene *NR4A3* is required for diagnosis (Flucke et al. 2012). Additional entities in the differential diagnosis of myoepithelioma include ossifying fibromyxoid tumor and chordoma, neither of which contains *EWSR1* translocations. Additionally, all chordomas stain with the specific notochordal marker brachyury, which is negative in myoepitheliomas (Tirabosco et al. 2008).

Nodular fasciitis

Nodular fasciitis was until very recently considered a reactive process rather than a neoplasm and termed pseudosarcomatous fibromatosis due to its cellularity. However, newly discovered molecular events have been demonstrated confirming its neoplastic nature. Nodular fasciitis can occur at any age but is most frequent in adults aged 20–40 years. It is a rapidly growing self-limited solitary nodule most commonly located on the volar aspect of the forearms. In addition to a predilection for the upper extremities, nodular fasciitis can also occur on the chest and back and head/neck, the latter being the most common location in infants and children and termed

cranial fasciitis if located on the scalp. Nodular fasciitis is composed of fibroblasts and myofibroblasts that resemble those seen in tissue culture or granulation tissue. The cells are arranged in short fascicles in a vague storiform growth pattern. There is ample intervening hyaluronidase and ground substance giving the lesion a loose feathery texture. There are usually scattered inflammatory cells, mitoses and focal areas of microhemorrhage. While the borders can be infiltrative, the lesion is overall well defined. Smooth muscle actin is consistently positive throughout the tumor, whereas desmin and smooth muscle myosin are negative or only weakly positive. Molecular changes had previously been reported in isolated cases. However, a recent study from the Mayo Clinic found 44 of 48 (92%) cases of nodular fasciitis had a t(17;22)(p13;q12) translocation leading to the fusion product *MYH9-USP6* (Erickson-Johnson et al. 2011). Other myxoid and fibrous lesions in the differential diagnosis were negative for the translocation. Despite the awareness of nodular fasciitis as a benign reactive lesion, it remains one of the most misdiagnosed soft tissue lesions and its confusion with myxofibrosarcoma can lead to unnecessary wide surgical excision. As such, strong consideration should be given to looking for the distinct translocation in cases in which both nodular fasciitis and a malignant sarcoma are in the differential diagnosis.

Prognosis and management

Whether evaluating soft tissue tumors or melanocytic neoplasms, FISH is not currently used for the purposes of prognostication. There is still a lack of data in the areas of risk stratification and clinical outcomes. In soft tissue tumors, with very few exceptions, alternate translocations within the same tumor type have not yet been found to correlate to differences in prognosis. For this reason, the presence or absence of translocations is not incorporated into standard TMN staging for soft tissue tumors. One of these exceptions is in synovial sarcoma. Patients with *SS18-SSX2* tumors have a better outcome than patients with *SS18-SSX1* tumors (5-year survival 73% vs 53%) (Ladanyi et al. 2002). In melanoma standard risk stratification and ultimate prognosis continues to rely on depth of tumor, ulceration, mitoses and nodal status. There is an active field devoted to molecular analysis of sentinel lymph nodes in melanoma patients in an attempt to detect micrometastasis more accurately. An early FISH study showed gains in 11q13 (*CCND1*) and 8q24 (*MYC*) were linked to poor prognosis and were second only to ulceration in their ability to predict metastasis (Gerami et al. 2011). In the field of theranostics, identification of kinase fusions by FISH in Spitzoid neoplasms mentioned above may become important in the future for selection of kinase inhibitor therapy. There are additional applications of molecular tests in dermatology not only for diagnosis but for prognosis and theranostic as well, which are reviewed in more detail in Hosler & Murphy's Molecular Diagnostics for Dermatology (Hosler 2014).

Conclusion

This is an exciting time to be a dermatopathologist. We now have more powerful and practical tools such as FISH to help us in some of the most diagnostically challenging areas of dermatopathology. For histologically ambiguous melanocytic lesions, FISH allows us to provide clinicians with information on biologic behavior. For soft tissue tumors we can now feel more confident in our diagnosis after identification of a characteristic translocation. In the hands of a proficient lab, FISH is a technically feasible test with rapid turnaround time and covered by most health insurance carriers. As such, our threshold for ordering FISH on difficult cases should be low, particularly for cases including large benign lesions and deep malignancies in the same histologic differential diagnosis.

References

Antonescu CR, Dal Cin P, Nafa K, et al. EWSR1-CREB1 is the predominant gene fusion in angiomatoid fibrous histiocytoma. Genes Chromosomes Cancer 2007; 46:1051–1060.

Antonescu CR, Le Loarer F, Mosquera JM, et al. Novel YAP1-TFE3 fusion defines a distinct subset of epithelioid hemangioendothelioma. Genes Chromosomes Cancer 2013; 52:775–784.

Antonescu CR, Nafa K, Segal NH, et al. EWS-CREB1: a recurrent variant fusion in clear cell sarcoma–association with gastrointestinal location and absence of melanocytic differentiation. Clin Cancer Res 2006; 12:5356–5362.

Antonescu CR, Zhang L, Chang NE, et al. EWSR1-POU5F1 fusion in soft tissue myoepithelial tumors. A molecular analysis of sixty-six cases, including soft tissue, bone, and visceral lesions, showing common involvement of the EWSR1 gene. Genes, Chromosomes Cancer 2010; 49:1114–1124.

Arrigoni G, Doglioni C. Atypical lipomatous tumor: molecular characterization. Curr Opin Oncol 2004; 16:355–358.

Bahrami A, Dalton JD, Krane JF, et al. A subset of cutaneous and soft tissue mixed tumors are genetically linked to their salivary gland counterpart. Genes Chromosomes Cancer 2012; 51:140–148.

Busam KJ, Fang Y, Jhanwar SC, et al. Distinction of conjunctival melanocytic nevi from melanomas by fluorescence in situ hybridization. J Cutan Pathol 2010; 37:196–203.

Crozat A, Aman P, Mandahl N, et al. Fusion of CHOP to a novel RNA-binding protein in human myxoid liposarcoma. Nature 1993; 363:640–644.

Dalton SR, Gerami P, Kolaitis NA, et al. Use of fluorescence in situ hybridization (FISH) to distinguish intranodal nevus from metastatic melanoma. Am J Surg Pathol 2010; 34:231–237.

de Alava E, Pardo J. Ewing tumor: tumor biology and clinical applications. Int J Surg Pathol 2001; 9:7–17.

Delattre O, Zucman J, Plougastel B, et al. Gene fusion with an ETS DNA-binding domain caused by chromosome translocation in human tumours. Nature 1992; 359: 162–165.

Doyle LA, Möller E, Cin PD, et al. MUC4 Is a highly sensitive and specific marker for low-grade fibromyxoid sarcoma. Am J Surg Pathol 2011; 35:733–741.

Erickson-Johnson MR, Chou MM, Evers BR, et al. Nodular fasciitis: a novel model of transient neoplasia induced by MYH9-USP6 gene fusion. Lab Invest 2011; 91:1427–1433.

Errani C, Zhang L, Sung YS, et al. A novel WWTR1-CAMTA1 gene fusion is a consistent abnormality in epithelioid hemangioendothelioma of different anatomic sites. Genes Chromosomes Cancer 2011; 50:644–653.

Evans HL. Low-grade fibromyxoid sarcoma. A report of two metastasizing neoplasms having a deceptively benign appearance. Am J Clin Pathol 1987; 88:615–619.

Fernandez AP, Sun Y, Tubbs RR, et al. FISH for MYC amplification and anti-MYC immunohistochemistry: useful diagnostic tools in the assessment of secondary angiosarcoma and atypical vascular proliferations. J Cutan Pathol 2012; 39:234–242.

Flucke U, Tops BJ, Verdijk MJ, et al. NR4A3 rearrangement reliably distinguishes between the clinicopathologically overlapping entities myoepithelial carcinoma of soft tissue and cellular extraskeletal myxoid chondrosarcoma. Virchows Archiv 2012; 460:621–628.

Fodor J, Orosz Z, Szabo E, Sulyok Z, et al. Angiosarcoma after conservation treatment for breast carcinoma: our experience and a review of the literature. J Am Acad Dermatol 2006; 54:499–504.

Folpe AL, Hill CE, Parham DM, et al. Immunohistochemical detection of FLI-1 protein expression: a study of 132 round cell tumors with emphasis on CD99-positive mimics of Ewing's sarcoma/primitive neuroectodermal tumor. Am J Surg Pathol, 2000; 24:1657–1662.

Gammon B, Beilfuss B, Guitart J, et al. Fluorescence in situ hybridization for distinguishing cellular blue nevi from blue nevus-like melanoma. J Cutan Pathol 2011; 38:335–341.

Gammon B, Beilfuss B, Guitart J, et al. Enhanced detection of spitzoid melanomas using fluorescence in situ hybridization with 9p21 as an adjunctive probe. Am J Surg Pathol 2012; 36:81–88.

Gerami P, Beilfuss B, Haghighat Z, et al. Fluorescence in situ hybridization as an ancillary method for the distinction of desmoplastic melanomas from sclerosing melanocytic nevi. J Cutan Pathol 2011; 38:329–334.

Gerami P, Jewell SS, Morrison LE, et al. Fluorescence in situ hybridization (FISH) as an ancillary diagnostic tool in the diagnosis of melanoma. Am J Surg Pathol 2009; 33:1146–1156.

Gerami P, Jewell SS, Pouryazdanparast P, et al. Copy number gains in 11q13 and 8q24 [corrected] are highly linked to prognosis in cutaneous malignant melanoma. J Mol Diagn 2011; 13:352–358.

Gerami P, Li G, Pouryazdanparast P, et al. A highly specific and discriminatory FISH assay for distinguishing between benign and malignant melanocytic neoplasms. Am J Surg Pathol 2012; 36:808–817.

Gerami P, Mafee M, Lurtsbarapa T, et al. Sensitivity of fluorescence in situ hybridization for melanoma diagnosis using RREB1, MYB, Cep6, and 11q13 probes in melanoma subtypes. Arch Dermatol 2010; 146:273–278.

Gerami P, Wass A, Mafee M, et al. Fluorescence in situ hybridization for distinguishing nevoid melanomas from mitotically active nevi. Am J Surg Pathol 2009; 33:1783–1788.

Gleason BC, Fletcher CDM. Myoepithelial carcinoma of soft tissue in children: an aggressive neoplasm Analyzed in a Series of 29 Cases. Am J Surg Pathol 2007; 31:1813–1824.

Goldblum JR, Folpe AL, Weiss SW. Enzinger & Weiss's Soft Tissue Tumors (6 ed.): Elsevier; 2014.

Guo T, Zhang L, Chang NE, et al. Consistent MYC and FLT4 gene amplification in radiation-induced angiosarcoma but not in other radiation-associated atypical vascular lesions. Genes Chromosomes Cancer 2011; 50:25–33.

Ha SY, Lee SE, Kwon MJ, et al. PDGFB rearrangement in dermatofibrosarcoma protuberans: correlation with clinicopathologic characteristics and clinical implications. Hum Pathol 2013; 44:1300–1309.

Harker D, Jennings M, McDonough P, et al. c-MYC amplification in angiosarcomas arising in the setting of morbid obesity. J Cutan Pathol 2016 (in press).

Hornick JL, Bosenberg MW, Mentzel T, et al. Pleomorphic liposarcoma: clinicopathologic analysis of 57 cases. Am J Surg Pathol 2004; 28:1257–1267.

Hosler GA, Murphy KM. Molecular Diagnostics for Dermatology. Berlin: Springer-Verlag, 2014.

Isaac AK, Lertsburapa T, Pathria Mundi J, et al. Polyploidy in spitz nevi: a not uncommon karyotypic abnormality identifiable by fluorescence in situ hybridization. Am J Dermatopathol 2010; 32:144–148.

Italiano A, Bianchini L, Keslair F, et al. HMGA2 is the partner of MDM2 in well-differentiated and dedifferentiated liposarcomas whereas CDK4 belongs to a distinct inconsistent amplicon. Int J Cancer 2008; 122:2233–2241.

Kawamura-Saito M, Yamazaki Y, Kaneko K, et al. Fusion between CIC and DUX4 up-regulates PEA3 family genes in Ewing-like sarcomas with t(4;19)(q35;q13) translocation. Hum Mol Genet 2006; 15:2125–2137.

Kuroda M, Ishida T, Takanashi M, et al. Oncogenic transformation and inhibition of adipocytic conversion of preadipocytes by TLS/FUS-CHOP type II chimeric protein. Am J Pathol 1997; 151:735–744.

Ladanyi M, Antonescu CR, Leung DH, et al. Impact of SYT-SSX fusion type on the clinical behavior of synovial sarcoma: a multi-institutional retrospective study of 243 patients. Cancer Res 2002; 62:135–140.

Leach FS, Tokino T, Meltzer P, et al. p53 Mutation and MDM2 amplification in human soft tissue sarcomas. Cancer Res 1993; 53:2231–2234.

Levsky JM, Singer RH. Fluorescence in situ hybridization: past, present and future. J Cell Sci 2003; 116:2833–2838.

Manner J, Radlwimmer B, Hohenberger P, et al. MYC high level gene amplification is a distinctive feature of angiosarcomas after irradiation or chronic lymphedema. Am J Pathol 2010; 176:34–39.

Marchal C, Weber B, de Lafontan B, et al. Nine breast angiosarcomas after conservative treatment for breast carcinoma: a survey from French comprehensive Cancer Centers. Int J Radiat Oncol Biol Phys 1999; 44:113–119.

Mentzel T, Beham A, Katenkamp D, et al. Fibrosarcomatous ('high-grade') dermatofibrosarcoma protuberans: clinicopathologic and immunohistochemical study of a series of 41 cases with emphasis on prognostic significance. Am J Surg Pathol 1998; 22:576–587.

Mertens F, Fletcher CD, Antonescu CR, et al. Clinicopathologic and molecular genetic characterization of low-grade fibromyxoid sarcoma, and cloning of a novel FUS/CREB3L1 fusion gene. Lab Invest 2005; 85:408–415.

Ozdemirli M, Fanburg-Smith JC, Hartmann DP, et al. Differentiating lymphoblastic lymphoma and Ewing's sarcoma: lymphocyte markers and gene rearrangement. Mod Pathol 2001; 14:1175–1182.

Panagopoulos I, Hoglund M, Mertens F, et al. Fusion of the EWS and CHOP genes in myxoid liposarcoma. Oncogene 1996; 12:489–494.

Patel KU, Szabo SS, Hernandez VS, et al. Dermatofibrosarcoma protuberans COL1A1-PDGFB fusion is identified in virtually all dermatofibrosarcoma protuberans cases when investigated by newly developed multiplex reverse transcription polymerase chain reaction and fluorescence in situ hybridization assays. Hum Pathol 2008; 39:184–193.

Patel RM, Downs-Kelly E, Weiss SW, et al. Dual-color, break-apart fluorescence in situ hybridization for EWS gene rearrangement distinguishes clear cell sarcoma of soft tissue from malignant melanoma. Mod Pathol 2005; 18:1585–1590.

Pouryazdanparast P, Newman M, Mafee M, et al. Distinguishing epithelioid blue nevus from blue nevus-like cutaneous melanoma metastasis using fluorescence in situ hybridization. Am J Surg Pathol 2009; 33:1396–1400.

Reid R, de Silva MV, Paterson L, et al. Low-grade fibromyxoid sarcoma and hyalinizing spindle cell tumor with giant rosettes share a common t(7;16)(q34;p11) translocation. Am J Surg Pathol 2003; 27:1229–1236.

Rose B, Tamvakopoulos GS, Dulay K, et al. The clinical significance of the FUS-CREB3L2 translocation in low-grade fibromyxoid sarcoma. J Orthop Surg Res 2011; 6:15.

Rutkowski P, Van Glabbeke M, Rankin CJ, et al. Imatinib mesylate in advanced dermatofibrosarcoma protuberans: pooled analysis of two phase II clinical trials. J Clin Oncol 2010; 28:1772–1779.

Salgado R, Llombart B, R MP, Fernandez-Serra A, et al. Molecular diagnosis of dermatofibrosarcoma protuberans: a comparison between reverse transcriptase-polymerase chain reaction and fluorescence in situ hybridization methodologies. Genes Chromosomes Cancer 2011; 50:510–517.

Shibuya R, Matsuyama A, Shiba E, et al. CAMTA1 is a useful immunohistochemical marker for diagnosing epithelioid hemangioendothelioma. Histopathology, 2015.

Shimizu A, O'Brien KP, Sjoblom T, et al. The dermatofibrosarcoma protuberans-associated collagen type Ialpha1/platelet-derived growth factor (PDGF) B-chain fusion gene generates a transforming protein that is processed to functional PDGF-BB. Cancer Res 1999; 59:3719–3723.

Shing DC, McMullan DJ, Roberts P, et al. FUS/ERG gene fusions in Ewing's tumors. Cancer Res 2003; 63:4568–4576.

Simon MP, Pedeutour F, Sirvent N, et al. Deregulation of the platelet-derived growth factor B-chain gene via fusion with collagen gene COL1A1 in dermatofibrosarcoma protuberans and giant-cell fibroblastoma. Nat Genet 1997; 15:95–98.

Sirvent N, Coindre JM, Maire G, et al. Detection of MDM2-CDK4 amplification by fluorescence in situ hybridization in 200 paraffin-embedded tumor samples: utility in diagnosing adipocytic lesions and comparison with immunohistochemistry and real-time PCR. Am J Surg Pathol 2007; 31:1476–1489.

Sirvent N, Maire G, Pedeutour F. Genetics of dermatofibrosarcoma protuberans family of tumors: from ring chromosomes to tyrosine kinase inhibitor treatment. Genes Chromosomes Cancer 2003; 37:1–19.

Sorensen PH, Lessnick SL, Lopez-Terrada D, et al. A second Ewing's sarcoma translocation, t(21;22), fuses the EWS gene to another ETS-family transcription factor, ERG. Nat Genet 1994; 6:146–151.

Stacchiotti S, Pedeutour F, Negri T. Dermatofibrosarcoma protuberans-derived fibrosarcoma: clinical history, biological profile and sensitivity to imatinib. Int J Cancer 2011; 129:1761–1772.

Tanas MR, Rubin BP, Montgomery EA, et al. Utility of FISH in the diagnosis of angiomatoid fibrous histiocytoma: a series of 18 cases. Mod Pathol 2010; 23:93–97.

Tanas MR, Sboner A, Oliveira AM, et al. Identification of a disease-defining gene fusion in epithelioid hemangioendothelioma. Sci Transl Med 2011; 3:98ra82.

Tirabosco R, Mangham DC, Rosenberg AE, et al. Brachyury expression in extra-axial skeletal and soft tissue chordomas: a marker that distinguishes chordoma from mixed tumor/myoepithelioma/parachordoma in soft tissue. Am J Surg Pathol 2008; 32:572–580.

Turc-Carel C, Aurias A, Mugneret F, et al. Chromosomes in Ewing's sarcoma. I. An evaluation of 85 cases of remarkable consistency of t(11;22)(q24;q12). Cancer Genet Cytogenet 1988; 32:229–238.

Waters BL, Panagopoulos I, Allen EF. Genetic characterization of angiomatoid fibrous histiocytoma identifies fusion of the FUS and ATF-1 genes induced by a chromosomal translocation involving bands 12q13 and 16p11. Cancer Genet Cytogenet 2000; 121:109–116.

Wiesner T, He J, Yelensky R, et al. Kinase fusions are frequent in Spitz tumours and spitzoid melanomas. Nat Commun 2014; 5:3116.

Yang J, Zhang W. New molecular insights into osteosarcoma targeted therapy. Curr Opin Oncol 2013; 25:398–406.

Yusifli Z, Kosemehmetoglu K. CAMTA1 immunostaining is not useful in differentiating epithelioid hemangioendothelioma from its potential mimickers. Turk Patoloji Derg 2014; 30:159–165.

Zucman J, Delattre O, Desmaze C, et al. EWS and ATF-1 gene fusion induced by t(12;22) translocation in malignant melanoma of soft parts. Nat Genet 1993; 4:341–345.

15 T/B gene rearrangement assays

Gregory A. Hosler

The diagnosis of cutaneous hematolymphoid tumors remains one of the more challenging endeavors for the dermatopathologist. Molecular testing is fairly new to the diagnostic armamentarium but offers no magic bullet. The technical and biological limitations of the T-cell receptor (TCR) and immunoglobulin (Ig) gene rearrangement assays, in their current form, prevent their use as effective stand-alone tests. The presence or absence of a detectable clone must therefore be integrated with the clinical, histomorphological, and immunohistochemical data to establish a meaningful interpretation.

Despite their limitations, TCR and Ig gene rearrangement assays can be powerful when used correctly. They are used by many in diagnostic algorithms for mycosis fungoides (MF) and Sézary syndrome (SS). Similarly, they are routinely used in the diagnosis of non-MF/SS T-cell lymphomas, B-cell lymphomas, various B-cell and T-cell leukemias, and to exclude various non-B/T-derived hematolymphoid tumors. Moreover, these molecular assays can be effective at monitoring leukemia/lymphoma patients undergoing therapy for therapeutic responses and relapses, and may provide some valuable prognostic data.

TCR and Ig gene rearrangement assays have evolved over the past few decades and will undoubtedly improve further. Southern blots have been largely replaced by complex multiplex polymerase chain reaction (PCR) assays coupled with capillary electrophoresis. Some laboratories are now experimenting with complete sequencing of these recombined loci (via next-generation sequencing, for example), and the additional data offered by these newer techniques may ultimately lead to the replacement of current methods.

Historical perspective

The cutaneous lymphoma literature can be traced back to L'Hôpital Saint-Louis in France (Steffen, 2006; Willemze & Meijer, 2006). This hospital was one of the first, if not the first, hospital solely devoted to dermatological disease. It was here, in 1806, that Jean-Louis-Marc Alibert (1768-1837) first described mycosis fungoides. Later, in 1870, Pierre-Antoine-Ernest Bazin (1807-1878) furthered Alibert's descriptions by writing on the natural progression of mycosis fungoides, from patch to plaque to tumor stage (Bazin 1862). Only much later, in the 1970s, would it become clear that mycosis fungoides, or Alibert-Bazin disease, was due to a clonal proliferation of the T cell. Following Alibert's and Bazin's tenure, Louis-Anne-Jean Brocq (1856-1928) became one of the 'big 5' at L'Hôpital Saint-Louis – along with Ferdinand-Jean Darier (1856-1938) – and first described the related disorder parapsoriasis in 1902 (Broqc 1902).

By the latter part of the 19th century, tissue processing and staining were sufficiently developed to the point that many human diseases would become characterized at the microscopic level. Prior to this era, cutaneous lymphoma was diagnosed by clinical and autopsy findings alone. By the early 20th century, the histomorphologic features of cutaneous lymphoma were more fully developed and became part of the diagnostic criteria for MF. In 1938, Albert Sézary (1880-1956), working with the French cardiologist Yves Bouvrain (1910-2002), wrote on an erythrodermic patient (Sezary & Bouvrain 1938). This patient's skin biopsy showed epidermotropism and the blood smear had 'monster cells'. Sézary named this disorder paramycosis hémotrope and incorporated skin and blood findings into his diagnostic criteria. Paramycosis hémotrope would later be declared Sézary-Bouvrain lymphoma, and now almost exclusively goes by the name of Sézary syndrome.

The 20th century saw a shift in the diagnostic criteria of cutaneous lymphoma with the advent of ancillary tests. The mid-20th century introduced immunohistochemistry (IHC) to the pathologist's repertoire, credited to work by Albert Coons (1912-1978). IHC was used first used to characterize cutaneous lymphoma in the 1970s and 1980s (Barr et al. 1980; Kung et al. 1981). IHC made clear that MF and SS were due to clonal proliferations of CD3+ T cells, most commonly with the CD4+ helper T-cell phenotype. This new technology also allowed for the development of revised classification schemes to include non MF/SS T-cell lymphomas and leukemias, B-cell lymphomas and leukemias, and non-B/T lymphomas and leukemias (natural killer, or NK, cell tumors, for example).

Around the same period as IHC development, the first TCR and Ig gene rearrangement assays were developed and used to help diagnose lymphomas (Willemze et al. 1983). These assays arguably became the first molecular assays used in dermatopathology. Southern blots were the first assays used for detecting clonal lymphoid populations, but have limitations (**Figure 15.1**). In the Southern blot technique, genomic and recombined DNA is digested by restriction endonucleases and the products are separated using agarose gel electrophoresis. Clonal bands are detected using radioactive or fluorescent probes. Most modern laboratories have replaced Southern blots with multiplex PCR coupled with separation of the PCR products by size and/or charge, such as using capillary gel electrophoresis. Interpretation is performed by sophisticated software. Even newer technologies attempt to completely sequence the recombined genes of the TCR and Ig loci in cutaneous lymphoma in hopes to improve overall diagnostic accuracy and better understand lymphoma biology.

Principles of clonality testing

B- and T-cell molecular clonality assays are unique in molecular diagnostics because they

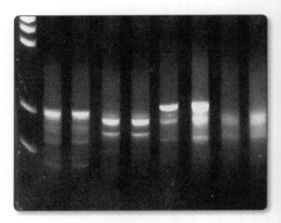

Figure 15.1 Southern blot. In this Southern blot, DNA was extracted from four tissue samples and T-cell gene rearrangement (TRG) PCR was performed. The PCR products were separated by gel electrophoresis and stained with ethidium bromide (left lane is size ladder, samples 1-4 run in duplicate). Sample 1 is a lymphoma, and samples 2-4 are negative controls, challenging to distinguish on the gel alone. The results were confirmed by probe analysis, highlighting only the bands in sample 1 (not shown).

take advantage of a normal biologic process – the somatic recombination of DNA within the developing lymphocyte. This differs from the more typical oncologic molecular assay designed to detect tumorigenic activating mutations (see Chapter 16). Because clonal expansion is a normal lymphocyte response to antigen, clonality does not always equal malignancy. The identification of a clone must be interpreted within the context of all available data, including the clinical presentation.

Somatic recombination

The role of the lymphocyte is to combat foreign antigen. How are the lymphocytes able to recognize millions, if not billions, of foreign pathogens, and not attack their host, given only 25,000 genes in the entire human genome (Lander et al., 2001)? The answer lies with a process unique to the lymphocyte termed somatic recombination. Somatic recombination uses a cut-and-paste method with a finite number of **V**ariable, **D**iversity, and **J**oining gene segments at TCR and Ig gene loci to logarithmically increase the antigen-recognition diversity of the corresponding receptor proteins.

Developing lymphocytes rearrange their V, D, and J gene segments in an attempt to create an immunologic army armed with a wide repertoire of different surface antigen receptors capable of combating an equally wide array of potential pathogens. T-cell development occurs in the thymus, and B-cell development occurs in the bone marrow. If a lymphocyte rearranges its receptor genes to create a non-functional receptor or a receptor that recognizes itself, it is programmed to die.

T-cell somatic recombination and generation of TCR

For developing T cells, there are four rearrangeable loci: *TRD* (δ), *TRG* (γ), *TRB* (β), and *TRA* (α) (**Figure 15.2**). *TRB* (β) and *TRG* (γ) are the most important for clonality assays (see below). These four genes rearrange in sequential order until a functional surface TCR is produced (Hosler & Murphy, 2014; Strominger, 1989). The TCR-γ chain pairs with the TCR-δ chain to form

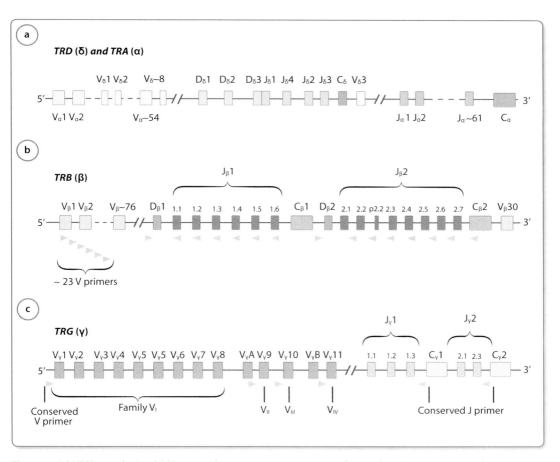

Figure 15.2 (a) TCR gene loci and PCR primer design strategy. TRA (α), TRD (δ), TRB (β), and TRG (γ) loci are shown, along with a primer design strategy for TRB and TRG. TRD (upper labels) resides within TRA (lower labels) at the same locus. (b) TRB contains approximately 76 V gene segments, followed by almost a duplication of D-J-C segments. (c) TRG has 14 V gene segments. An example of a primer design strategy is also depicted (arrowheads). For TRG (γ), there is good sequence homology among family members. For example, Vγ1-Vγ8 (family V I) can be potentially covered by a single primer. By designing primers to conserved regions flanking V and J gene family members, most if not all possible TRG rearrangements can be amplified. In contrast, the TRB (β) locus has many more gene segments and less sequence homology in the flanking regions. To cover all potential rearrangements, many more primers are required.

TCR$^{\gamma/\delta}$ on γ/δ T cells, and the TCR-α chain pairs with the TCR-β chain to form TCR$^{\alpha/\beta}$ on CD4+ or CD8+ α/β T cells. These receptors couple with CD3 on the T-cell surface membrane, to form functional TCR complexes. *TRB* (β) and *TRD* (δ) have variable, diversity, and joining (V-D-J) gene segments, adjacent to constant (C) regions. The *TRA* (α) and *TRG* (γ) loci are made up of only variable and joining (V-J) gene segments, adjacent to constant (C) regions. Therefore, the complete TCR$^{\alpha/\beta}$ and TCR$^{\gamma/\delta}$ contain an antigen-binding domain dictated by exactly one V-J sequence and one V-D-J sequence (**Figure 15.3**).

During T-cell development, the first loci to attempt rearrangement are *TRD* (δ) and *TRG* (γ). At the *TRG* (γ) locus, a random V region gene segment and a random J region gene segment recombine, splicing out the interval DNA. This newly formed recombined DNA is transcribed to primary RNA transcripts and modified to mRNA by splicing out all the interval genetic material, ultimately combining the V-J and C segments. The V-J-C mRNA transcripts are translated to the TCR-γ chain protein. At virtually the same time, *TRD* (δ) recombines V-D-J-C segments to form the TCR- δ chain protein. If the recombination events of *TRG* (γ) and *TRD* (δ) are successful at forming a functional surface TCR$^{\gamma/\delta}$, the γ/δ T cell leaves the thymus seeking its antigen. If not, the lymphocyte attempts to rearrange its other allele at the failed recombination locus. If recombination of both alleles fails for either the *TRG* (γ) or *TRD* (δ) locus, the cell becomes committed to the more common TCR$^{\alpha/\beta}$ lineage and segments from the TCR-β chain attempt to rearrange. At the *TRB* (β) locus, randomly selected D and J gene segments recombine, and then that D-J recombines with a randomly selected V segment. The recombined V-D-J DNA is transcribed to primary RNA transcripts. These transcripts are modified to V-D-J-C mRNA and translated into the TCR-β chain protein. Meanwhile, the lymphocyte rearranges V-J on the *TRA* (α) locus (splicing out all of *TRD*), ultimately forming the TCR-α chain protein. Similar to the other loci, if recombination fails to generate a functional TCR protein, rearrangement of the other allele is attempted.

B-cell somatic recombination and generation of Ig

The creation of immunoglobulin (Ig) in the developing B cell is analogous to the creation of

TCR in the developing T cell. For B cells, *IGH*, *IGK*, and *IGL* encode the proteins of Ig. *IGH* encodes the IgH heavy chain and *IGK* and *IGL* encode the kappa and lambda light chains, respectively (**Figure 15.4**). Each Ig is made up of the heavy chain and either kappa or lambda.

The Ig heavy chain locus, *IGH*, is the first to rearrange (**Figure 15.5**). It has V, D, and J gene segments, similar to the *TRB* (β) and *TRD* (δ) TCR loci. A randomly selected D gene segment recombines with a randomly selected J gene segment, splicing out the interval DNA. D-J then recombines with a randomly selected V gene segment to form V-D-J. A primary RNA transcript is formed and modified to mRNA, creating the V-D-J-C transcript, which is translated to the IgH heavy chain protein. If a functional IgH is not produced, the other *IGH* allele attempts rearrangement.

Similar to the *TRA* (α) and *TRG* (γ) TCR loci, the kappa *IGK* and lambda *IGL* light chain loci rearrange their V and J (no D) gene segments. *IGK*, is the first of the light chain loci to rearrange. A randomly selected V and J segment recombine at the DNA level. These are transcribed into primary RNA transcripts, which are modified/spliced into V-J-C mRNA, and translated into the kappa light chain. This light chain binds with its heavy chain counterpart to form a surface immunoglobulin. If a functional kappa light chain protein is not formed, the other allele begins rearrangement. If that also fails, rearrangement of the lambda locus, *IGL*, proceeds. Similar to *IGK*, *IGL* randomly recombines its V and J segments and creates V-J-C mRNA transcripts to get translated into lambda light chains, which bind with heavy chains to form surface immunoglobulin. Similar to the other loci, *IGL* has two attempts (two alleles) to generate a functional protein.

Generating diversity of TCR and Ig

Because there is an apparent random selection of V, D, and J gene segments during somatic recombination, the total number of permutations of unique receptor proteins is logarithmically increased. This process is termed combinatorial diversity (**Table 15.1**). Combinatorial diversity is just one mechanism, however, contributing to total receptor diversity. Other contributing

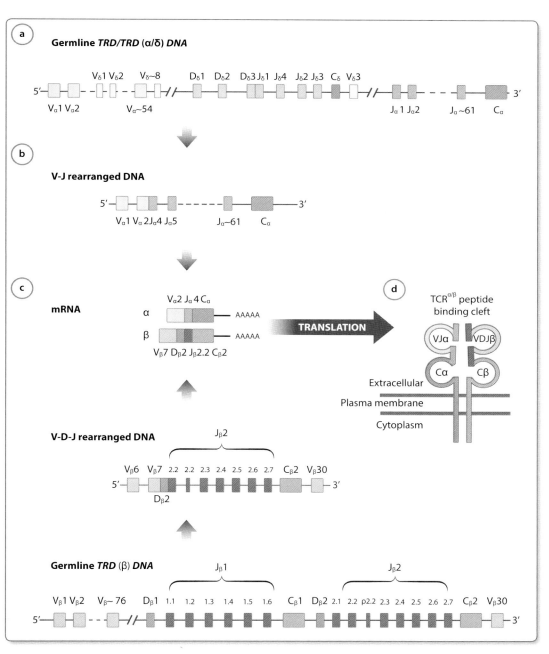

Figure 15.3 T-cell receptor somatic recombination. This schematic highlights the steps involved in rearrangement of the TRA (α) and TRB (β) loci to form a surface TCRα /β protein. (a) TRA (α) contains V and J gene segments, interrupted by the TRD (δ) locus. (b) During somatic recombination, a randomly selected Vα gene segment recombines with a Jα gene segment, deleting the interval genetic material. (c) The primary RNA transcripts are modified to mRNA, splicing out all interval genetic material to achieve the V-J-C union (with a poly-A tail). A similar process is taking place at the TRB (β) locus. TRB (β) is slightly different in that it also must recombine a D gene segment, first to a J segment, and then to a V segment (bottom half of figure). (d) Once mRNA transcripts for the TCR-α and TCR-β chains are generated, they are translated into the TCR-α and TCR-β proteins and expressed on the surface of the TCRα/β T cell.

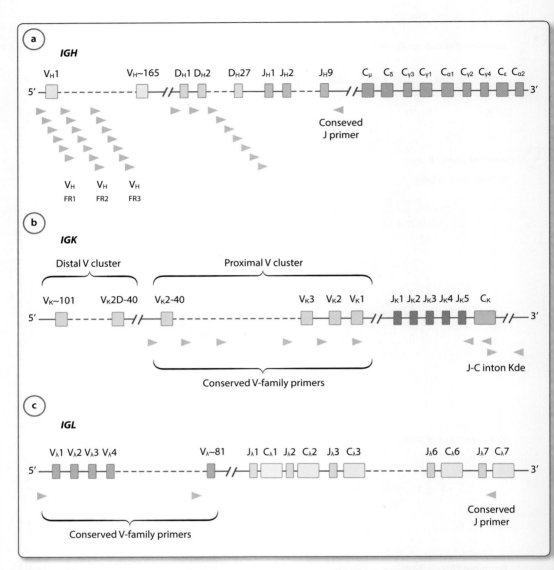

Figure 15.4 Immunoglobulin gene loci and PCR primer design strategy. IGH (heavy chain), IGK (kappa light chain), and IGL (lambda light chain) loci are shown, as well as primer design strategies. (a) IGH has many V, D, and J gene segments along with many constant (C) region gene segments. The C gene segments play a role in isotype switching. (b) IGK has V, J, and C gene segments. The V gene segments are arranged in two large duplicated clusters designated proximal and distal. (c) The IGL locus has V, J, and C gene segments. The IGL locus has a J-C cluster with approximately 11 total genes each. Primer design takes into account sequence homology. For IGH, the VH gene segments are arranged into three groups – framework regions 1, 2 and 3 (FR1, FR2, FR3). Multiple primers, up to 28, are required to cover most-to-all possible V-D-J rearrangements. For the IGK locus, most assays require up to 6 Vκ primers and two Jκ consensus primers (and a distal Kde primer and a primer to the Jκ-Cκ intron) to cover all possible V-J rearrangements. For the IGL locus, this can be accomplished by 2 Vλ primers and 1 Jλ primer, greatly simplifying the assay.

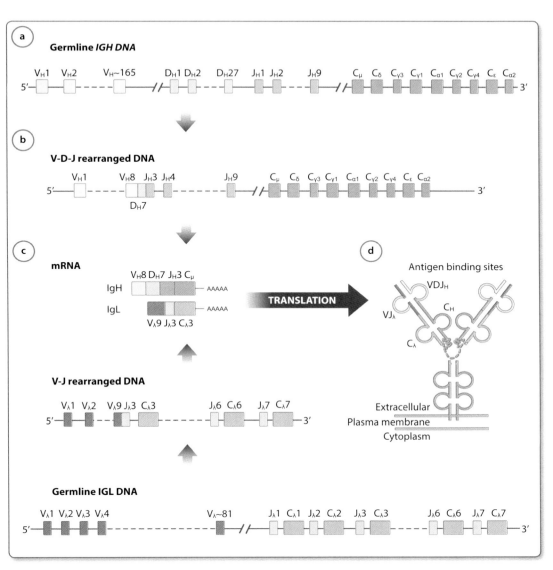

Figure 15.5 Immunoglobulin somatic recombination. This schematic highlights the steps involved in rearrangement of the IGH and IGL loci to form a surface immunoglobulin protein. (a) IGH contains V, D, J, and C gene segments. (b) During somatic recombination, a randomly selected DH gene segment first recombines with a JH gene segment, then a VH gene segment, deleting the interval genetic material. (c) The primary RNA transcripts are modified to mRNA, splicing out all interval genetic material to achieve the V-D-J-C union (with a poly-A tail). A similar process is taking place at the IGL locus (after IGK failed its recombination attempts). IGL is slightly different in that has no D gene segments (bottom half of figure). (d) Once mRNA transcripts for the heavy and light chains are generated, they are translated into the heavy and light chain proteins and expressed as an immunoglobulin on the surface of the B cell.

Table 15.1 Combinatorial diversity generated from TCR and Ig loci

Locus		Total genes	Functional rearrangeable genes	Combinatorial diversity (max) V × D × J
TCR				
TRA (α)	V	54	45	
	J	61	50	2250
	C	1	1	
TRB (β)	V	76	48	
	D	2	2	1248
	J	14	13	
	C	2	2	
TRG (γ)	V	14	6	
	J	5	5	30
	C	2	2	
TRD (δ)	V	8	8	
	D	3	3	
	J	4	4	96
	C	1	1	
Ig				
IGH	V	165	46	6348
	D	27	23	
	J	9	6	
	C	11	9	
IGK	V	101	38	190
	J	5	5	
	C	1	1	
IGL	V	81	33	165
	J	11	5	
	C	11	5	

a vast array of complex and distinct intruders (Davis & Chien, 2013). For completeness, somatic hypermutation is another diversity-generating process, occurring over the life of B cells but not T cells. In this process, as clonal populations of B cells expand, point mutations occur in the VDJ region, allowing minor alterations over time (or 'fine tuning') at the antigen-recognition site.

Allelic exclusion, clonal expansion and clonal selection of lymphocytes

Following somatic recombination, the body has an army of lymphocytes, each with a unique surface receptor capable of recognizing foreign antigen. Each lymphocyte expresses only one receptor due to allelic exclusion (only one but not both alleles of each chain are expressed due to the sequential nature of recombination). During a normal inflammatory response to antigen, lymphocytes that have their surface antigen-receptor engaged (Ig for B cells and TCR for T cells) will undergo clonal expansion. Therefore, any lymphocyte that recognizes its antigen will proliferate, creating a clonal army capable of recognizing this same antigen. Because only the cells that recognize antigen become activated and multiply, these cells become over-represented among the entire body's population of lymphocytes, a process termed clonal selection. In most infections or benign inflammatory diseases, there are numerous antigens, many of which are complex with multiple epitopes, resulting in numerous clonal expansions, or, effectively, a polyclonal response.

Testing for clonality

The meaning of clonality

The clonal proliferations described above are normal responses to antigen. In lymphocytic neoplasia, there is also a clonal expansion, but it is due to molecular oncogenic events and not receptor engagement with antigen. In neoplasia, all cells harbor virtually identical gene rearrangement sequences, and may or may not express a functional surface TCR or Ig. If any single V-J or V-D-J rearrangement appears overrepresented among a population of an infiltrate, this is evidence for clonality. It should be clear from the above discussion that clonality

factors include the coupling of proteins from two separate loci to form a functional receptor (the product of combinatorial diversity of IGH and IGK, for example) and the imprecise joining of gene segments (with single nucleotide insertions or deletions, for example), potentially altering the entire amino acid sequence of the protein chain. Using these various mechanisms, lymphocytes are able to use a few hundred gene segments to create a diverse repertoire: 10^{15} unique permutations for TCR$^{\alpha/\beta}$, 10^{18} for TCR$^{\gamma/\delta}$, and 10^{18} for Ig – apparently sufficient to combat does not necessarily equal malignancy. Over-representation of V-J or V-D-J recombination sequences by molecular analysis could potentially occur in reactive processes when the number of recognized antigens/epitopes is few and finite, resulting in clonal expansion of only one or few clones. Over-represented V-J or V-D-J recombination sequences may be true clonal populations, but biologically normal. If the sample assayed is focal enough to pick up a small clonally-expanded population of cells (such as a single germinal center, or, taken to an extreme, only 1 cell), this will give the appearance of a neoplastic clone, or pseudoclone. Clonality may also be present and detected in pre-neoplastic but biologically irrelevant processes, as these conditions may never progress to true malignancy. For T-cell processes, these latter examples of detectable clones in non-malignant conditions have been assigned various terms over the years, including clonal dermatitis, abortive or latent lymphoma, and T-cell dyscrasia.

Sensitivity of molecular testing

One of the main challenges of diagnosing lymphoma is receiving samples from early stages of the disease. The neoplastic cells are often cloaked by numerous companion normal inflammatory cells, requiring sensitive detection methods. Studies that have looked at the longitudinal progression of lymphoma have noted that clones are detected with increased frequency in skin, blood, and lymph nodes as the disease progresses, supporting the notion that false negative results are, at least in part, a function of limits of detection. Molecular tools are attractive because of their inherent high analytical sensitivity (low limits of detection). Southern blot and PCR techniques have reported limits of detection of 5% and 1% neoplastic cells, respectively, and these limits can be pushed even further by certain manipulations of the sample, such as manual microdissection (Hosler & Murphy 2014). Pushing the limits too far will ultimately lead to detection of a pseudoclone, and therefore, there is a 'molecular sweet-spot' in clonality testing, with the test being very sensitive, but not too sensitive. Most PCR-based assays recommend 0.5–2 μg of total DNA (with a significant portion from lymphocytes) as a template per reaction to ensure a sufficient number of cells are represented in the assessment.

Limitations of the molecular assay and performance characteristics

Molecular tools have been available and used for the diagnosis of cutaneous lymphoma for several decades and have been an important addition to diagnostic checklists, but not without controversy (Hosler & Murphy 2014; Ponti et al. 2005; van Dongen et al. 2003; Wood et al. 1994). It is well known that clonal analysis for early lymphoma suffers from less-than-ideal sensitivity and specificity parameters. Unambiguous lymphoma, confirmed by progression or other means, does not always have a detectable clone, and, conversely, clones are commonly reported in inflammatory dermatoses. For example, regarding the latter, clones have been detected in 10–32% of benign inflammatory conditions – pityriasis lichenoides et varioliform acuta (PLEVA), pityriasis lichenoides chronica (PLC), lichen planus, psoriasis, eczema, and drug eruptions – all considered in the clinical and histological differential diagnosis of MF (Hosler & Murphy 2014).

For MF/SS, the overall sensitivity of molecular testing has been reported as high as 90% in established MF/SS patients and as low as 10% in early MF. Wide variations in performance characteristics have prevented widespread implementation of molecular assays. Newer-generation standardized assays have helped reduce variability from laboratory to laboratory. Standardization not only offers the benefit of being able to compare data across studies, but is imperative for clearly defining diagnostic criteria, staging, as well as accurately assessing responses to therapy with recurrence and minimal residual disease. One of the more widely used molecular clonality assays for B-cell and T-cell lymphomas was developed in a European BIOMED-2 Concerted Action collaborative study (van Dongen et al., 2003). This study reported excellent performance characteristics and, subsequently, versions of these assays, including the EuroClonality / BIOMED-2 multiplex PCR kit have become commercially available and are widely used (InVivoScribe Technologies, Inc., San Diego, CA). In the BIOMED-2 study, for T-cell malignancies, the authors report a sensitivity of 89% for *TRG* (γ) and 94% for *TRB* (β) (van Dongen et al. 2003). Of note, these performance characteristics correspond to analysis of fresh or cryopreserved tissue. Other studies on formalin-fixed paraffin embedded material have been able to push the sensitivity to 90% and keep specificity in the mid-80s with specific adaptations (Hosler & Murphy 2014; Zhang et al. 2010). The performance characteristics of the molecular clonality assays will continue to vary from laboratory to laboratory depending on the methods used and their interpretative criteria.

Variations in assays

Southern blot (see **Figure 15.1**) is an older technique for clonality assessment, still used in select laboratories, but has largely been replaced by multiplex PCR-based assays. The main variables between PCR-based methods include the sample selection (frozen vs. FFPE, +/- microdissection), the targeted locus (γ vs. β, for example), primer selection (primer design and number required), and the detection method of PCR amplicons. This is not a complete list, however, as variations exist at pretty much any point in pre-analytical → analytical → post-analytical process. A few of these of these variables are pertinent to this discussion and are discussed below. For a more detailed account, the reader is directed elsewhere (Hosler & Murphy, 2014). For a discussion on emerging technologies, such as high-throughput (next generation) sequencing, refer to Chapter 16.

The quality of the specimen is one of the more important pre-analytic variables. Most dermatopathology specimens are formalin-fixed and paraffin embedded (FFPE). Current assays are now optimized on this material, but there are still potential pitfalls. The DNA in FFPE material can be of variable quality, depending on its age, how the tissue was processed, presence of inhibitors, how it was transported, etc. Many laboratories will perform a test of DNA integrity by amplifying control targets of different amplicon size. The ability to amplify 300 base pairs predicts sufficient DNA quality to perform most PCR gene rearrangement assays. Additionally, most laboratories will use at least two concentrations of DNA from the FFPE sample in amplification reactions to assess for the presence of inhibitors. These procedures can reduce the number of false-negative and ambiguous results. Laboratories also vary on the degree of enrichment of the sample. Some laboratories use complete full-slide tissue sections, others manually microdissect the specimens. Manual microdissection offers several

benefits. During re-evaluation of the slide for microdissection, the dermatopathologist has an opportunity to review the biopsy and eliminate any unnecessary testing for inappropriate specimens. Cases with low lymphocyte counts can be flagged in the event of a possible pseudoclone. Also, by dissecting out the atypical population in potential lymphoma cases, the neoplastic population is enriched compared to the background polyclonal infiltrate, improving assay sensitivity. High levels of non-target DNA have been known to inhibit PCR reactions, and therefore, eliminating non-lymphoid DNA from the reaction may have added benefit.

The PCR targets may also vary between assays. All gene rearrangement assays are predicated on the events of somatic recombination during normal lymphocyte development (refer back to **Figures 15.2–15.5**). These assays amplify DNA by using primers to conserved sequences in the V, D, and/or J regions that flank the recombined DNA. For T-cell clonality testing, the four candidate targets are *TRA* (α), *TRB* (β), *TRG* (γ), and *TRD* (δ). *TRG* (γ) is now the most commonly used target for the following reasons: *TRG* (γ) is not too complex, and therefore, the total number of possible recombinations is manageable to assay; *TRG* (γ) has relatively good sequence homology flanking the gene segments, therefore minimizing the number of PCR primers and reactions required in a multiplex assay; the PCR amplicon is less than 500 base pairs (smaller than *TRB* (β)), minimizing DNA degradation issues from FFPE samples; *TRG* (γ) is rearranged before *TRB* (β) during development, and is therefore present in a higher percentage of tumors (whether or not TCR$^{\gamma/\delta}$ is actually expressed); and the performance characteristics of the *TRG* (γ) assay have an attractive combination of high sensitivity and specificity relative to the other loci. The *TRB* (β) clonality assay is more complex than the *TRG* (γ) assay, but still used alone or in a *TRB* (β)/*TRG* (γ) combination algorithm to maximize test performance (van Dongen et al. 2003; Zhang et al. 2010). *TRD* (δ) can be used as a target in select scenarios, such as with γ/δ T-cell lymphomas and certain leukemias. *TRD* (δ) is not a good choice as a target for other T-cell tumors, including MF/SS, since it is spliced/removed during the rearrangement of *TRA* (α). For B-cell clonality testing, the three candidate loci are *IGH* (Ig heavy chain), *IGK* (Ig kappa light chain), and

IGL (Ig lambda light chain). It is logical that the *IGH* locus is the most common target as it is the first of the loci to rearrange and rearrangement is required for the survival and propagation of B-cell neoplasms. *IGK* and *IGL* loci are also often assayed, either in parallel or as a reflex to a negative *IGH* assay, to increase the overall sensitivity.

Selection of primers for a rearrangement assay is a balancing act. On the one hand, enough primers must be included in the assay to detect as many possible V-D-J recombination events (one primer may be used for more than one gene segment if there is sequence homology). If the clone recombined its DNA using a gene segment unrecognized by the primer cocktail, the result will be false-negative. On the other hand, if too many primers are included in the assay, it may not be possible to achieve reaction conditions for all primers to optimally amplify the interval DNA, also resulting in a false-negative result. As opposed to previous generations of tests which limited primer coverage to more commonly rearranged genes, most modern clonality assays use a multiplex approach that can detect most all gene segment rearrangement combinations. Primers are designed to bind 5' to all the possible V gene segments (or D segments in some settings) and 3' to all possible J segments. Therefore, regardless of which random segments recombine, one set of primers will be juxtaposed enough to create a detectable PCR product less than a few hundred base pairs in length. Of course, the total number of primers needed to cover all possible rearrangements is dependent on the sequence homology flanking the gene segments. For the commonly used InVivoScribe assays, only six primers are needed to cover most all rearrangements of *TRG* (γ) (see **Figure 15.2**) (van Dongen et al., 2003). The same company's kit targeting *TRB* (β) requires 38 different primers. The Ig loci are particularly challenging for primer design due to their relatively large number of V-D-J gene segments and lack of complete sequence homology flanking those gene segments (see **Figure 15.4**). For the *IGH* locus, there are three V framework regions (FR1, FR2, FR3), each requiring multiple primers to 'cover' all possible rearrangements. In the InVivoScribe assay, 28 different primers divided into five different reaction tubes are used (tubes A-E) to reduce the complexity of any single reaction mix. *IGK* and *IGL* are less complex with more sequence homology, requiring 10 total primers in two reaction tubes for *IGK* and 3 total primers in a single reaction tube for *IGL*. There is a trade-off between designing primers capable of detecting as many permutations as possible, to increase sensitivity, and minimizing the complexity of the assay. The more primers in the reaction mix, the more risk for competing reactions and failed reactions due to suboptimal annealing conditions.

Impact of using different assay methods

Despite efforts to standardize clonality assays, different testing centers may employ different methods, and therefore results cannot necessarily be correlated. For example, a positive clone detected on a diagnostic biopsy using *TRG* (γ) as a target at testing center A may be followed up by a negative clonality assay using *TRB* (β) as a target (or using a different *TRG* (γ) assay) at testing center B, even though the disease is progressing. Moreover, even when the same assay and target are used (even on the same exact biopsy), results vary widely from laboratory-to-laboratory and technician-to-technician.

Interpretation

When using a gene rearrangement assay to assess for clonality, there are different levels of interpretation. The reaction data must first be interpreted (individually as well as a collective interpretation of all reaction mixes/tubes for a given sample), and then the result must be assimilated with other data on the patient in order to establish a diagnosis. False positive and false negative results are common and must be considered at all interpretation tiers. There may be biologic or technical reasons for these misleading results (**Table 15.2**).

Most PCR-based assays use multiple primer sets in multiplex reactions, generating multiple sets of data for each sample. Each reaction should yield one of the following results (assuming no reaction failure): clonal (positive), polyclonal (negative), or some indeterminate category, such as 'peak noted' or 'suspicious'. Failed reactions occasionally occur and are mostly due to poor quality DNA or variations in sample preparation (fixation, inhibitors, etc.).

With polyclonal populations, the amplicons will vary in size, in a vague Gaussian distribution,

Table 15.2 Potential technical and biological sources of false positive and false negative gene rearrangement studies

	False positives	False negatives
Technical	• Carry-over contamination • Switched specimen	• Contaminated or poor quality DNA, poor amplification* • Inhibitors causing inefficient or failed PCR* • Specific targeted gene rearrangements undetectable due to primer selection • Tumor below limit of detection • Switched specimen
Biological	• Limited DNA sample: pseudoclonality and oligoclonality • Clonal expansion of normal, non-malignant inflammatory process • Oligoclonality/pseudoclonality in patients with immunodeficiency (elderly, immunocompromised, etc.) • Pre-malignant but stable disease • Other biologically irrelevant clones • Incorrect clinical diagnosis (follow-up too short, patient actually has lymphoma)	• Ig/TCR loci unrearranged (germline) • Ig/TCR locus with trans-rearrangement (Vγ-Jβ, for example) • Targeted gene rearrangement and/or primer sites deleted or absent during lymphocyte development • Somatic hypermutation of IGH, IGK, and/or IGL loci • Translocation (with IGH , for example) prohibiting amplification • Antitumor response resulting in oligoclonality • Tumor with secondary rearrangement, resulting in oligoclonality • Biclonality • Incorrect clinical diagnosis (patient doesn't have lymphoma)

*Results in failed reaction, not false negative result

due to the numerous and random V-J and V-D-J rearrangements represented in the mix (**Figure 15.6a** and **15.6b**). Clonal populations have an overrepresented specific rearrangement, and when present, the PCR amplification of this clone dominates within the mix (**Figure 15.6c** and **15.6d**). In these cases, there is little or no background polyclonal tracing. It should be noted that different laboratories use different criteria for what constitutes a clonal peak, and therefore, a 'clonal' call can be quite subjective. Moreover, neoplastic populations may have rearrangement of one allele, causing a single peak, or, in approximately 40% of tumors, rearrangement of two alleles, resulting in two peaks. True biclonality may occur, but is considered rare. Often times, the tracings do not clearly separate into clonal or polyclonal categories (**Figure 15.6e** and **15.6f**). For example, there may be a spike or spikes rising above a polyclonal tracing. This could be a spurious, biologically irrelevant finding but may also represent a true low-level clone within a background polyclonal population. Pseudoclonality is another interpretive challenge. Pseudoclonality refers to the detection of a biologically irrelevant 'clone', possibly by

amplifying DNA from a single cell or small population of cells. This spurious finding can often be identified by its lack of reproducibility in duplicated or repeated reactions. Sometimes clonal peaks are also observed just outside of the normally acceptable amplicon size range. In all these circumstances, interpretation can be challenging, and may lead to the unsatisfactory reporting of 'peak noted' or 'suspicious', requiring further studies.

Once the individual reactions are interpreted, the results are incorporated into a final molecular report. The final report takes into account the quantity and quality of all potential clonal peaks, as well as possible additional data, such as the clinical, histologic, and immunophenotypic findings. Similar to the interpretation of individual reactions, the final molecular report will result into one of at least three categories: clonal (positive), polyclonal (negative), and a middle category. This middle category may include 'indeterminate' (for cases with conspicuous populations but do not otherwise meet the laboratory's criteria for clonality), or possibly 'oligoclonal' (>2 clonal-appearing peaks).

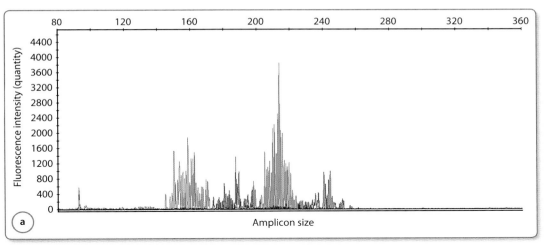

a

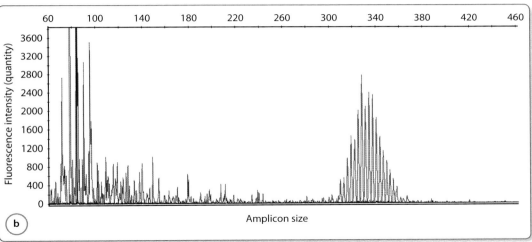

b

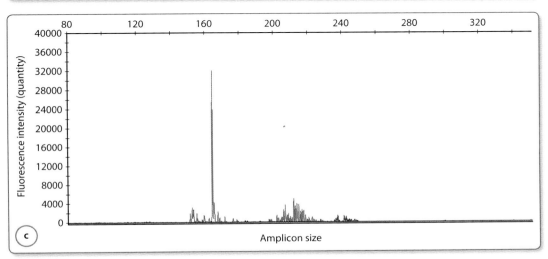

c

Figure 15.6 *(continues overleaf)*

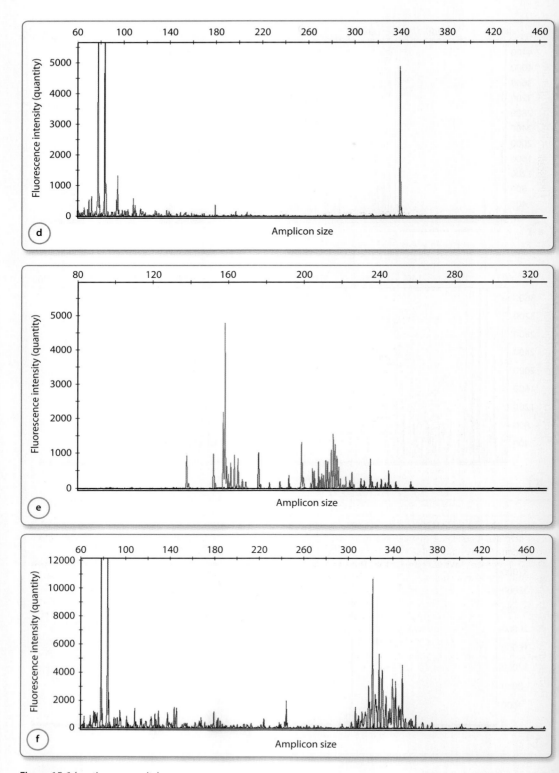

Figure 15.6 *(continues opposite)*

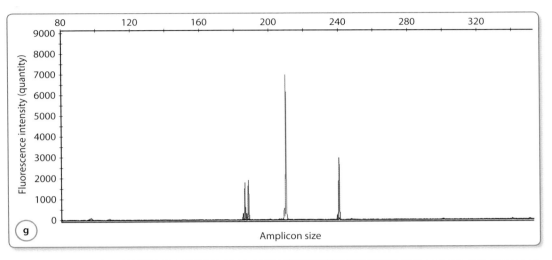

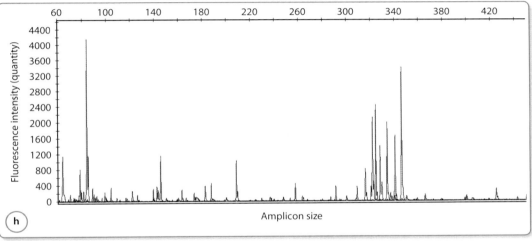

Figure 15.6 *continued*. Interpretation of TCR and Ig gene rearrangement studies. In these examples, DNA is extracted from microdissected FFPE tissue from suspected lymphoma patients. Fluorescently-labeled primers are grouped into two separate PCR reactions (mix A and mix B, BIOMED-2 protocol, InVivoScribe) for TRG and five reactions (mix A-E, BIOMED-2 protocol, InVivoScribe) for IGH. The amplicons are separated by capillary electrophoresis based on amplicon size (with GeneScan technology). Only mix/tube A results are shown for clarity. Blue and green tracings correspond to different groups of fluorescently-labeled primers within the multiplex reaction. The X-axis corresponds to amplicon size and the Y-axis to fluorescence intensity (quantity). A polyclonal population of cells will have Gaussian spread of amplicon sizes due to the numerous different rearrangements represented in the reaction [(a), TRG; (b), IGH]. A clonal population of T cells will have an overrepresented rearrangement, indicated by a peak, or spike, with a low level or suppressed polyclonal background [(c), TRG; (d), IGH]. Often, a prominent spike or spikes is present with a background polyclonal component, requiring integration of all available clinical and pathologic data to render a final interpretation [(e), TRG; (f), IGH]. The oligoclonal pattern has multiple (>2) peaks [(g), TRG; (h), IGH], which may occur in reactive or truly malignant processes, also requiring integration of other available data.

While true neoplastic clonal processes will often have one (one allele rearranged) or two (both alleles rearranged) discrete peaks, sometimes there are more than two. Oligoclonality refers to the presence of multiple discrete peaks, which would be interpreted as clonal if there were only one or two per tracing (**Figure 15.6g** and **15.6h**). There are several possible reasons for oligoclonality. It could be a 'false positive', resulting from sampling, limited DNA input, or DNA degradation. However, oligoclonality may be a sign of true clonality. Multiple clones may exist in bi-lineage tumors or if the tumor has a secondary rearrangement of their TCR/Ig locus. This latter event certainly occurs in the case of T-cell leukemia, and likely in MF/SS, albeit more rare of an event as these are neoplasms of post-thymic T cells. Another possibility for oligoclonality is the presence of a 'clonal' anti-tumor response in the tested tissue. While the anti-tumor T-cell clone may not be a true neoplasm, its presence may still aid in the identification of underlying lymphoma. Laboratories will often report oligoclonality as such, but due to the uncertainty of its meaning, final interpretations may differ in their level of concern for a neoplasm.

Final molecular interpretations often rely upon analysis of molecular data only. This is especially true for reference laboratories that usually receive no additional information on the patient. While it is important for all laboratories to analyze the data in isolation initially (similar to an examining as H&E slide prior to biasing oneself with the clinical history), final interpretation can be enhanced, or shaped, in light of the entire patient picture. This practice may resolve a subset of cases in the less-than-desirable 'indeterminate' category. For example, in patients with a very low pre-test probability of having MF/SS (clinician thought eczema, biopsy unimpressive, etc.), a borderline 'indeterminate' case can be downgraded to 'negative'. This clinical–pathologic correlation is good practice for molecular interpretation, but it is a requirement for rendering a final biopsy interpretation. Submitting samples for clonality analysis without screening for pre-test probability will yield an increased number of false-positive results.

It should be clear from the discussion that molecular analysis of rearranged Ig or TCR loci should never be a standalone test. There are technical and biological reasons for false positive and false negative results (see **Table 15.2**), requiring incorporation of all available data – clinical, histologic, immunophenotypic, and molecular – to reach an accurate diagnosis. The power of the molecular test can be enhanced by the following:

1. Limitation of testing to cases with a high pre-test probability
2. Communication between clinician, pathologist, and molecular diagnostician on the differential diagnosis and relative level of concern for each possibility
3. Preparation of the sample by enriching area of interest through manual microdissection
4. Assessment of DNA quality by quantifying extracted DNA and performing control amplifications
5. Performing the rearrangement assay with appropriate targets based on the sample characteristics
6. Interpreting the results in the context of all available data for the individual patient

When incorporating the molecular data into the evaluation of a biopsy for lymphoma, there is no single or right way, as any way is acceptable so long as the basic principles are applied: molecular analysis is not a stand-alone test, molecular data concordant with the pre-test probability should carry significant diagnostic weight, and, accordingly, molecular data discordant with the pre-test probability should carry significantly less diagnostic weight.

Regarding MF/SS, because the clonality tests are not infallible with respect to performance parameters, the power of testing is highly dependent on the pre-test probability for disease (**Figure 15.7**). Pre-test probability can be determined by a variety of means, including using algorithmic approaches for evaluating histologic and immunophenotypic data (see *Applications* below). One effective approach to interpreting a biopsy with molecular data is to first establish a pre-test probability of MF, and then perform TRG (γ) rearrangement studies. The interpretive weight of the TRG (γ) rearrangement test result is guided by the pre-test probability. Discordant results may advocate a second round of molecular testing, using a different target, like TRB (β). In the event the results remain discordant (or TRB

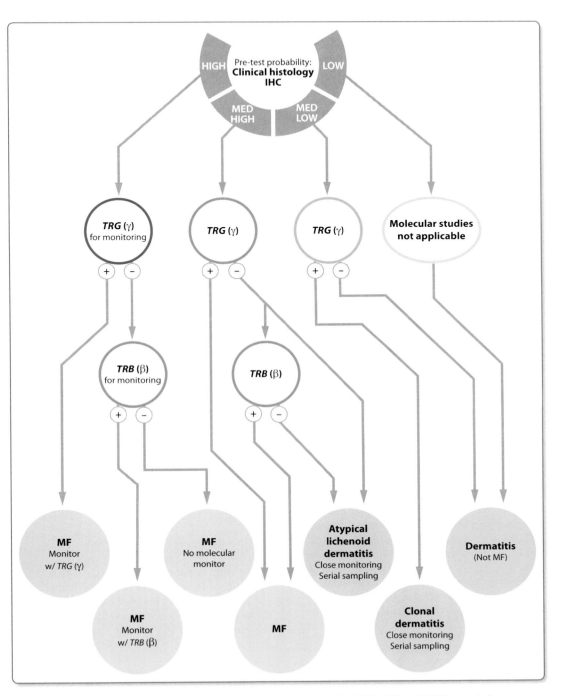

Figure 15.7 Algorithm for incorporating molecular data when evaluating for MF. For MF, the TRG (γ) assay is the preferred initial molecular test due to its performance parameters and relatively low complexity. TRB (β) testing may have utility in some scenarios. Pre-test probability for the disease will shape the testing strategy and interpretation of data.

(β) testing not performed at all), diagnoses such as 'atypical lichenoid dermatitis' (high pre-test probability but no clone) or 'dermatitis with detectable T-cell clone' (low pre-test probability but positive for clone) would be appropriate. In these cases, recommendations would include the following: close monitoring of the patient, serial sampling with molecular studies (at 6 month intervals from untreated areas), and sampling multiple anatomic sites (which has been shown to increase sensitivity/specificity (Thurber et al., 2007)). Similar diagnostic algorithms have been proposed (Hosler & Murphy, 2014; Langerak et al., 2012; Zhang et al., 2010).

For non-MF/SS samples, a similar approach may be used (**Figure 15.8**). For these tumors, well-established algorithms are not available for the dermatology patient, requiring pre-test probability assessments to rely on subjective data. Once an initial assessment is made, however, molecular testing can proceed, with the molecular target dictated by the tumor's immunophenotype (B cell or T cell). For B-cell tumors, testing would begin with *IGH* (could even start with just the *IGH* V-J reactions). If this is negative but there is a high index of suspicious for lymphoma, test *IGK*, and if that is negative, test *IGL*. Performing these tests in parallel may be appropriate when there are time constraints and less concern for cost. For suspected non-MF/SS T-cell neoplasms, the testing algorithm should be similar to suspected MF/SS samples. An exception is the option to use *TRD* (δ) as a target for suspected γ/δ and primitive (lymphoblastic) T-cell tumors, for the reasons described above (see *Variations* in assays section). Again, the molecular result should not trump the other available data. If there are discordant results, there is no shame in the diagnosis of 'atypical lymphoid hyperplasia' (high pre-test probability but no clone) or 'atypical clonal infiltrate' (low pre-test probability with clone) and recommending close follow-up with repeat sampling.

Applications

The primary dermatopathology application for T-cell and B-cell gene rearrangement studies is to aid in the diagnosis of lymphoma. In the vast majority of cases, more specifically, they are used to help diagnosis early mycosis fungoides and differentiate reactive B-cell proliferations from low grade B-cell lymphoma. Less commonly, testing is used to distinguish reactive infiltrates from non-MF/SS low-grade T-cell tumors, high grade B-cell and T-cell tumors from reactive processes, and B/T-cell tumors from other mimickers, such as NK or histiocytic tumors. There are also some specific prognostic applications. The most common applications are listed in **Table 15.3**.

Diagnosis of MF/SS

Diagnoses of MF and SS are made by assimilating the clinical, histomorphologic, immunohistochemical and molecular data. As discussed above (see Interpretation on page 215), for clonality studies to be useful for diagnosis, there must be a relatively high pre-test probability. For example, in patients with clear benign inflammatory conditions, such as eczema and psoriasis, T-cell clonality studies will only cloud the picture, as 10–30% of these patients will have a PCR-detectable clone (Langerak et al., 2007; Plaza et al., 2008). After all, if the test is positive, it must be explained. Similarly, in patients with clear or known MF/SS, either by clinical or histomorphologic criteria, up to one-third will not have a PCR-detectable clone, also requiring explanation. In cases of tumor stage or erythrodermic MF, or SS, clonality detection approaches 100% (Ponti et al., 2005). In these latter patient groups, molecular testing for diagnosis may not be indicated but may be useful for other purposes, such as determining prognosis or tracking a patient's response to therapy.

MF is the most common cutaneous T-cell lymphoma, often progressing through patch, plaque, and tumor stages. Patch stage MF is comprised of multiple, variably-sized (usually >5 cm) erythematous plaques, most commonly located on skin with low ultraviolet exposure, or a 'bathing suit' distribution. Skin lesions may have epidermal atrophy, telangiectasias, and variable pigmentation (poikilodermatous). As the disease progresses, skin lesions become larger and thicker with possible ulceration and tumor formation. Erythroderma, lymphadenopathy, and visceral organ involvement are late findings. SS is related to MF, with a leukemic component. SS is defined by circulating neoplastic cells (specifically,

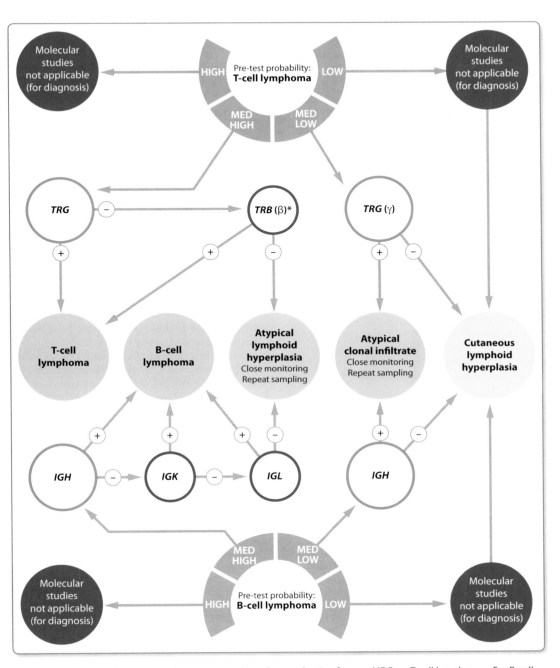

Figure 15.8 Algorithm for incorporating molecular data when evaluating for non-MF B- or T-cell lymphomas. For B-cell and T-cell infiltrates, the molecular diagnostic strategy and interpretation of results will be dependent on the pre-test probability for lymphoma. The algorithm uses tests in sequence, not in parallel, for cost considerations. Assays can be performed in parallel if there are time constraints.
*TRD testing may also be performed in suspected primitive (lymphoblastic) or γ/δ T-cell tumors

Table 15.3 Applications for TCR and immunoglobulin rearrangement studies

Category	Application
Diagnosis	Diagnosis of MF/SS Diagnosis of low grade B-cell lymphoma versus pseudolymphoma Diagnosis of other primary cutaneous B-cell and T-cell lymphomas Diagnosis of B-cell versus T-cell lymphoma Diagnosis of other hematopoietic tumors primarily and secondarily involving the skin
Prognosis	Evaluating blood, lymph node, and bone marrow for molecular evidence of disseminated tumor Evaluate for same clone from multiple biopsy sites
Other	Evaluate for therapeutic efficacy (minimal residual disease) Evaluate for relapse/recurrence

>1000 Sézary cells/mm^3 and/or >20% Sézary cells) resulting in erythroderma and generalized lymphadenopathy. SS patients have generalized disease at presentation. SS is rare, accounting for <5% of cutaneous T-cell malignancies.

By histology and immunohistochemistry, MF has characteristic features. In the most conventional type, early lesions have a mild lichenoid or band-like infiltrate, often with characteristic stromal changes (**Figure 15.9**). Cytologically atypical cells tag along the epidermal-dermal junction and migrate into the epidermis, forming Pautrier microabscesses. These cells are cytologically atypical, with enlarged, irregular nuclei and perinuclear halos. At times, the nuclei fold upon themselves, creating a cerebriform appearance. More advanced lesions will have denser and deeper infiltrates and may transform into larger cells. SS infiltrates are often histologically subtle, with variable perivascular, interstitial, and epidermal infiltrates. By immunohistochemistry, in most cases, the neoplastic cell of MF and SS is a post-thymic CD4+/CD45RO+ helper T cell. A subset of MF cases will be CD8+/CD4-. Aberrant loss of normal T-cell markers, such as CD7, CD5, and/or CD2 is helpful when present. Transformed cases of MF may express CD30.

When classic clinical, morphologic, and immunohistochemical features are present, a diagnosis of MF/SS can usually be made without requiring molecular analysis (although molecular testing may be prudent for other means, as discussed below). Early MF diagnosis is plagued by its vague clinical presentation, which can be quite protean, overlapping with many reactive inflammatory dermatoses. These include eczema, psoriasis, lymphomatoid papulosis, pityriasis lichenoides et varioliform acuta (PLEVA), and drug eruptions, among other papulosquamous disorders. The histology can be equally ambiguous, and there is often interpretation variability, even among panels of experts. There are many well-described histologic mimickers of MF, mirroring the clinical differential diagnosis. Immunohistochemical evaluation of T-cell populations remains limited by subjective assessment of CD4:CD8 ratios (the best available immunosurrogate for clonality) and variable T-cell antigen loss. Further compounding problems with diagnosis are well-described clinical and pathologic variants of MF - hypopigmented, purpuric, bullous, follicular, palmoplantar, granulomatous, pagetoid reticulosis, and others – all of which clinically and histologically deviate from conventional MF. There are also various poorly defined, nebulous chronic conditions, like small- and large-plaque parapsoriasis, which may or may not be precursors to MF.

In order to more clearly define early MF, facilitate its diagnosis, and perhaps reduce inter-observer variability intrinsic to early MF,

Figure 15.9 Histologic and immunohistochemical features of MF. (a) In MF, lymphocytes extend into the epidermis, in a pattern of epidermotropism (left-hand panel, H&E, 200×). These cells align along the epidermal-dermal junction as well as extend into more superficial layers of the epidermis, forming Pautrier microabscesses. The lymphocytes are cytologically atypical, with enlarged hyperchromatic and convoluted (cerebriform) nuclei, and perinuclear halos. (b) By immunohistochemistry, the epidermal infiltrate is positive for CD3 (not shown) and CD4 (CD4, 200×). (c) There are virtually no epidermal CD8+ cells (CD8, 200×), and (d) CD7 expression appears aberrantly lost (CD7, 200×). An example of a less-clear-cut case of MF, requiring molecular studies, is shown on the right-hand panels.

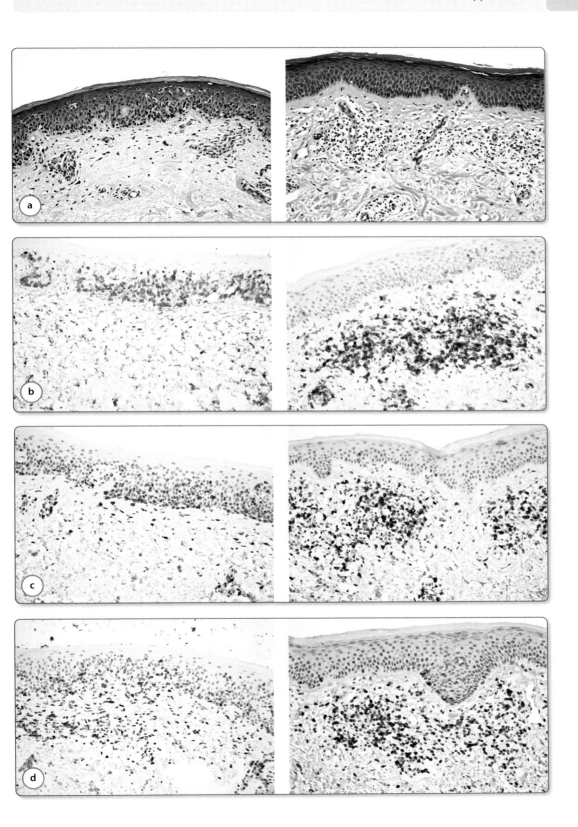

algorithmic methods have been proposed (Guitart et al., 2001; Pimpinelli et al., 2005; Santucci et al., 2000). These are often based upon various weighted combinations of clinical, histologic, immunophenotypic and sometimes molecular findings. One example is from the International Society for Cutaneous Lymphoma (ISCL) (Pimpinelli et al., 2005). They use a point-based system, requiring 4 points for a diagnosis of MF. There are two major criteria – one clinical and one histological – each awarded 2 points. For the clinical criteria, 2 points are awarded if the patient has persistent and/or progressive patches or thin plaques with two of the following: non-sun-exposed location, size/shape variation, poikiloderma. If only one, not two, from this list is met, only 1 point is awarded. For the major histological criteria (2 points), there must be a superficial lymphoid infiltrate with two (i.e. both) of the following: epidermotropism without spongiosis, and lymphoid atypia. If there is only one of these present, 1 point is awarded. An additional 1 point could be 'earned' if a molecular clone is detected. A further 1 point is scored if immunophenotypic criteria are met, as defined by any or all of the following:

1. <50% CD2+, CD3+, and/or CD5+ T cells
2. <10% CD7+ T cells

3. Epidermal/dermal discordance of CD2, CD3, CD5, or CD7 (antigen loss confined to epidermis)

Comprehensive algorithmic approaches may help standardize the diagnosis of early MF/SS, or, at minimum, can be used to establish a pre-test probability for MF/SS prior to molecular testing (see **Figure 15.7**).

Diagnosis of low grade B-cell lymphoma versus pseudolymphoma

The second most common application for molecular clonality testing is distinguishing reactive/pseudolymphomatous infiltrates from low grade B-cell lymphomas. The clinical presentations offer little insight and there is significant overlap in the histologic and immunophenotypic features. Combining the histological features with immunohistochemistry and molecular studies can often lead to the correct diagnosis (**Table 15.4**).

Pseudolymphoma

The term pseudolymphoma refers to a reactive lymphocytic infiltrate and is synonymous with cutaneous lymphoid hyperplasia. Any persistent

	Clinical	Histology	IHC	Cytogenetics	Molecular
Pseudolymphoma	Wide age range and presentations	Dense infiltrate, usually mixed, reactive germinal centers common	Mixture of CD20+ and CD3+ cells, Bcl-6-, Bcl-2-, CD43-, CD5-, κ/λ mixed, ↑↑Ki67	Normal	Polyclonal
PCMZL	Wide age range, usually older adults, trunk and extremities, head/neck, usually solitary, can be grouped papules, plaques and nodules	Nodular and diffuse, can have plasmacytoid and/or monocytoid morph, germ centers common	CD20+, κ/λ restricted, CD43var, CD23var, Bcl-2var, Bcl-6-, CD10-, CD5-	t(14;18) IGH-MALT1 rare t(11;18) API2-MALT1 rare t(3;14) rare	Clonal
PCFCL	Elderly, head/neck, solitary or grouped papules, plaques and nodules	Nodular and diffuse, may have large irregular germinal centers, variable proportions of centroblasts and centrocytes	CD20+, Bcl-6+, Bcl-2var, CD10var, CD43var, CD5-, ↑Ki67, CD21/CD23 dendritic cell lysis	t(14;18) IGH-BCL2 rare	Clonal
CLL/SLL	Elderly, localized papules/nodule or generalized	Diffuse, interstitial, monomorphous small mature-appearing lymphocytes	CD20+, CD5+, CD23+, κ/λ restricted, CD43+, Bcl-2var, Bcl-6-	Trisomy 12 13q abnormalities	Clonal

Table 15.4 Pseudolymphoma versus low grade B-cell lymphoma

antigen-presenting state (arthropod assault, penetrating injury, drug, etc.) can lead to a pseudolymphoma. Discrete lesions of known inflammatory conditions, such as tumid lupus erythematosus, can also mimic lymphoma. Because, by definition, pseudolymphomnas are reactive conditions, the infiltrates are often mixed. This can be demonstrated by morphology (mix of lymphocytes, histiocytes, plasma cells, granulocytes), and immunohistochemistry (mix of CD3+ and CD20+ cells). Molecular analysis will yield a polyclonal tracing. As discussed, however, lack of a detectable clone does not exclude malignancy (see **Table 15.2**). Additionally, because many pseudolymphomas are due to chronic antigen stimulation in a focal area, the occasional detection of a clone should not be surprising. If the molecular test sample contains a single germinal center, for example, a clonal result is likely.

Primary cutaneous marginal zone lymphoma (PCMZL)

Primary cutaneous marginal zone lymphoma (PCMZL) is the cutaneous counterpart of the mucosa-associated lymphoid tissue (MALT) lymphoma, which is most commonly observed in the gastrointestinal tract. PCMZL is extremely difficult to differentiate from pseudolymphoma, and, in fact, many cases arise within a backdrop of pseudolymphoma. On histology, PCMZL is usually a dense nodular infiltrate, with an overlying grenz zone. There may be germinal centers, but they are reactive-appearing and not the prominent feature. Most of the infiltrate consists of small, mature-appearing lymphocytes. Occasionally, there may be a prominent plasmacytoid population or monocytoid (fried egg)-appearing cells. Immunohistochemistry is sometimes helpful. For plasmacytoid populations, light chain (kappa/lambda) restriction is a surrogate for clonality, suggestive of PCMZL. The aberrant expression of CD43, normally a T-cell marker, is also helpful but not diagnostic nor specific. Because PCMZL may only minimally deviate from pseudolymphoma using histologic and immunophenotypic criteria, molecular testing for clonality can be very helpful for distinguishing these two entities.

Primary cutaneous follicle center cell lymphoma (PCFCL)

Primary cutaneous follicle center cell lymphoma

(PCFCL) is the most common primary cutaneous B-cell lymphoma, accounting for approximately 40–50% of cases. Follicular lymphoma may arise in the lymph node, but these are now considered separate entities. On histology, PCFCL can have a follicular pattern or a more nodular/diffuse pattern without follicles. Cases with the classic follicular pattern may be diagnosed without immunohistochemistry or molecular studies. These cases have large irregular germinal centers without the typical reactive features such as polarization and numerous tingible-body macrophages. Immunohistochemistry is very helpful in the diagnosis of PCFCL. The follicle center cell has a CD20+/Bcl-6+ immunophenotype. Bcl-2 staining is variable, but when diffusely positive, may suggest nodal lymphoma involving the skin. The t(14;18)(q32;q21) translocation that results in the *IGH-BCL2* fusion, which promotes a cellular anti-apoptosis signal, is observed in up to 90% of nodal follicular lymphomas but is present in only a minority of PCFCL cases. In Bcl-2+/Bcl-6+/CD10+ tumors, there should be high suspicion for nodal follicular lymphoma secondarily involving the skin. At times, PCFCL can be difficult to distinguish from pseudolymphoma as both may have prominent follicles. The follicles will share the same immunophenotype requiring the subjective determination of reactive versus neoplastic. Moreover, the PCFCL without the follicular pattern can have significant histologic overlap with pseudolymphoma (bcl-6 staining is particularly useful in this setting). Molecular clonality studies may be useful in these ambiguous cases and should be incorporated into diagnostic algorithms (see **Figure 15.8**).

Diagnosis of other primary cutaneous B-cell and T-cell lymphomas

Other primary cutaneous B-cell lymphomas in the most recent classification system include diffuse large B-cell lymphoma, leg type, and diffuse large B-cell lymphoma, other (which includes intravascular large B-cell lymphoma) (Willemze et al., 2005). The non-MF/SS primary cutaneous T-cell lymphomas include the CD30+ lymphoproliferative disorders (primary cutaneous anaplastic large cell lymphoma and lymphomatoid papulosis), subcutaneous panniculitis-like T-cell lymphoma, primary cutaneous CD4+ small/medium pleomorphic T-cell lymphoma (provisional entity), adult T-cell leukemia/lymphoma, primary cutaneous NK/T-cell lymphoma, nasal type, primary cutaneous aggressive CD8+ T-cell lymphoma (provisional entity), primary cutaneous γ/δ T-cell lymphoma (provisional entity), and primary cutaneous peripheral T-cell lymphoma, unspecified. All of these entities are often clonal by molecular studies (**Table 15.5**). In many cases, however, the infiltrates are readily recognized as malignant and do not require molecular analysis. Ig/TCR rearrangement studies can be useful in early lesions or other diagnostically ambiguous scenarios, and the molecular data should be incorporated into diagnostic algorithms (see **Figure 15.8**).

Diagnosis of B-cell versus T-cell lymphoma

On rare occasion, the dermatopathologist is confronted with an atypical infiltrate of uncertain lineage. Immunohistochemistry may reveal a mixture of B cells and T cells, but the etiology of

the malignant population cannot be determined with certainty. Performing both Ig and TCR clonality studies may help in this scenario. Interpretation of the molecular results should not be performed in a vacuum, however. B-cell neoplasms can have rearranged TCR and T-cell neoplasms can have rearranged Ig (Chen et al., 1988). Fortunately, these rare events are much more common in acute leukemia and would be considered extremely rare in more mature post-thymic and post-bone marrow leukemias/lymphomas, such as those commonly encountered in the skin.

Diagnosis of other hematopoietic tumors primarily and secondarily involving the skin

Other primary non-lymphocyte-derived cutaneous hematopoietic tumors such as blastic plasmacytoid dendritic cell neoplasm, tumors of natural killer (NK) cells and Langerhans cells (and others of monocytic/dendritic lineage) do not undergo gene rearrangement. Although rare cases exist, as a rule, tumors

Table 15.5 TCR and Immunoglobulin rearrangement in primary cutaneous lymphomas			
Tumor			**Tumor cases with Ig/TCR rearrangement (%) (Hosler & Murphy 2014)**
T cell	Indolent	Reactive/pseudolymphoma	10–30
		Mycosis fungoides and variants	80–90
		Anaplastic large cell lymphoma	Most
		Lymphomatoid papulosis	60–70
		Subcutaneous panniculitis-like T-cell lymphoma	Most
		CD4+ small/medium pleomorphic T-cell lymphoma	Most
	Indolent/aggressive	Adult T cell leukemia/lymphoma	40–60
	Aggressive	NK/T-cell lymphoma, nasal type	Low, but up to 30%
		Aggressive CD8+ T-cell lymphoma	Most
		γ/δ T-cell lymphoma	Most
		Sézary syndrome	>95
		Peripheral T-cell lymphoma, unspecified	Most
B cell	Indolent	Reactive/pseudolymphoma	10–25
		Marginal zone lymphoma	50–80
		Follicle center cell lymphoma	60–90
	Intermediate	Diffuse large B-cell lymphoma, leg type	50–90
		Diffuse large B-cell lymphoma, other	Most
		Intravascular large B-cell lymphoma	Most

derived from a non-lymphocyte lineage maintain the TCR and Ig loci in germline configuration, and thus clonality studies will be negative.

Of course, T- and B-cell leukemias can secondarily involve the skin and will be positive by Ig/TCR clonality studies. Many leukemias have already been diagnosed by the time there is cutaneous involvement, limiting the utility of molecular testing. The indolent leukemias, however, may reach the skin and clinically mimic other processes, requiring biopsy. Of these, chronic lymphocytic leukemia (CLL)/small cell lymphocytic lymphoma (SLL) is the most common. Cutaneous involvement by CLL/SLL may be the primary reason for a skin biopsy, but CLL/SLL also is commonly identified in biopsies of elderly individuals as an incidental finding (biopsies of skin cancers, inflammatory processes, etc.). CLL/SLL may mimic the primary cutaneous B-cell lymphomas or pseudolymphoma, but ancillary testing can lead to the correct diagnosis (**Table 15.4**). Hodgkin lymphoma, now considered a B-cell process (and many cutaneous cases re-classified as EBV mucocutaneous ulcers), will also have a rearranged *IGH* locus. T-cell large granular lymphocytic leukemia (T-LGL) is indolent and a challenging diagnosis, possibly requiring TCR clonality testing to confirm its presence in the skin.

Evaluating prognosis in the MF/ SS patient

The above-mentioned applications for clonality testing all focus on diagnosis. There are several ways clonality testing can potentially impact prognosis in the lymphoma patient:

- Detecting clones in the blood, lymph nodes, or visceral organs at diagnosis
- Detecting clones in multiple, anatomically separate skin biopsies at diagnosis

Tumor involving blood, lymph nodes and/ or visceral organs (bone marrow) at diagnosis predicts a worse patient outcome. Flow cytometric analysis and histopathology remain the standard for these types of evaluations, but molecular analysis may also play a role. More multivariate analyses are needed to determine the independent prognostic value of a molecularly-detected clone in these settings, but, for now, molecular data are required for complete staging

in the Tumor-Node-Metastasis-Blood (TNMB) staging system, even if only for data-collecting purposes (Edge et al., 2011; Olsen et al., 2007; Willemze et al., 2005).

While staging remains the primary focus for utilizing molecular data for the purposes of stratifying patients based on risk of progression, there are other potential uses. For example, there is evidence that patients with multiple skin biopsies harboring the same T-cell clone have a higher risk of progression (Vega et al., 2002).

Following patients longitudinally

Molecular testing may also be used for disease monitoring, for example searching for minimal residual disease, therapeutic responses, or recurrences in patients who achieve clinical remission (Kandolf Sekulović et al., 2007). These applications argue for molecular testing at diagnosis even when testing is not required to establish the diagnosis. These scenarios are often challenging to characterize by histology and immunohistochemistry alone, as the tumor population may be overshadowed by the preponderance of normal cells Comparing tracings from cutaneous biopsies at diagnosis with those from blood, lymph node, and bone marrow specimens can help when looking for occult disease. Moreover, longitudinally monitoring the patient for disease recurrence is much easier if there is a previous clonality test with a 'clonal signature' on that patient to use for comparison. In these cases, a correctly-sized peak, no matter how prevalent within a polyclonal background, can be meaningful. Patients with a known signature clone are more easily monitored for minimal residual disease or recurrence by following a specific rearrangement amplicon size (**Figure 15.10**).

Other molecular assays

As with other areas of molecular diagnostics, next-generation (high throughput, massive parallel) sequencing assays will likely play a prominent role in the diagnosis of MF/SS in the future. Complete sequencing of the TCR genes and other areas of the T-cell genome (or transcriptome) will generate much more data, perhaps more quickly and cheaper and reproducible than

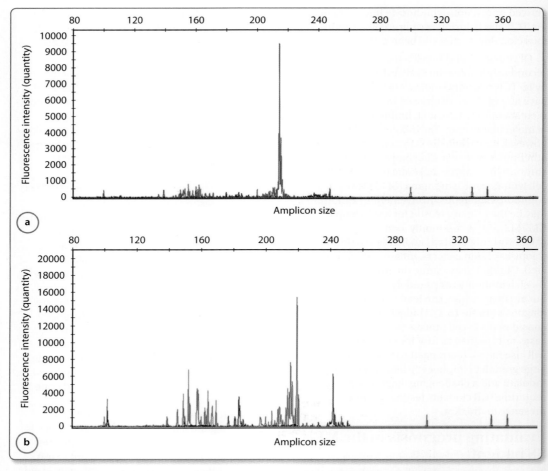

Figure 15.10 Interpretation of gene rearrangement studies – disease monitoring. DNA is extracted from microdissected FFPE tissue from a suspected MF patient and two time points – (a) at diagnosis and (b) following therapy. Fluorescently-labeled primers are grouped into two separate PCR reactions (mix A and mix B, BIOMED-2 protocol, InVivoScribe) for TRG. The amplicons are separated by capillary electrophoresis based on amplicon size (with GeneScan technology). Only mix/tube A results are shown for clarity. Blue and green tracings correspond to different groups of fluorescently-labeled primers within the multiplex reaction. The X-axis corresponds to amplicon size and the Y-axis to fluorescence intensity (quantity). Spikes within a polyclonal background can be difficult to interpret. If the primary tumor's signature rearrangement is known (a), spikes with an identical size, even with a significant background polyclonal population (b), are likely significant. This particular patient had been in remission and developed a new skin eruption with a clinical differential diagnosis of recurrent MF versus eczema versus drug eruption. Knowing the signature clone may also be helpful in the evaluation of occult tumor in lymph nodes or bone marrow, the evaluation of cutaneous recurrence (as in this case), and/or the evaluation of therapeutic efficacy.

current gene rearrangement assays, likely inserting next-generation sequencing into future diagnostic algorithms. Commercial offerings of next-generation sequencing for this purpose are beginning to surface, but are not yet mainstream assays.

Summary

Gene rearrangement analysis is arguably the first molecular diagnostics assay used in dermatology, and it continues to play an integral part in diagnostic algorithms for mycosis fungoides and Sézary syndrome, despite its limitations. The scope of clonality testing in dermatology has increased, now including diagnosis of non-MF/SS cutaneous tumors and expanding beyond diagnosis to provide data on prognosis and disease monitoring following therapy. The evolution of the gene rearrangement assay is proceeding as follows: Southern blot → PCR-based assay → high throughput (next-gen) sequencing. Southern blot techniques have largely been replaced by PCR-based methods, and high-throughput sequencing will likely dominate by the next decade. The data garnered by next-gen sequencing, including the characterization of oncogenic molecular driving events in lymphoma, may ultimately make gene-rearrangement analysis obsolete. Until then, however, gene-rearrangement assays will continue to be a staple in the multi-pronged diagnostic algorithms for cutaneous lymphoma.

References

Barr RJ, Sun NC, King DF. Immunoperoxidase staining of cytoplasmic immunoglobulins. A diagnostic aid in distinguishing cutaneous reactive lymphoid hyperplasia from malignant lymphoma. J Am Acad Dermatol 1980; 3:58–62.

Bazin PAE. Lecons théoriques et cliniques sur les affections cutanées artificielles. Paris: Delahaye, 1862.

Broqc LAJ. Les parapsoriasis. Ann Dermatol Syph 1902; 3:313–343.

Chen Z, Font MP, Loiseau P, et al. The human T-cell V gamma gene locus: cloning of new segments and study of V gamma rearrangements in neoplastic T and B cells. Blood 1988; 72:776–83.

Davis MM, Chien YH. T-cell Antigen Receptors. In: W. E. Paul (Ed.), Fundamental Immunology (7th ed., pp. 279-305). Philadelphia: Wolters Kluwer, Lippincott Williams & Wilkins, 2013.

Edge SB, Byrd DR, Compton CC, et al (Eds.). Primary Cutaneous Lymphomas. In: AJCC Cancer Staging Manual (7th ed., pp. 615–617, 627–630). London: Springer, 2011.

Guitart J, Kennedy J, Ronan S, et al. Histologic criteria for the diagnosis of mycosis fungoides: proposal for a grading system to standardize pathology reporting. J Cutan Patho 2001; 28:174–83.

Hosler GA, Murphy KM. Molecular Diagnostics for Dermatology. Springer Berlin Heidelberg, 2014.

Kandolf Sekulović L, Cikota B, Stojadinović O, et al. TCRgamma gene rearrangement analysis in skin samples and peripheral blood of mycosis fungoides patients. Acta Dermatovenerologica Alpina, Panonica, et Adriatica 2007; 16:149–55.

Kung PC, Berger CL, Goldstein G, et al. Cutaneous T cell lymphoma: characterization by monoclonal antibodies. Blood 1981; 57;2:261–266.

Lander ES, Linton LM, Birren B, et al. Initial sequencing and analysis of the human genome. Nature 2001; 409:860–921.

Langerak AW, Groenen PJTA, Brüggemann M, et al. EuroClonality/BIOMED-2 guidelines for interpretation and reporting of Ig/TCR clonality testing in suspected lymphoproliferations. Leukemia 2012; 26:2159–71.

Langerak AW, Molina TJ, Lavender FL, et al. Polymerase chain reaction-based clonality testing in tissue samples with reactive lymphoproliferations: usefulness and pitfalls. A report of the BIOMED-2 Concerted Action BMH4-CT98-3936. Leukemia 2007; 21:222–9.

Olsen E, Vonderheid E, Pimpinelli N, et al. Revisions to the staging and classification of mycosis fungoides and Sezary syndrome: a proposal of the International Society for Cutaneous Lymphomas (ISCL) and the cutaneous lymphoma task force of the European Organization of Research and Treatment of Ca. Blood 2007; 110:1713–22.

Pimpinelli N, Olsen EA, Santucci M, et al. Defining early mycosis fungoides. J Am Acad Dermatol 2005; 53:1053–63.

Plaza JA, Morrison C, Magro CM. Assessment of TCR-beta clonality in a diverse group of cutaneous T-Cell infiltrates. J Cutan Pathol 2008; 35:358–65.

Ponti R, Quaglino P, Novelli M, et al. T-cell receptor gamma gene rearrangement by multiplex polymerase chain reaction/heteroduplex analysis in patients with cutaneous T-cell lymphoma (mycosis fungoides/Sézary syndrome) and benign inflammatory disease: correlation with clinical, histological and immunophenotypical findings. Br Dermatol, 2005; 153:565–73.

Santucci M, Biggeri A, Feller AC, et al. Efficacy of histologic criteria for diagnosing early mycosis fungoides: an EORTC cutaneous lymphoma study group investigation. European Organization for Research and Treatment of Cancer. Am J Surg Pathol, 2000; 24:40–50.

Sezary A, Bouvrain Y. Erythrodermie avec pesence de cellules monstrueuses dans le derme et le sang circulant. Bull Soc Fr Dermatol Syphiligr 1938; 45:254–260.

Steffen C. The man behind the eponym dermatology in historical perspective: Albert Sézary and the Sézary syndrome. Am J Dermatopathol 2006; 28:357–67.

Strominger JL. Developmental biology of T cell receptors. Science 1989; 244;4907: 943–50.

Thurber SE, Zhang B, Kim YH, et al. T-cell clonality analysis in biopsy specimens from two different skin sites shows high specificity in the diagnosis of patients with suggested mycosis fungoides. J Am Acad of Dermatol 2007; 57:782–90.

Van Dongen JJ M, Langerak AW, Brüggemann M, et al. Design and standardization of PCR primers and protocols for detection of clonal immunoglobulin and T-cell receptor gene recombinations in suspect lymphoproliferations: report of the BIOMED-2 Concerted Action BMH4-CT98-3936. Leukemia 2003; 17:2257–317.

Vega F, Luthra R, Medeiros LJ, et al. Clonal heterogeneity in mycosis fungoides and its relationship to clinical course. Blood 2002; 100:3369–73.

Willemze R, de Graaff-Reitsma CB, Cnossen J, et al. Characterization of T-cell subpopulations in skin and peripheral blood of patients with cutaneous T-cell lymphomas and benign inflammatory dermatoses. The Journal of Investigative Dermatology 1983; 80:60–6.

Willemze R, Jaffe ES, Burg G, et al. WHO-EORTC classification for cutaneous lymphomas. Blood 2005; 105:3768–85.

Willemze R, Meijer CJLM. Classification of cutaneous T-cell lymphoma: from Alibert to WHO-EORTC. J Cutan Pathol 2006; 33:18–26.

Wood GS, Tung RM, Haeffner AC, et al. Detection of clonal T-cell receptor gamma gene rearrangements in early mycosis fungoides/Sezary syndrome by polymerase chain reaction and denaturing gradient gel electrophoresis (PCR/DGGE). J Invest Dermatol 1994; 103;1:34–41.

Zhang B, Beck AH, Taube JM, et al. Combined use of PCR-based TCRG and TCRB clonality tests on paraffin-embedded skin tissue in the differential diagnosis of mycosis fungoides and inflammatory dermatoses. J Mol Diagn 2010; 12:320–7.

PCR, sequencing, and gene expression profiling

Gregory A. Hosler

Molecular assays are still underutilized in dermatology and dermatopathology, compared to other fields, but are quickly becoming more relevant (Hosler & Murphy, 2014). Prior to the 21st century, only few dermatopathology applications existed, including the Ig/TCR clonality assays and in situ hybridization methods discussed in the preceding chapters. Recent technological advances in DNA sequencing and RNA preservation have opened the door for new molecular assays. These assays have not only improved diagnostics but have also transformed the entire management of the dermatology patient by providing prognostic information and data used to guide therapeutic decisions.

History of sequencing

Modern DNA sequencing began in the 1970s when the British biochemist Frederick Sanger (1918-2013) developed his 'di-deoxy' chain termination and capillary electrophoresis-based method (Sanger et al., 1977). This method allowed, for the first time, investigators to sequence portions of the human genome in a reliable and reproducible manner. Sanger sequencing, as it would eventually be called, became automated and more efficient in the 1980s. During this time, Kary Mullis developed the polymerase chain reaction (PCR), a new DNA amplification technology with many applications including enhancement of the Sanger method (Mullis et al., 1986). Variations of automated Sanger sequencing were the workhorses behind The Human Genome Project, which completed sequencing of the entire human genome in 2003 (Lander et al., 2001). The next decade witnessed a revolution of the sequencing world, and, hence, all of molecular biology, with the advent of a new technique termed massively parallel sequencing, or 'next-generation' sequencing (NGS). A description of the first NGS sequencer, Life Sciences' 454 GS-20, was published in 2005 (Margulies et al., 2005). In 2013, the FDA paved the way for NGS use in clinical care (Collins & Hamburg, 2013).

It is truly amazing to think about the advances and evolution in sequencing technology over the past few decades (**Figure 16.1**). The Human Genome Project took 15 years to complete, used hundreds of sequencers, and cost roughly $3 billion. Today, using NGS technology, a single sequencer can sequence over 40 different entire human genomes in 24 hours for roughly $1000 each. As the cost per base sequenced continues to plummet, opportunities to use sequencing

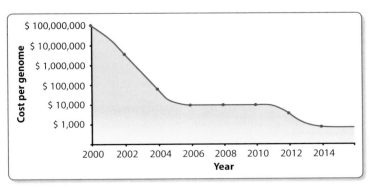

Figure 16.1 The evolution of sequencing. The cost of sequencing the human genome has precipitously dropped since the Human Genome Project, outpacing Moore's law.

technology in the diagnosis and management of disease continue to rise. Indeed, NGS is replacing more traditional methods for detecting germline mutations, detecting and quantifying somatic mutations, characterizing RNA expression levels, and identifying epigenomic alterations in the context of human disease, including dermatologic disease.

Examples of molecular techniques

Polymerase chain reaction (PCR)

Method

PCR is a genetic amplification assay. To perform PCR, small DNA primers are designed such that they hybridize to regions flanking the DNA (or RNA/cDNA) template of interest. The addition of a DNA polymerase and single nucleotides allows for replication of the template between the primer sequences. By cycling through temperatures (thermocycling), the DNA template strands separate, replicate by the polymerase, and reanneal. This process continues, logarithmically increasing copies of the template, until cycling ceases or the reagents are exhausted (**Figure 16.2**). The PCR product can be detected and isolated based on its size and/or sequence. PCR products can be separated by size using capillary electrophoresis (by applying an electric current, DNA migrates a distance through the gel depending on the size of its fragment). Labeled probes can be used to identify PCR fragments based on sequence homology.

PCR can be performed on RNA, using a technique called reverse-transcription PCR, or RT-PCR. In this method, the RNA is isolated and converted to cDNA prior to thermocycling. The rest of the process is the same as regular PCR. Newer generations of PCR are quantitative (qPCR). Real-time PCR allows for quantifying amplification products using fluorescent binders to DNA. The fluorescent signal can be traced in real time. Other variations of PCR also exist, including nested PCR, allele-specific PCR, qRT-PCR, and others (Hosler & Murphy, 2014).

Advantages/disadvantages

PCR has been a staple in molecular research and diagnostics for decades. It is an extremely simple yet powerful technique to amplify genetic material, serving many purposes (detecting small quantities of DNA/RNA, characterizing mutations, cloning, etc.). It is inexpensive, offers remarkable sensitivity and specificity, and has broad applications in dermatology (mutational analysis, pathogen detection, clonality testing, microsatellite instability testing, identity testing, and more). Because of these features, PCR-based assays are endeared by small clinical and research laboratories. If the genetic sequence of a target or flanking a target is known, a PCR assay can be developed. The main limitations for PCR are the following: the genetic sequence of the target must be known and the targeted area is limited (usually) to a few hundred basepairs. PCR methodology can be used as a stand-alone assay but its true power may lie in its incorporation into newer technologies, such as high-throughput sequencing and gene expression profiling.

Sanger sequencing

Method

Sanger sequencing has been the gold standard for sequencing DNA in clinical and research laboratories for over 30 years. In the Sanger method, a small segment of DNA is sequenced. This target DNA is first amplified by PCR. After this template is created, a DNA polymerase begins replicating the strands using a mixture of 'normal' nucleotides (A, T, C, G, or dNTPs) and 'chain-terminating' nucleotides (di-deoxy A, T, C, G, or ddNTPs). The chain terminating nucleotides, ddNTPs, are fluorescently labeled, each nucleotide a different color, and immediately halt the replication procedure once incorporated into the newly forming DNA strand. This effectively produces a mixture of DNA containing strands of all possible lengths of the target template, each labeled by the last nucleotide incorporated (which is the first ddNTP incorporated). These strands can be separated by capillary electrophoresis, and based on the color of the chain-terminating ddNTP, a sequence is generated (**Figure 16.3**).

Advantages/disadvantages

Sanger sequencing has several advantages. Because it has been around for decades, many laboratories have experience with this method and are comfortable interpreting the data. The

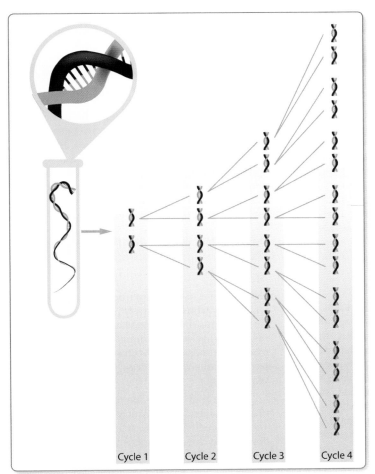

Figure 16.2 PCR. PCR is a powerful technique used to amplify nucleic acid, causing logarithmic increases in copy numbers via temperature cycling (thermocycling), which optimizes DNA separation, annealing and polymerase activity.

Cycle 1   Cycle 2   Cycle 3   Cycle 4

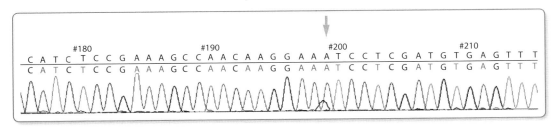

Figure 16.3 Sanger sequencing data. Fluorescently labeled chain termination ddNTPs can be detected and plotted in order to create a sequence read. A point mutation (arrow) will often show two differently colored peaks at the same position using this commonly employed readout.

data are provided in analog form, allowing the user to scrutinize each peak in order to make a final base call. Other methods, such as NGS, do not have this luxury. The error rate of Sanger sequencing is very low, estimated at one error per 10,000 base calls. Because of these very high performance characteristics, Sanger sequencing is still used by many laboratories as a primary sequencing platform or to verify mutations detected by other, newer methods.

Unfortunately for Sanger lovers, Sanger sequencing is becoming too slow and too costly to accommodate today's molecular demands. It can only sequence short DNA segments (one exon of one gene, for example) for a given run. This limits its clinical use to only well-characterized and tightly localized mutational analysis. The fluorescence requirement keeps costs elevated. Another disadvantage is Sanger's limit of detection, which is approximately 40% of mutant cells (20% mutant alleles). This analytic sensitivity is fine for detecting germline mutations (homozygous or heterozygous mutations) and somatic mutations in fairly pure tumor samples, but is inadequate for samples with low tumor burden and/or molecularly heterogeneous tumor populations.

Pyrosequencing

Method

Pyrosequencing was developed in the 1990s. Like Sanger sequencing, it uses a PCR-amplified target DNA template. Instead of fluorescently-labeled nucleotides, pyrosequencing detects the incorporation of a nucleotide into the replicating strand by the generation and detection of a light ('pyro') signal. The nucleotides are added one at a time, so the detector can identify which nucleotide (A, T, C, or G) was incorporated by whether or not it produced a signal. Of course, this process is happening very quickly. Based on

the light signals, the computer software generates a plot depicting the light signal for each base added (**Figure 16.4**).

Advantages/disadvantages

The main advantages of pyrosequencing compared with the Sanger method are the lower cost and lower limits of detection. Because fluorescence is not required, the cost per run is markedly reduced. The limit of detection is approximately 10% mutant cells (5% alleles). Pyrosequencing is excellent for targeted mutation detection, similar to Sanger sequencing, but is not practical for detecting mutations that span multiple exons of a gene or multiple genes.

Next-generation sequencing (NGS)

Method

NGS is a term used to describe a new sequencing technology which effectively performs numerous simultaneous sequencing reactions and aligns the results to create a summative single-sequence read. This process is also termed 'massively parallel' sequencing or 'deep' (or 'ultra-deep') sequencing.

There are several variations of NGS, but all maintain several basic principles (**Figure 16.5**). The first step in NGS is to create a sequencing library. The type of library depends on the

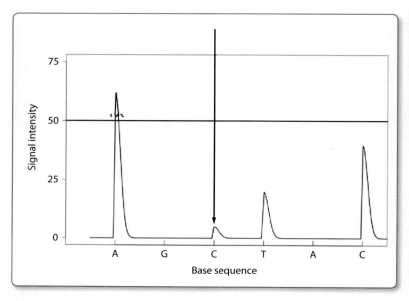

Figure 16.4 Pyrosequencing data. Point mutations will often result in the loss of peak height for one base (germline configuration) and the gain of peak height corresponding to the mutation (T to C mutation, see arrow).

strategy or purpose of the assay (see Strategies on page 238). The library is made by fragmenting the genomic DNA (or other template) and preparing it for sequencing. In most methods, this preparation consists of ligating adaptors to the library fragments followed by fragment amplification. Actual sequencing can be performed by various means, including, but not limited to, detecting the addition of each fluorescently-labeled dNTPs (Illumina method), pyrosequencing (454 method), or detecting the released hydrogen ions with each dNTP added (Ion Torrent method). Once all the small fragments are fully sequenced, sophisticated software aligns them with each other and with reference genetic material using an alignment algorithm, and makes base calls to generate a sequence read. For a given base, the 'depth' can be anywhere from 7 to 1000 aligned sequences. The depth of the read can be adjusted based on the purpose of the assay. Low read depths may be all that is needed when analyzing genomic DNA for germline mutations, as they will be highly represented (heterozygous or homozygous) in the sample. Deeper depths are required to analyze somatic mutations in tumors, for example, as these samples may have low tumor burden and the tumor DNA may be molecularly heterogeneous. Deeper depth reads are also required for sequencing the complex RNA transcriptome.

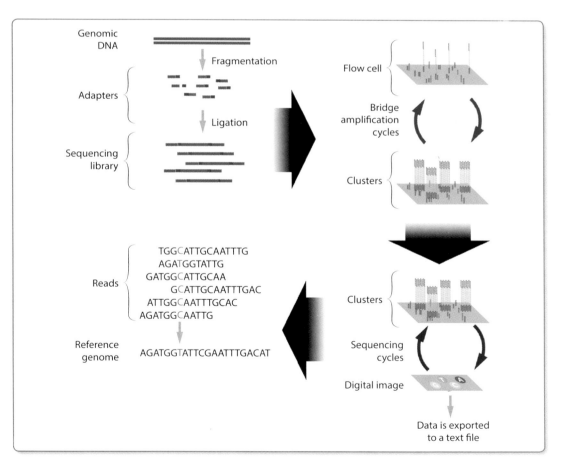

Figure 16.5 Next-generation sequencing (NGS). Depicted is just one example of NGS methodology (see main text for details).

Strategies

Depending on the purpose of the assay, different strategies of NGS may be employed. NGS can be used in discovery of new mutations, detection of known mutations, and characterization of gene expression. The technology behind these applications is quite similar, differing mainly in the generation of the initial library. Infrequently, NGS is also used to characterize epigenomic alterations (methylation, histone modification, etc.) and identify genetic material of pathogens.

DNA libraries: There are different tiers of 'magnification' (degree of genomic coverage) when sequencing DNA. The most comprehensive method is whole-genome sequencing, which, as the name implies, will sequence the entire 3.2 billion bases of the human genome, including coding and non-coding areas. Because the resolution of sequencing is very high (one base, in fact), whole-genome sequencing is replacing other methods, such as microarray platforms, to examine the entire genome. Whole genome sequencing may be useful when screening for an unknown genetic cause for disease, for example. The next tier is whole-exome sequencing. Whole exome sequencing analyzes the entire genomic coding region, and therefore, focuses on areas that impact protein expression and function. The exome accounts for approximately 2% of the total genome, and therefore may be a cost-effective approach to broadly examine the entire breadth of the genome. The third magnification tier is targeted sequencing. Targeted sequencing usually targets a subset of the exome, often a specific mutational hotspot, an entire single gene or group of related genes. Targeted sequencing may serve the same function as Sanger or pyrosequencing, but usually has an expanded target to include multiple exons of a single gene or group of genes.

RNA libraries: RNA libraries are made by isolating the RNA, removing ribosomes, inactivating or eliminating nucleases, and converting the RNA to cDNA. Similar to DNA libraries, RNA libraries for NGS will depend upon the purpose of the assay. NGS can be used to analyze the entire transcriptome or targeted RNA transcripts, providing both qualitative and quantitative information. Whole transcriptome analysis allows for the comprehensive examination of gene expression by tumors or other populations at a given point in time.

Targeted RNA sequencing analyzes the expression of a pre-selected gene or group of genes. NGS is just one method for performing this gene expression profiling (GEP, see page 239), and has several current applications in dermatopathology. NGS may also be used to evaluate other RNA forms - mRNA, microRNA, and non-coding RNA, for example - but primarily in the research setting.

Advantages/disadvantages

The advantages of NGS technology are significant and have elevated NGS to the forefront of molecular diagnostics, both in research/discovery and clinical medicine. As already discussed, it is cheaper and faster than other sequencing and array-based technologies. NGS has a broader scope, able to detect point mutations, insertions, deletions, and genetic copy number changes, all in a cost-effective, qualitative and quantitative manner. This diversity allows NGS to detect alterations in tumor suppressor genes. If adapted for RNA analysis, NGS can be used for gene expression profiling, not possible for Sanger or pyrosequencing.

While the excitement for NGS is clear, there remain some limitations. The largest barrier for its widespread use is the interpretation and storage of data. While the entire genome may be sequenced for $1000, providing adequate interpretation of these data may logarithmically elevate the cost (Mardis, 2010). Analysis is so expensive because individuals may have over 20,000 genetic variants, and distinguishing these variants from biologically-relevant mutations can be a challenge. Moreover, when studying tumors, there can be immense genetic instability, and tumor populations may be molecularly heterogeneous, also providing an interpretive challenge. NGS data are not easily scrutinized as with other sequencing methods since the base calls are already highly processed by software prior to receiving a final sequence read. The error rate of NGS varies depending on how deep the runs are, but can be up to one error per 1,000 base calls, one log higher than Sanger sequencing. For this reason, may laboratories still confirm NGS findings by Sanger sequencing. The complexity of NGS and interpretation of its data require considerable effort to ensure the results are effectively communicated to the clinician for appropriate patient management. And finally, there are costs associated with storage of this newly-generated colossal amount of sequencing data.

Gene expression profiling

Method

Gene expression profiling (GEP) is used to assess cellular function (usually tumor) at a given point in time. By identifying and quantifying different RNA transcripts, GEP can provide diagnostic information, prognostic information, and other features of cellular function in the tested population. To perform GEP, RNA is isolated from the test sample (a microdissected paraffin block, for example) (**Figure 16.6**). There are different ways to analyze the type and quantity of RNA transcripts. In most assays, the RNA is labeled (by fluorescence, for example) and hybridized to a cDNA microarray chip. Once a scanner identifies the location of the hybridizations, software can interpret the result using sophisticated algorithms. Quantitative reverse-transcription PCR (qRT-PCR) can be used to amplify transcripts of interest, either as a stand-alone test or in conjunction with chip-based platforms. And as mentioned above, NGS is another option. NGS and chip-based assays can evaluate the entire transcriptome or focus on a small collection of genes/transcripts designed for a specific purpose (melanoma chip, for example).

Advantages/disadvantages

GEP is a new, very powerful technology. Recent advances in the ability to extract and assay RNA before degradation has made it possible for GEP to enter clinical molecular diagnostics. By examining the transcriptome, GEP is the next step in progression from DNA sequencing, providing functional information.

GEP has limitations. While RNA extraction technologies have dramatically improved, the rate of failed tests due to quality or quantity of RNA remains high. The complexity of the transcriptome makes data interpretation very challenging. There are numerous genes, including housekeeping genes, expressed at any given time. Identifying relevant alterations in otherwise

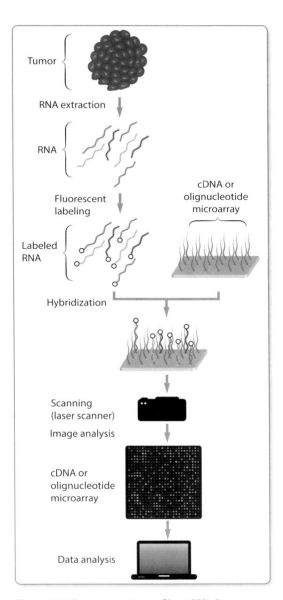

Figure 16.6 Gene expression profiling (GEP). For microarray-based GEP, RNA is extracted from either fresh tumor, or more commonly, from paraffin-embedded tumor. The RNA is labeled and allowed to bind to oligonucleotides on a microarray. Based on the position and quantity of bound RNA, a gene expression profile can be computer generated. GEP can also be performed by quantitative RT-PCR, among other methods.

normal gene expression patterns can be difficult. Moreover, GEP provides only a snapshot of the expression of genes in the entire studied population of cells. These data are clouded if the population of interest represents only a fraction of the total population and/or the functional status of the cells of interest is significantly changing over time.

Clinical applications

While use of these technologies is rampant in the research world, there remain only few current clinical applications in dermatology (**Table 16.1**). There are even fewer tangible applications for the dermatopathologist, since germline testing does not require a skin biopsy (it is usually performed off peripheral blood leukocytes from a blood draw). Nonetheless, the list of molecular applications continues to grow, covering diagnostic, prognostic, and theranostic (predicting sensitivity/resistance to therapy) applications.

Genomic (DNA) sequencing for assessing germline variants/mutations

Sequencing continues to be the best modality for identifying or confirming heritable disease. For the genodermatoses, there are different strategies. Rarely, genome-wide (whole-genome or whole-exome) screening is performed to search for mutations in patients with polygenic disorders or disorders with an unknown cause (or undescribed disorders within families). Commercial tests covering 4–5,000 disorder-specific mutations are now available to evaluate afflicted patients or as carrier screens. More commonly, targeted sequencing is performed to confirm a suspected genodermatosis. If there is a concern the patient has a genodermatosis characterized by a localized mutational hotspot, any sequencing modality may suffice. However, most genodermatoses involve mutations that span an entire exon or multiple exons, making NGS a better choice. At times, little is known

Table 16.1 Current clinical applications for PCR, sequencing and gene expression profiling in dermatology

Dermatologic condition	Assay
Genodermatoses	PCR for known and targeted mutations (diagnostic) Complete gene sequencing by Sanger or NGS (diagnostic) Genome-wide screening by NGS (diagnostic)
Melanoma	Gene expression profiling (diagnostic and prognostic) Mutational analysis by PCR +/- various sequencing platforms (therapy) BRAF NRAS KIT others
Non-melanoma skin cancers (metastatic)	Mutational analysis by NGS sequencing (therapy)
Cutaneous metastases	Gene expression profiling Cancers with unknown primary (diagnostic) Mutational analysis by NGS sequencing (therapy)
Cutaneous lymphoma	Clonality (TCR/Ig) assays by PCR or NGS (diagnostic and prognostic)
Soft tissue tumors	Translocation and amplification detection by RT-PCR or NGS (diagnostic)
Infectious disease	PCR-based pathogen detection (diagnostic) NGS pathogen-specific (metagenomics) gene sequencing (diagnostic) NGS for predicting organism drug susceptibility/resistance (therapy)
Other	PCR or NGS for pharmacogenetic gene variant analysis (therapy)

about the patient except they have a condition within a category of disorders (some bullous disease or ichthyosis, for example), and in these circumstances, it may be prudent to use NGS on a panel of genes.

Pharmacogenetics is defined by how variations in a single gene predict response to a drug (some use the term pharmacogenomics interchangeably or when referring to the entire genome). The genes impact drug efficacy in different ways, including encoding proteins that alter absorption, metabolism, and binding. By better understanding how a patient will respond to taking a certain drug, based on their genome, dosages can be modified, adverse drug events can be minimized, and the cost of unnecessary or ineffective drugs can be reduced. The best characterized examples in pharmacogenetics/pharmacogenomics are not primary dermatologic drugs (warfarin, for example) (Hosler & Murphy, 2014), but dermatology patients may be taking these drugs, and the future addition of dermatologic drugs (biologics, immunosuppressants, antibiotics) on this growing list seems likely.

Genomic (DNA) sequencing for assessing somatic mutations in melanoma and other tumors

In recent years, knowledge of tumorigenesis has grown leaps and bounds (**Figure 16.7**). The list of somatic mutations leading to constitutively activated oncogenes and/or deactivated tumor suppressor genes, both of which cause uninhibited cell proliferation, continues to grow. Moreover, the specific functions of these altered genes are better understood and have led to therapeutic strategies to negate their tumorigenic properties. Theranostics refers to the use of molecular assays to predict therapeutic efficacy and help design regimens based on the tumor's genetic makeup. Pathologists, including dermatopathologists, are playing an integral role in theranostics. Accurate histologic diagnoses and, in many cases, purification of tumor by the dermatopathologist, are required for obtaining meaningful molecular data (**Figure 16.8**). A dermatopathologist's review for molecular testing can enhance performance of the molecular test by purifying tumor and may also prevent unnecessary testing by eliminating inadequate samples or samples with incorrect diagnoses.

It should be noted that, interestingly, as opposed to theranostic assays, there are no routinely-performed molecular diagnostic mutational assays in dermatopathology (an exception to this is translocation detection used for soft tissue tumors). Diagnostic mutational assays have been elusive in dermatopathology for the following reasons: a consistent and strong correlation between a specific mutation and a specific tumor has not been identified, the mutation is present in both benign and malignant counterparts (*BRAF* V600E in nevi and melanoma, for example), and/or the mutation does not have an effective assay (tumor suppressor gene defects, for example). Newer technologies will undoubtedly alter this trend.

The prototype for a theranostic application in dermatopathology is melanoma. In 2011, following a series of pre-clinical and clinical trials, the FDA approved the B-Raf[V600E] inhibitor vemurafenib for the treatment of advanced stage melanoma patients with tumors carrying the *BRAF* V600E gene mutation (Chapman et al., 2011). Vemurafenib joined a very short list of available drugs for patients with metastatic disease. Because the *BRAF* V600E mutation is present in approximately half of all melanomas, and patients without the mutation did not respond to inhibitor therapy, testing for the mutation began almost immediately and on almost all patients with metastatic disease following the drug's approval. *KIT* mutations occur in a relatively high percentage of acral lentiginous melanomas, primary mucosal melanomas, and melanomas of chronically sun-damaged skin. Because there are available c-kit inhibitors, molecular testing in patients with these histologic subtypes is often performed. The role of mutations in other genes, such as *NRAS* and *PI3KCA*, are less well defined in melanoma, but due to their known role in oncogenesis, possible role in resistance mechanisms, and possible role in paradoxical activation of the MAP-kinase pathway in patients on B-Raf-inhibitors, testing, particularly for *NRAS* mutations, is often performed.

Because the *BRAF* V600E mutation is so localized, targeted approaches, such as Sanger sequencing or pyrosequencing (or PCR-based assays) can be effective. *NRAS* mutational analysis is slightly more complex, but can still be performed using a targeted approach. Q61 on exon 2 is the most common mutation, and there

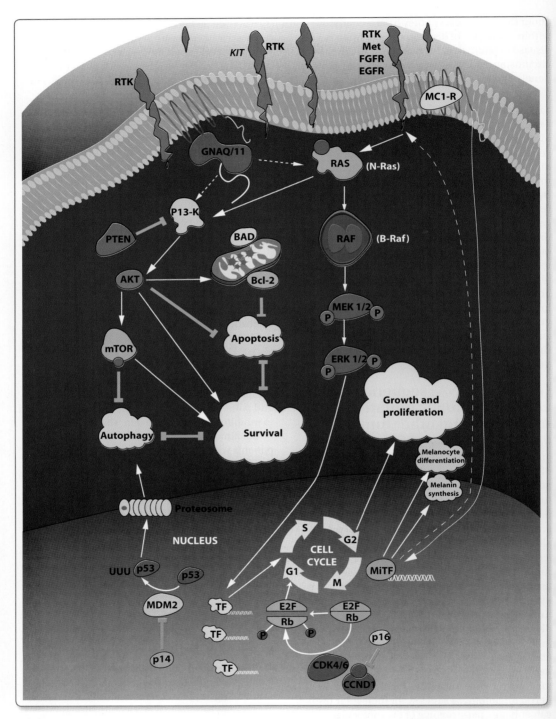

Figure 16.7 Cellular signaling pathways and therapeutic targets in melanoma. This schematic is an oversimplified depiction of the complex signaling pathways involved in melanomagenesis. Recent develop of inhibitor therapies to constitutively activated proteins (B-Raf, KIT, others) have led to therapeutic responses.

complete-gene sequencing (usually by NGS) is the preferred approach. Indeed, with the emergence of NGS, many laboratories are moving towards 3-gene *(BRAF, NRAS* and *KIT)* or multi-gene melanoma theranostics panels, regardless of histologic subtype.

Theranostic testing is, by far, more commonly performed on melanoma than other primary cutaneous tumor types. This is not to say that a similar approach cannot be used on metastatic non-melanoma skin cancers. Moreover, many tumors metastasize to the skin, and the cutaneous sample may be the only or best sample for theranostic testing. The evidence for *BRAF* testing in melanoma is strong, but there is an argument for testing many other genes for melanoma and other metastatic cancers based on the availability of target-specific inhibitor therapy. These patients have dire prognoses and their oncologists look for any molecular evidence to support use of specific targeted therapy, even as part of a clinical trial. The NGS multi-gene theranostic screen is attractive since it can be performed independent of tumor type. In fact, several laboratories now offer comprehensive NGS panels for the purpose of driving therapeutic decision-making. These NGS assays range from 15-gene panels, to 150-gene panels, to 500-gene mega-panels, to whole-exome sequencing. Negative results from smaller panels may reflex to more broad coverage of the genome.

Gene expression profiling in melanoma and cancers of unknown primary

As discussed above, GEP can be performed using qRT-PCR, cDNA microarrays or by NGS technology. GEP with dermatopathology applications has recently moved from the research setting to commercially available assays. Several applications exist.

For melanoma, commercially available GEP assays exist for both diagnostic (myPath, Myriad Genetics) and prognostic (DecisionDX – Melanoma, Castle Biosciences) purposes. Both assays are qRT-PCR based. The diagnostic assay is designed to aid in the diagnosis of atypical melanocytic lesions (Clarke et al., 2015). It is an ancillary test to aid, not supplant, routine histomorphologic analysis. There are no guidelines on its use as an adjunct or replacement for FISH analysis. In the diagnostic assay, RNA transcripts are analyzed from 23 target genes.

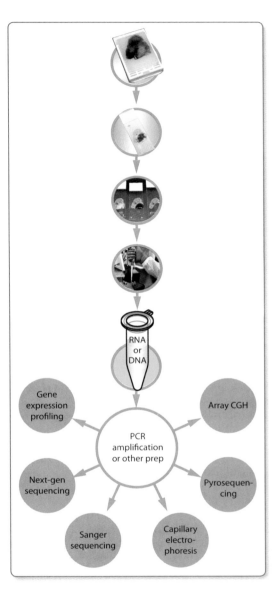

Figure 16.8 Preparation of tumor samples for molecular analysis. Tumor DNA or RNA can be extracted from paraffin-embedded tissue to perform a variety of different molecular assays. The dermatopathologist plays an important role for isolating and evaluating quality and quantity of tumor prior to the extraction step.

is a second hot-spot on exon 1. *KIT* is even more complex as mutations, although concentrated in the juxtamembrane domain, can span the entire gene. A targeted approach can be used for the juxtamembrane domain of the gene, but

The genes of interest are involved in melanocyte differentiation, immune regulation, and immune signaling. The data are analyzed by software, which generates a score and reports out a result of benign, malignant, or indeterminate based on that score. The assay has a reported 90% sensitivity and 91% specificity. The prognostic assay is very similar in principle, but targets a slightly different makeup of 31 genes (Gerami et al., 2015). It is designed to provide prognostic information for thin (Stage I/II) melanomas. Following analysis, the proprietary software labels the sample as Class 1 or Class 2. Reportedly, Class 1 cases have a 97% 5-year disease-free survival versus 31% for Class 2, and new data suggest GEP may identify patients with a high risk of disease progression despite a negative sentinel lymph node biopsy. This prognostic information can be informative for the patient and clinician, but its role in guiding management (determining whether or not to perform a sentinel lymph node biopsy or whether or not to give the patient adjuvant therapy, for example) is yet to be realized.

GEP may also be used to identify cancers of unknown primary (CUP). CUP is not an uncommon problem for the dermatopathologist. Prior to GEP assays, the workup of CUP was relegated to extensive and expensive immunohistochemical analysis only. With GEP, immunohistochemical panels can be modified to same-gene expression panels and performed in a single assay.

Other PCR, sequencing, and GEP applications

There are other applications for PCR, GEP, and sequencing technology in dermatopathology.

These applications have been discussed elsewhere and/or are rarely used, typically restricted to unique settings. Examples include the following:

- Translocation and gene amplification testing by qRT-PCR or NGS (see Chapter 13)
- Clonality testing for lymphoma by PCR or NGS (see Chapter 15)
- Metagenomic screening for infections with unknown pathogens
- PCR or sequencing for esoteric and/or culture-resistant pathogens (mycobacteria, for example)
- NGS screening for organism drug susceptibility/resistance gene variants

Summary

Molecular assays in dermatopathology are no longer a technology seeking an application. Extremely powerful tools, such as NGS and GEP, allow for the targeted or completely comprehensive examination of genomic sequence and cellular function, capable of providing both qualitative and quantitative data. These technologies will only get better and cheaper, opening more doors to new and currently unconceived clinical applications, potentially infiltrating the realms of diagnostics, prognostics, and theranostics for all dermatologic conditions. The dermatopathologist is and will remain a centerpiece in this process, providing diagnoses with the aid of these assays, procuring tumor for molecular triage, and interpreting and communicating results in the context of the whole patient with the entire care team.

References

Chapman PB, Hauschild A, Robert C, et al. Improved survival with vemurafenib in melanoma with BRAF V600E mutation. New Eng J Med 2011; 364:2507–2516.

Clarke LE, Warf BM, Flake DD, et al. Clinical validation of a gene expression signature that differentiates benign nevi from malignant melanoma. J Cutan Pathol 2015; 42:244–252.

Collins FS, Hamburg MA. First FDA Authorization for Next-Generation Sequencer. New Eng J Med 2013; 369:2369–2371.

Gerami P, Cook RW, Wilkinson J, et al. Development of a prognostic genetic signature to predict the metastatic risk associated with cutaneous melanoma. Clinical Cancer Research 2015; 21:175–183.

Hosler GA, Murphy KM. Molecular Diagnostics for Dermatology. Berlin: Springer Science & Business Media, 2014.

Lander ES, Linton LM, Birren B, et al. Initial sequencing and analysis of the human genome. Nature 2001; 409:860–921.

Mardis ER. The $1,000 genome, the $100,000 analysis? Genome Medicine 2010; 2:84.

Margulies M, Egholm M, Altman WE, et al. Genome sequencing in microfabricated high-density picolitre reactors. Nature 2005; 437:376–380.

Mullis K, Faloona F, Scharf S, et al. Specific enzymatic amplification of DNA in vitro: The polymerase chain reaction. Cold Spring Harbor Symposia on Quantitative Biology. 1986; 51:263–273.

Sanger F, Nicklen S, Coulson AR. DNA sequencing with chain-terminating inhibitors. Proceedings of the National Academy of Sciences of the United States of America 1977; 74:5463–5467.

Section 8

Conclusion

17 Final thoughts

Gregory A. Hosler

'The keen eyesight of the investigator and his ingenuity should be able to do something still greater in histology... For otherwise we would, in fact, degenerate into manual laborers and our results would be wholly dependent upon good stains.'

Gierke, from *Färberei zu mikroscopischen Zwecken* (Conn, 1933; Gierke, 1884)

As this author evaluates a melanoma through his Olympus BX40, there is a touch of guilt. The H&E protocol is optimized with discriminating pinks and blues. In the event of uncertainty, immunohistochemistry, fluorescence in situ hybridization, and gene expression profiling are patiently waiting. A consultation is an internet connection away. It is hard not to marvel at the diagnostic abilities by the pathology (e.g. Virchow, Merkel, Welch, et al.), dermatology (e.g. von Hebra, Darier, et al.), and dermatopathology (e.g. Simon, Unna, et al.) giants of yore using such a different and seemingly primitive tool set.

The hematoxylin and eosin (H&E) stain has been used by pathologists for over two centuries. Hematoxylin came to pathology in an amazing journey via Europe via the Campeche region of Mexico with the aid of pirates of the textile industry. The H&E stain has proven inexpensive, reliable, and easy to interpret, which has made the H&E a true champion of diagnostics, reaching the far corners of pathology's Earth. H&E is not infallible, however, and its shortcomings have spurred the development of new, more sophisticated techniques in medicine's continual quest for improvements in diagnosis and characterization of disease.

Supplementary tools for the dermato–pathologist continue to evolve, and many have come and gone. The current quiver contains subjects of the preceding chapters – histochemistry, immunohistochemistry, immunofluorescence, electron microscopy, and now a growing regimen of molecular tests (**Table 17.1**). Some of these assays have been adapted to improve upon patient care by allowing for point of care, or bedside, diagnostic testing as well as rapid turnaround for on-the-spot diagnosis and definitive treatment by Mohs micrographic surgery, for example.

Histochemical ('special') stains were and continue to be an important addition to the H&E. Primitive staining of tissue began in the 18th century with use of natural dyes but the technology and repertoire of stains exploded with the discovery of aniline dyes and their importance for textiles in the mid-to-late 19th century. Advances in the understanding of biochemistry and technological improvements in fixation and slide prep allowed for the creation of slide murals with disparate colors and intensities, which could highlight otherwise invisible elements and discern the various tissue substances. Special stains are perhaps not as sexy as newer antibody- or molecular-based tests, but they continue to be developed and optimized, and remain relatively inexpensive and useful.

The early 20th century brought electron microscopy (EM), opening up a previously unchartered subcellular world. During its hay day, EM played a large role in the reification of subcellular organelles and infectious organisms. It allowed for direct visualization of cell-cell interactions and intracellular substance. EM's role in the advancement of dermatopathology cannot be overstated but its high cost has prevented its use in the diagnostic mainstream. Many EM applications largely have been replaced by other more inexpensive techniques, such as immunohistochemistry, but for the foreseeable future, EM will continue to have a role in research and in niche diagnostic testing at large laboratories and tertiary care centers when direct visualization is required.

Test		Applications
Histochemistry ('special stains')		Pathogens Deposition disease Metabolic disease Autoimmune disease Connective tissue disease Pigmentary disorders Mast cell disorders Tumors
Electron microscopy		Mechanobullous disease Metabolic disease CADASIL Tumors
Immunohistochemistry		Tumors* Pathogens Various inflammatory processes
Immunofluorescence	Direct immunofluorescence (DIF)	Immunobullous disease Connective tissue disease Vasculitis Oral disease Mechanobullous disease
	Indirect immunofluorescence (IIF)	Immunobullous disease
Point of care		Pathogens Pustular dermatoses Tumors (Mohs) Exfoliative dermatitis
Molecular	ISH	Infectious disease HPV/EBV-driven tumors Lymphoma (κ/λ)
	FISH	Soft tissue tumors* Melanocytic tumors†
	Ig/TCR clonality	Leukemia/lymphoma§
	GEP	Melanocytic tumors† Cancers of unknown primary
	Sequencing	Genodermatoses Pathogens§ Pharmacogenomics§ Tumor profiling* Clonality testing§
Other	Teledermatopathology	Teaching/education Tumor board Remote consultation Technical/professional services
	Social media medicine	Education Consultation

Table 17.1 Modern dermatopathology testing and common applications, 'beyond the H&E'

*Diagnostic, prognostic, and therapy selection/monitoring applications
†Diagnostic and prognostic applications
§Diagnostic and therapy selection/monitoring applications

Immunohistochemistry (IHC) and immunofluorescence (IF) both take advantage of the hugely specific antigen-antibody interaction and are extremely important additions to any modern dermatopathology laboratory. The importance of IHC in today's practice of dermatopathology is highlighted by the girth of Chapter 6. With the development of IHC in the mid-20th century, it became the 'next generation' of histochemical stains. The antigen-antibody interaction created a new level of sensitivity and specificity as compared to special staining techniques. Monoclonal and polyclonal antibodies potentially can be generated to any cell-specific or tissue-specific antigen, further improving upon diagnostic capabilities and solving more mysteries of disease. IF uses a similar technology as IHC but with the fluorescence component allowing for an enhanced signal. In dermatopathology, direct IF (DIF) evaluates for the presence of antibodies bound to skin elements. It is often required for diagnosis of immunobullous disease, and can be confirmatory for diagnoses of connective tissue disease and vasculitis. Indirect IF (IIF) evaluates for circulating (as opposed to tissue-bound) autoantibodies and can help diagnose challenging immunobullous diseases. The cost of immunofluorescence remains high and ultimately may lead to replacement of tissue-based IF (especially IIF) with serologic or other assays.

Molecular testing is no longer just style over substance. It is encroaching upon all aspects of management of the dermatologic patient. Until recently, most dermatopathologists' exposure to molecular testing was from board exam studying or attendance of a rare molecular talk at national meetings. Today, one cannot escape the reality of molecular testing in dermatopathology as assays such as in situ hybridization (ISH), fluorescence in situ hybridization (FISH), comparative genomic hybridization (CGH), Ig/TCR clonality testing, gene expression profiling (GEP), and sequencing continue to improve and/or find new validated applications. Commercial kits continually emerge, and dermatopathologists are more than ever being forced to make the decision to bring up these tests, bear the costs of sending them out to reference laboratories, or be tempted to bury their head in the sand and ignore them. ISH continues to be a sensitive and specific technique for detection of viral DNA, such as HPV and EBV, aiding in the diagnosis of infection and virally-driven tumors, and newer applications (light-chain restriction, for example) are continually being developed. FISH has been around since the 1980s and is the primary assay for detecting tumor-defining macrogenetic defects, such as translocations, deletions, and amplifications. Newer applications include characterizing melanocytic lesions, such as melanoma and spitzoid tumors, as well as offering prognostic data. TCR/Ig clonality testing was developed in the late 20th century as an effective ancillary tool for diagnosing lymphoproliferative disease. The technology has evolved from Southern blots to multiplex PCR-based assays to possible complete Ig/TCR sequencing, with all platforms capitalizing on the unique biological properties of Ig and TCR gene rearrangement in lymphocyte development. GEP is a recently developed assay, using tumor- and milieu-specific RNA transcripts to provide diagnostic and prognostic information for melanoma. Direct sequencing of genomes has also evolved with respect to technology, from classic Sanger sequencing to next-generation (massively parallel, or NGS) sequencing, which also has entered the diagnostic scene in the 21st century. With technological improvement, costs of sequencing have plummeted, allowing for new exciting applications in dermatopathology. NGS is arguably the biggest 'needle-mover' of the molecular assays, lionized by leaders in the field, with the potential to replace all others in this class. NGS has the ability to detect and characterize patient genomes, infectious agents genomes, tumor genomes, and all the corresponding transcriptomes in a relatively rapid and inexpensive manner. With this capability, NGS can and will be used for diagnosis of germline defects in the genodermatoses, infectious disease, and somatic defects in tumors and other dermatologic disease. It can transcend 'mere' diagnostic capabilities and evaluate biomarkers for prognosis and optimizing therapy (tumor profiling, pharmacogenomics, etc.).

In addition to the numerous above-mentioned assays and their ever-changing applications, new technologies outside the diagnostic realm are changing the field of dermatopathology.

Teledermatopathology has become a reality and may be the biggest most immediate threat to the microscope. Slide preparation remains a requisite, but with the availability of high-throughput slide scanners and diminishing costs of hardware and memory, biopsy interpretation can bypass the microscope and be performed on a monitor. Virtual slides are becoming increasingly used for teaching, standardized exams, tumor boards, and for technical and professional clinical services including consultation, all of which can be performed remotely. Social media has entered medicine by storm, with the creation of innumerable posts and information-gathering and discussion groups run by academic institutions, foundations, health care providers, and patients. Examples of dermatopathology-related groups include Facebook's *The Dermpath Forum* and *Dermatopathology*, with logarithmic growth of members and dermatopathology-related posts on these sites and other social media platforms. The complete impact of social media has yet to be realized, but at a minimum, has transformed how patients and providers gather information and connect with each other to further education, research, and clinical care.

The von Gierke quote at the opening of this chapter was made in the context of a 25-year tribute to the history of histological staining. This message holds true to current times as dermatopathologists struggle to stay relevant in an ever-changing landscape. The future of dermatopathology depends on perspective. For some, it appears dim and out of focus, as traditional roles for dermatopathologists appear to narrow – in some cases becoming outsourced or commoditized. The H&E stain is time-tested and remains the bread and butter for the dermatopathologist, but those tethered to the microscope with complete reliance on the H&E will cause the field to degenerate into perfunctory analysis by replaceable manual laborers. Contrarily, for others on the right side of this schism, the future is bright with clarity as new technologies expand the scope of dermatopathology. Dermatopathologists, who respect the H&E but embrace new technologies and abandon their stale practices, will find themselves in a more prominent role. These dermatopathologists will not be marginalized but have the tools to become a focal point of the entire dermatologic care team, leading this great specialty into the future.

References

Conn HJ, ed. History of Staining. Geneva, NY: The WF Humphrey Press, 1933.

Gierke H. Färberei zu mikroscopischen Zwecken. Zits Wis Mikr 1884; 1:62–100.

Index